Manual of Surgical
Treatment of
Atrial Fibrillation

Manual of Surgical Treatment of Atrial Fibrillation

EDITED BY

Hauw T. Sie, MD

Department of Thoracic Surgery
Isala Klinieken
Zwolle, The Netherlands

Giuseppe D'Ancona, MD

Department of Cardiac Surgery
ISMETT @ UPMC
Mediterranean Institute for Transplantation
and Advanced Specialized Therapies
Palermo, Italy

Fabio Bartolozzi, MD

Chief CT Surgeon
Galway Clinic
Galway, Ireland

Willem P. Beukema, MD

Department of Cardiology
Isala Klinieken
Zwolle, The Netherlands

Donald B. Doty, MD

Chief of Thoracic Surgery
University of Utah Medical Center
Salt Lake City, UT, USA

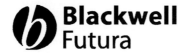

© 2008 by Blackwell Publishing
Blackwell Futura is an imprint of Blackwell Publishing

Blackwell Publishing, Inc., 350 Main Street, Malden, Massachusetts 02148-5020, USA
Blackwell Publishing Ltd, 9600 Garsington Road, Oxford OX4 2DQ, UK
Blackwell Science Asia Pty Ltd, 550 Swanston Street, Carlton, Victoria 3053, Australia

First published 2008

1   2008

ISBN: 978-1-4051-4032-4

Library of Congress Cataloging-in-Publication Data

Manual of surgical treatment of atrial fibrillation / edited by Hauw T. Sie . . . [et al.].
      p. ; cm.
    Includes bibliographical references and index.
    ISBN-13: 978-1-4051-4032-4 (alk. paper)
    ISBN-10: 1-4051-4032-1 (alk. paper)
1. Atrial fibrillation–Treatment.   2. Heart–Surgery.   3. Heart–Surgery–Complications–Prevention.   I. Sie, Hauw T.
    [DNLM: 1. Atrial Fibrillation–physiopathology.   2. Atrial Fibrillation–surgery.   3. Cardiac Surgical
Procedures–methods.   4. Intraoperative Complications–prevention & control.

WG 330 M2945 2008]
RC685.A72M36 2008
617.4′120592–dc22   2007038432

A catalogue record for this title is available from the British Library

Commissioning Editor: Gina Almond
Development Editor: Beckie Brand
Editorial Assistant: Victoria Pittman
Production Controller: Debbie Wyer

Set in 9.5/12pt Minion by Aptara Inc., New Delhi, India
Printed and bound in Singapore by Fabulous Printers Pte Ltd

For further information on Blackwell Publishing, visit our website:
www.blackwellcardiology.com

The publisher's policy is to use permanent paper from mills that operate a sustainable forestry policy, and which has been manufactured from pulp processed using acid-free and elementary chlorine-free practices. Furthermore, the publisher ensures that the text paper and cover board used have met acceptable environmental accreditation standards.

Designations used by companies to distinguish their products are often claimed as trademarks. All brand names and product names used in this book are trade names, service marks, trademarks or registered trademarks of their respective owners. The Publisher is not associated with any product or vendor mentioned in this book.

The contents of this work are intended to further general scientific research, understanding, and discussion only and are not intended and should not be relied upon as recommending or promoting a specific method, diagnosis, or treatment by physicians for any particular patient. The publisher and the author make no representations or warranties with respect to the accuracy or completeness of the contents of this work and specifically disclaim all warranties, including without limitation any implied warranties of fitness for a particular purpose. In view of ongoing research, equipment modifications, changes in governmental regulations, and the constant flow of information relating to the use of medicines, equipment, and devices, the reader is urged to review and evaluate the information provided in the package insert or instructions for each medicine, equipment, or device for, among other things, any changes in the instructions or indication of usage and for added warnings and precautions. Readers should consult with a specialist where appropriate. The fact that an organization or Website is referred to in this work as a citation and/or a potential source of further information does not mean that the author or the publisher endorses the information the organization or Website may provide or recommendations it may make. Further, readers should be aware that Internet Websites listed in this work may have changed or disappeared between when this work was written and when it is read. No warranty may be created or extended by any promotional statements for this work. Neither the publisher nor the author shall be liable for any damages arising herefrom.

Contents

Contributors

Niv Ad, MD
Inova Heart and Vascular Institute,
Falls Church, VA, USA

Ottavio Alfieri, MD
Division of Cardiac Surgery,
San Raffaele Hospital, Milan, Italy

Maurits Allessie, MD, PhD
Department of Physiology,
Faculty of Medicine, Maastricht University,
Maastricht, The Netherlands

Robert H. Anderson, MD, FRCPath
Cardiac Unit, Institute of Child Health,
University College, London, UK

Belhhan Akpınar, MD
Department of Cardiovascular Surgery,
Florence Nightingale Hospital, Sisli, Istanbul, Turkey

Osman Bayındır, MD
Department of Anesthesiology,
Florence Nightingale Hospital, Sisli,
Istanbul, Turkey

Stefano Benussi, MD
Division of Cardiac Surgery,
San Raffaele Hospital, Milan, Italy

Willem P. Beukema, MD
Department of Cardiology,
Isala Klinieken, Zwolle, The Netherlands

Ramon Brugada, MD, FACC
Associate Professor of Medicine,
Canadian Research Chair Genetics of Arrhythmias,
University of Montreal; *and* Director,
Clinical Cardiovascular Genetics Center,
Montreal Heart Institute, Montreal, Canada

Robert A. Byrne, MB, MRCPI
Specialist Registrar in Cardiology,
University College Hospital, Galway, Ireland

Kieran Daly, MB, DCh, FRCPI, FESC, FACC
Consultant Cardiologist/Senior Lecturer,
University College Hospital, Galway, Ireland

Virginia Dietel, MD
Department of Cardiac Surgery, Heart Center,
University of Leipzig, Leipzig, Germany

Nicolas Doll, MD, PhD
Department of Cardiac Surgery, Heart Center,
University of Leipzig, Leipzig, Germany

Arif Elvan, MD
Department of Cardiology,
Isala Klinieken, Zwolle, The Netherlands

Alexander M. Fabricius, MD
Department of Cardiac Surgery, Heart Center,
University of Leipzig, Leipzig, Germany

A. Marc Gillinov, MD
Surgical Director, The Center for Atrial Fibrillation,
The Cleveland Clinic Foundation, Cleveland, OH, USA

Maura Greiser, MD
Department of Physiology, Faculty of Medicine,
Maastricht University, Maastricht, The Netherlands

Mustafa Güden, MD
Department of Cardiovascular Surgery,
Florence Nightingale Hospital, Sisli, Istanbul, Turkey

Gerard M. Guiraudon, MD
Emeritus Professor of Surgery,
University of Western Ontario; *and* Consultant,
Department of Cardiac Surgery,
London Health Sciences Center;
and Scientist CSTAR and Lawson Health Science Institute;
and Associate Scientist, Imaging Department,
The Robarts Research Institute, London, Ontario, Canada

Jan F. Gummert, MD, PhD
Department of Cardiac Surgery, Heart Center,
University of Leipzig, Leipzig, Germany

Michel Haïssaguerre, MD
Hôpital Cardiologique du Haut-Lévêque;
and Université Victor Segalen Bordeaux II,
Bordeaux, France

Erik Harks, MD
Department of Physiology, Faculty of Medicine,
Maastricht University, Maastricht, The Netherlands

Siew Yen Ho, PhD, FRCPath
Paediatrics, National Heart & Lung Institute,
Imperial College and Royal Brompton and
Harefield NHS Trust, London, UK

Mélèze Hocini, MD
Hôpital Cardiologique du Haut-Lévêque;
and Université Victor Segalen Bordeaux II,
Bordeaux, France

Li-Fern Hsu, MBBS
Hôpital Cardiologique du Haut-Lévêque;
and Université Victor Segalen Bordeaux II,
Bordeaux, France

Pierre Jaïs, MD
Hôpital Cardiologique du Haut-Lévêque;
and Université Victor Segalen Bordeaux II,
Bordeaux, France

Anders Jonsson, MD
Hôpital Cardiologique du Haut-Lévêque;
and Université Victor Segalen Bordeaux II,
Bordeaux, France

Michael Knaut, MD
Department of Cardiac Surgery, Heart Center Dresden,
University of Technology Dresden, Dresden, Germany

Yoshio Kosakai, MD
President & Director of Takarazuka Municipal Hospital,
Supervisor of Cardiovascular Surgery,
Takarazuka, Hyogo, Japan

Anand Ramdat Misier, MD
Department of Cardiology, Isala Klinieken,
Zwolle, The Netherlands

Friedrich W. Mohr, MD, PhD
Department of Cardiac Surgery, Heart Center,
University of Leipzig, Leipzig, Germany

Antoon F. Moorman, PhD
Department of Anatomy and Embryology,
Academic Medical Center, University of Amsterdam,
Amsterdam, The Netherlands

Takashi Nitta, MD
Associate Professor, Cardiothoracic Surgery,
Nippon Medical School, Bunkyo-ku, Tokyo, Japan

Carlo Pappone, MD, PhD
Department of Cardiology,
Electrophysiology and Cardiac Pacing Unit,
San Raffaele University Hospital, Milan, Italy

Fernando Rosas, MD
Department of Pediatric Cardiac Surgery
and Electrophysiology,
Clínica A. Shaio and Fundación Cardio-Infantil,
Bogotá, Colombia

Thomas Rostock, MD
Hôpital Cardiologique du Haut-Lévêque;
and Université Victor Segalen Bordeaux II,
Bordeaux, France

Martin Rotter, MD
Hôpital Cardiologique du Haut-Lévêque;
and Université Victor Segalen Bordeaux II,
Bordeaux, France

Mark J. Russo, MD, MS
Surgical Arrhythmia Program,
College of Physicians and Surgeons of Columbia University,
Division of Cardiothoracic Surgery, Department of Surgery,
New York, NY, USA

Fréderic Sacher, MD
Hôpital Cardiologique du Haut-Lévêque;
and Université Victor Segalen Bordeaux II,
Bordeaux, France

Prashanthan Sanders, MBBS, PhD
Hôpital Cardiologique du Haut-Lévêque;
and Université Victor Segalen Bordeaux II,
Bordeaux, France

Nestor Sandoval, MD
Department of Pediatric Cardiac Surgery and
Electrophysiology,
Clínica A. Shaio and Fundación Cardio-Infantil,
Bogotá, Colombia

Vincenzo Santinelli, MD
Department of Cardiology,
Electrophysiology and Cardiac Pacing Unit,
San Raffaele University Hospital, Milan, Italy

Hacer Sen
Department of Cardiology,
Isala Klinieken, Zwolle, The Netherlands

Hauw T. Sie
Department of Thoracic Surgery,
Isala Klinieken, Zwolle, The Netherlands

Yvonne Smyth, MB, MRCPI
Specialist Registrar in Cardiology,
University College Hospital, Galway, Ireland

Piotr Suwalski, MD
Department of Cardiac Surgery, Heart Center,
University of Leipzig, Leipzig, Germany

Z.A. Szalay, MD
Division of Cardiothoracic Surgery and Cardiology,
Kerckhoff Clinic Foundation, Bad Nauheim, Germany

Yoshihide Takahashi, MD
Hôpital Cardiologique du Haut-Lévêque;
and Université Victor Segalen Bordeaux II,
Bordeaux, France

Andrew Taylor, MD
Cardiac Unit, Institute of Child Health,
University College, London, UK

Thomas van Brakel, MD
Department of Physiology, Faculty of Medicine,
Maastricht University, Maastricht, The Netherlands

Victor Manuel Velasco, MD
Department of Pediatric Cardiac Surgery and
Electrophysiology,
Clínica A. Shaio and Fundación Cardio-Infantil,
Bogotá, Colombia

Sander Verheule, MD
Department of Physiology,
Faculty of Medicine, Maastricht University,
Maastricht, The Netherlands

Thomas Walther, MD, PhD
Department of Cardiac Surgery, Heart Center,
University of Leipzig, Leipzig, Germany

Mathew R. Williams, MD
Surgical Arrhythmia Program,
College of Physicians and Surgeons of Columbia University,
Division of Cardiothoracic Surgery,
Department of Surgery, New York, NY, USA

Foreword

It is with great pleasure that I salute the publication of this textbook that resulted from the joint effort of many colleagues and friends.

As a clinical and interventional electrophysiologist that has diagnosed and treated cardiac arrhythmias for the last 30 years, I recognize that many aspects of atrial fibrillation remain poorly investigated or completely unexplored and, as a consequence, managed without the clarity that evidence-based medicine imposes. In this context, it is quite clear that atrial fibrillation harvests a steady number of yearly morbidities and mortalities that mostly remain unrecognized or simply unreported. In spite of that, the majority of the medical community continues, for some reason, to consider atrial fibrillation as a benign condition and, consequently, as a condition with an irrelevant clinical and scientific impact.

I believe in the power of scientific publications and in their ability to disseminate not only knowledge but also conscience of our ignorance. As we try to concentrate on what we know, further unanswered queries arise. It is our responsibility, as members of the medical community, to join forces and build the basis for further scientific inquiries.

It is in this setting that I would like to welcome this new publication in the field of atrial fibrillation with the auspice that it will provide the readers with a sound foundation to ease the interpretation of future information and to trigger further research in the field.

One major aspect to be commended in this publication is the multidisciplinary approach. This is not a simple "surgical manual for the treatment of atrial fibrillation", as the title says, but a complex textbook that ranges from the anatomic aspects of the problem, to its pathophysiology, etiologic hypothesis, and possible medical, cardiologic, and surgical solutions. We have to appreciate the efforts the authors have made to come out from their platonic "myth of the cave" and consider an approach that goes beyond the simple surgical correction. At the same time, having the expertise of authors working in at least 10 different nations around the globe, we can comfortably state the book's international aspiration.

In the first chapter, Dr Anderson sets and precisely defines those that are the anatomical basis for understanding, diagnosing, and treating cardiac arrhythmias. In the following chapters the pathophysiology and genetics (Dr Brugada) of atrial fibrillation are proposed to further emphasize the complexity of this condition. The pharmacological options in the treatment of atrial fibrillation are considered as well (Dr Daly), followed by two focal chapters on the electrical basis of atrial fibrillation written by two pioneers in the field (Dr Allessie and Dr Haissaguerre). In the next section, Dr Guiraudon and Dr Ad report on the first attempts to treat atrial fibrillation surgically and on the evolution of the Maze procedure, on which basis all the present surgical approaches should stand.

The third section of the book deals with the many different surgical approaches that have been proposed through the years to treat atrial fibrillation including the radial approach (Dr Nitta), the Minimaze (Dr Szalay), and data collected within the vast Japanese experience (Dr Kosakai). Particular attention is given to the use of new energy sources (Dr Williams) to create cardiac ablation patterns and experiences with radiofrequency (Dr Sie) and microwave (Dr Knaut) are reported. Through the chapters there is an evolution towards a less invasive surgical approach where the majority of cardiac lesions are performed with bipolar sources of energy to guarantee transmurality (Dr Gillinov), epicardially (Dr Benussi) and, in some cases, via minimally invasive procedures (Drs. Güden and Akpınar). The last two sections of the book are dedicated to the invasive cardiology approach (Dr Pappone) and include a summary of the surgical treatment of cardiac arrhythmias in the pediatric population (Dr Sandoval) and finally a report on the complications that may derive from the surgical treatment of atrial fibrillation (Dr Doll and Dr Mohr).

In spite of the complexity of some topics dealt with in the different chapters, this manual has kept a logical and quite simple structure that makes it easily readable and, for this reason, I hope it will be appreciated by a large plethora of medical professionals, including the non specialists.

To conclude with the words of Hippocrates: "...The physician must not only be prepared to do what is right himself, but also to make the patient, the attendants, and externals cooperate". And I think we should all recognize the ability of the authors in making such a large cooperation become a reality with this book that will hopefully have the deserved readership.

Prof. Luigi Padeletti
Full Professor of Cardiology
University of Florence Medical School

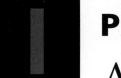

PART I

Anatomy, pathophysiology, and electrophysiologic basis of atrial fibrillation

CHAPTER 1

The morphology and development of the atrial chambers, with particular regard to atrial fibrillation

*Robert H. Anderson, Antoon F. Moorman,
Andrew Taylor, & Siew Yen Ho*

Introduction

In a previous review of the structure of the atrial chambers [1], we drew attention to the fact that, during the period 1996 through 2000, a search using the online facilities of the National Library of Medicine in the United States of America revealed 2695 articles on atrial arrhythmias, a threefold increase compared to the previous 5-year period. When the search was addressed specifically to atrial fibrillation, the number of hits was appreciably higher, at almost 5000 for the second period, albeit that this was less than a twofold increase. At that time, however, accounts of gross anatomy of the atrial chambers barely featured. We argued that this situation could be interpreted as indicating that all was known about the gross anatomy of the atrial chambers, but we went on to suggest that this was far from the case. Since that time, in the initial 5 years of the current century, our prognostications have proved well founded, since there has been an upsurge in interest not only in the structure of the atriums, but also in the location within the atrial musculature of potential arrhythmic substrates. These have sparked ongoing discussion with regard to the features permitting the histologic recognition of the so-called "specialized" tissues [2–6]. At the same time, the search for increased morphological knowledge by electrophysiologists has been accompanied by amazing improvements in diagnostic techniques, such that the atriums can now be reconstructed with remarkable accuracy. More importantly, the information can now be presented to the clinician in the context of the overall arrangement of the body [7]. This emphasizes the need for atrial structures to be described using attitudinally appropriate nomenclature [8], a need, which we have also done our best to champion [9], albeit still with relatively limited success. In this chapter, therefore, it is our task to provide the electrophysiologist, arrhythmologist, and cardiologist, with a review of atrial structure, emphasizing the relationship of the atriums to other structures within the thorax, the location of the components of the conduction system, and other potential arrhythmic substrates. We will also introduce the significant advances made in understanding the development of the atrial chambers [10], since this sheds considerable light on the location of the arrhythmic substrates, and also resolves some of the disputes concerning the nature of the musculature making up the pulmonary venous sleeves [3], now well recognized as significant in the genesis of atrial fibrillation [11].

Manual of Surgical Treatment of Atrial Fibrillation.
Edited by Hauw T. Sie *et al*. © 2008 Blackwell Publishing,
ISBN: 978-1-4051-4032-4.

The relationship of the heart within the body

Over the centuries, the basis for description of all structures within the body has been the agreement that they should be described as seen in the individual standing upright and facing the observer, the so-called "anatomical position" (Plate 1.1). It is surprising that this convention has been followed for virtually all the systems of organs, muscles, and nerves, yet ignored for the heart. Thus, almost all anatomic texts concerned with human anatomy, and all texts of clinical cardiology, continue to use adjectives for description of the heart that are based on its position as seen when removed from the body, and stood on its apex, the so-called "Valentine" configuration (Plate 1.2). In the past, when diagnosis depended on auscultation, or even on echocardiographic interrogation, these deficiencies were of relatively little significance, although the inconsistency of blockage of the "posterior" interventricular coronary artery producing inferior myocardial infarction cannot have gone unnoticed. With the proliferation of interventional techniques, particularly as used by the cardiologist to cure arrhythmias, these discrepancies became more significant. The conventional approach was recognized as being less than perfect when the interventionist realized it was necessary to describe a catheter inserted via the inferior caval vein as tracking anteriorly, when all the watchers could see the structure moving superiorly in the fluoroscopic screen [8]. Since the turn of the century, with the introduction of tomographic techniques that give the clinician the ability to reconstruct the heart in three dimensions, and to do so in the context of the other thoracic contents, the need to adopt an attitudinally appropriate nomenclature has become the more pressing [12]. In this chapter, therefore, we will describe all parts of the heart, including the atrial chambers as seen in their context of the living thorax (Plate 1.3), using adjectives as dictated by the anatomical position (Plate 1.1).

The basic arrangement of the heart within the thorax

The heart is positioned within the mediastinum, with its own long axis orientated from the right shoulder toward the left hypochondrium (Plate 1.4a). In the normal individual, two thirds of the bulk of the cardiac mass is usually to the left, with one third to the right. The overall cardiac silhouette projects to the anterior surface of the chest in trapezoidal fashion. It is convenient to consider the trapezoid itself in terms of atrial and ventricular triangles, the two meeting at the planes of the atrioventricular and ventriculoarterial junctions (Plate 1.4b and 1.5a). The relationships of the cardiac valves guarding the junctions are then well seen when the atrial myocardium and arterial trunks are removed, and the ventricular base is examined from its atrial aspect (Plate 1.5b). This dissection emphasizes, first, that the right atrium is positioned anteriorly relative to its alleged left-sided counterpart, and second, that the aortic valve forms the centerpiece of the cardiac short axis, being wedged between the mitral and tricuspid valves (Plate 1.5b). Examination of the cardiac structures in so-called "four chamber" orientation then shows how the heart is composed of the atrial and ventricular muscle masses, these two masses meeting at the atrioventricular junctions. Apart from the bundle of His, they are insulated electrically one from the other by the fibrofatty tissue planes of the junctions (Plate 1.6).

Relationship of the heart to the thoracic structures

The heart lies within the middle component of the mediastinum, enclosed within its pericardial sac, which functions as the cardiac "seat belt." Other important structures, of course, are also to be found within the thorax, and recent experience has shown that the interventionist needs to be well aware of their precise relationships to the heart. The location of the oesophagus has long been recognized as of clinical significance, since in the days prior to the advent of tomographic diagnostic techniques, the barium swallow was regularly used as a means of recognizing left atrial enlargement. Now, with the availability of magnetic resonance imaging, we are able to display the precise relationship of the oesophagus to the atrial components (Figures 1.1 and 1.2). As the section in the sagittal plane shows (Figure 1.1), the oesophagus runs within the posterior mediastinum directly behind the left atrium.

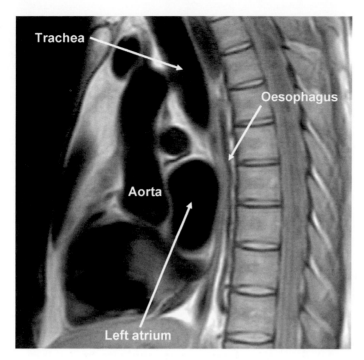

Figure 1.1 This magnetic resonance image is taken in the sagittal plane. It shows the intimate relationship between the oesophagus and the left atrium.

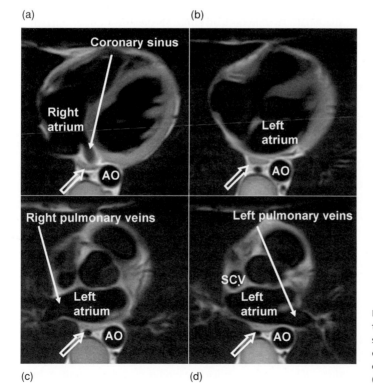

Figure 1.2 These resonance images, taken in the short axis of the body, show the relationship of the oesophagus (arrowed) to the atrial chambers at increasingly superior levels (a through d). AO, aorta.

Sections in the short axis then show that, just prior to its penetration through the diaphragm (Figure 1.2a), the oesophagus is directly related to the coronary sinus. When traced superiorly (Figure 1.2b–d) it comes into direct relationship with the posterior wall of the left atrium, running more-or-less along the middle of the chamber, albeit that reconstructions have shown that this relationship can vary with peristalsis even within the individual [7].

In addition to the oesophagus, and the aorta, albeit that the aorta is relatively distant from the atrial chambers (Figure 1.2), recent experience has shown that the interventionist also needs to take note of the relationship of the phrenic nerves as they pass through the thorax to innervate the diaphragm. In an elegant anatomic study, Sanchez-Quintana and colleagues [13] showed that the right phrenic nerve is intimately related to both the superior caval vein and the right pulmonary veins, running within millimeters of the lumens of these veins, whereas the left phrenic nerve was relatively safely located relative to the atrial chambers, albeit potentially at risk during implantation of leads into the great cardiac and obtuse marginal veins (Plate 1.7).

The phrenic nerves course through the mediastinum running anteriorly relative to the pulmonary hilums. Equally important are the vagus nerves, which extend through the mediastinum on both sides directly posterior to the hilums. These structures must also be at risk when ablations are carried out in the pulmonary venous orifices. The vagus nerves, along with the sympathetic chains, contribute numerous branches to the posterior cardiac plexus, which is intimately related to the left atrium and the interatrial groove. Thus far, the nerves have received relatively little attention, and a detailed account of their distribution is beyond the scope of this chapter, but it is likely that, in the near future, they will receive appreciably more attention [14].

The atrial components

Each of the atrial chambers is made up of comparable parts, albeit that the shape, orientation, and contribution of each component differ markedly between the two chambers. The basic components are the body, the appendage, the venous component, the vestibule, and the septum. Both the body and the appendage differentiate as working myocardium from the primary venous part of the linear heart tube. The body is placed in its larger part in the left atrium, with only a small part persisting in the right atrium between the venous component and the septum. We know, however, that the body forms a significant part of the left atrium, since this chamber retains a significant volume in the absence of its venous component, as seen in the congenital malformation of totally anomalous pulmonary venous connection (Plate 1.8). The two appendages also take their origin from the body, ballooning anteriorly during early development. Eventually, however, they come to form almost the entirety of the anterior wall of the right atrium, and a tubular extension from the body of the left atrium, both as anatomically discrete structures (Plate 1.9 and 1.10). Thus, the walls of the appendages are readily distinguished from the remaining atrial walls because of their pectinated appearance (Plate 1.9). The venous components are positioned posteriorly within both atriums. The venous sinus of the right atrium, derived from the initial bilaterally symmetrical systemic venous tributaries, receives the superior and inferior caval veins at its roof and floor, with the coronary sinus returning most of the venous drainage from the heart itself to the right atrium (Plate 1.9a). The venous component of the left atrium, a new developmental component, eventually receives one pulmonary vein at each of its four corners, and forms the roof of the left atrium, albeit with a degree of off-setting of the venous orifices (Plate 1.9b). The vestibules are the smooth atrial walls leading into, and attached at, the orifices of the atrioventricular valves (Plate 1.6 and 1.9). They are derived from the initial musculature of the atrioventricular canal. On the right side, the smooth vestibule is separated from the venous sinus throughout the extent of the atrioventricular junction by the pectinate muscles of the right appendage (Plate 1.9a). On the left side, in contrast, the smooth vestibule is confluent with the smooth walls of the pulmonary venous component and the body, the pectinate muscles being confined within the tubular appendage (Plate 1.9b). The septum is the wall separating the cavities of the two chambers (Plate 1.11). It is made up largely of the fibrous floor of the oval fossa, the fossa itself representing the site of embryonic interatrial communication. The larger parts of the superior, anterior, and posterior margins of the fossa are formed by infoldings of the atrial walls. It is only the anteroinferior rim, leading to the vestibule in the environs of the triangle of Koch (see below), that can be removed, along with the floor of the fossa, so as to create a direct communication between the atriums without encroaching on extracardiac space [15].

Description of the atriums

As will have become evident from all our discussions thus far, when the atriums are considered in the setting of the body, which is the only realistic way for the cardiologist to approach atrial morphology, the terms "right" and "left" are inappropriate for positional description. In reality, the right atrium is the anterior atrium, with hardly anything of the left atrium, other than the tip of its appendage, being visible when the cardiac chambers are projected onto the cardiac silhouette as seen in the frontal projection (Plate 1.4a). It is unlikely, however, that we will ever describe the atriums as being the anterior and posterior chambers. In the normal heart, it would be more appropriate to describe them as the systemic and pulmonary venous atriums, but even this convention would prove lacking when the heart is congenitally malformed (Plate 1.8). The better way of describing the two chambers, therefore, is to recognize them as being morphologically right and morphologically left, this convention holding good even when the chambers are mirror-imaged in the setting of congenital cardiac disease. It is the structure of the appendages that best distinguishes between the two atriums, this feature holding good even when the heart is grossly malformed as in the setting of visceral heterotaxy. Indeed, in this setting, careful examination of the extent of the pectinate muscles shows that the atrial chambers possess either two right appendages, or two left appendages, and hence are well described as having isomerism of the morphologically right or left atrial appendages [16]. In the setting of the normal heart, or the hearts in patients with atrial

arrhythmias, the important point is to appreciate that the atrial cavities are located more-or-less front to back. The atrial septum has a double oblique orientation, running posteriorly to anteriorly when traced from right to left, and at the same time, extending from anterior to posterior when traced from head to foot (Figure 1.2).

Positional arrangement of the components of the right atrium

In the right atrium, as their names suggest, the superior and inferior caval veins enter the roof and the floor of the systemic venous component, this part of the atrium being posterior to the extensive appendage. It is often thought that the appendage is no more than the triangular tip of the chamber abutting on the aorta (Plate 1.10). As is shown by the cast, nonetheless, the pectinated wall forms virtually the entirety of the front surface of the chamber (Plate 1.9a). When viewed from above, the pectinate muscles are seen to circle round the entirety of the vestibule of the tricuspid valve (Plate 1.12). Indeed, the muscles spill over and encroach on the diverticulum found beneath the coronary sinus (Plate 1.13 and 1.14), often described as the sub-Eustachian sinus. When the heart is positioned as it lies within the body, because this diverticulum is beneath the mouth of the coronary sinus, it is more appropriately described as being sub-Thebesian. The Eustachian and Thebesian valves, remnants of the right valve of the embryonic venous sinus [17], are found at the right boundary of the definitive systemic venous sinus, albeit being variably developed in different hearts. When extensive, they can become aneurysmal, particularly the Eustachian valve, and can form windsocks, which in extreme cases, can extend through the tricuspid valve and block the subpulmonary outflow tract.

More usually, the valves persist only as fibrous folds related to the openings of the inferior caval vein and the coronary sinus (Plate 1.14). It is then the commissure between the valves which is of more significance. This fibrous structure buries itself within the muscular posterior wall of the right atrium between the orifice of the coronary sinus and the depression formed by the oval fossa. This muscular area is known as the sinus septum, or the

Eustachian ridge. It is the fold between the walls of the coronary sinus, running in the left atrioventricular groove, and the margins of the oval fossa. The tendinous continuation of the fused venous valves extends throughout this musculature, burying itself in the anteroinferior rim of the atrial septum, and running anteriorly and superiorly to terminate in the so-called central fibrous body (Plate 1.14). We will return to discuss the central fibrous body when considering the location of the atrioventricular node and the bundle of His.

If we redirect our attention now to the appendage and the systemic venous sinus, an important groove is seen externally which marks the boundary between the two components. This is the terminal groove, or "sulcus terminalis." The superior extent of this groove is the crest of the atrial appendage, with the sinus node found subepicardially within the groove just inferior to this crest (Plate 1.15). Across the crest, the terminal groove becomes continuous with the anterior interatrial groove. Internally, the terminal groove corresponds with the location of the terminal crest, this being the prominent muscular bundle that forms the boundary between the appendage and the systemic venous sinus. The pectinate muscles extend like the teeth of a comb from the terminal crest to reach anteriorly as far as the smooth vestibule surrounding the tricuspid valvar orifice. In the anterior wall, the larger pectinate muscles are arranged nearly in parallel fashion, with thin branches in between, leaving areas of very thin atrial wall (Plate 1.13). Superiorly, at the tip of the appendage, the pectinate muscles lose their parallel arrangement. The terminal crest sweeps like a twisted "C," originating from the septal wall, passes anterior to the orifice of the superior caval vein, descends posteriorly and laterally, before turning anteriorly to skirt the right side of the orifice of the inferior caval vein. Close to its origin, the terminal crest is joined by a prominent bundle, the sagittal bundle, or "septum spurium," which extends anterolaterally toward the tip of the appendage. When traced inferiorly, the crest continues to form the boundary between the appendage and the systemic venous sinus, terminating in the region of the coronary sinus, where pectinate muscles continue to extend into the sub-Thebesian sinus. The inferior margin of the crest is of particular significance in the setting of atrial arrhythmias, since

this is part of the so-called cavo-tricuspid isthmus (Plate 1.14). This inferior isthmus is an extensive and complex structure, possessing posterior, middle, and anterior components. The posterior part is pectinated. The middle part is the thinnest, incorporating the floor of the sub-Thebesian sinus, while the anterior part is smooth, representing the vestibule of the tricuspid valve (Plate 1.16). The vestibular part of the inferior isthmus is itself confluent with a second area of crucial significance to the arrhythmologist. This is the septal isthmus, the area between the mouth of the coronary sinus and the hingeline of the septal leaflet of the tricuspid valve (Plate 1.14). As we will see, this area harbors the so-called "slow pathway" into the atrioventricular node, albeit that the precise anatomic substrate for this pathway has still to be determined. Both the septal isthmus and the anterior part of the cavo-tricuspid isthmus are part of the vestibule of the right atrium, this being the smooth-walled component of atrial musculature that inserts into the full circumference of the orifice of the tricuspid valve, apart from the small area occupied by the membranous septum, this being part of the central fibrous body (Plate 1.14).

The final atrial component, the septum, forms the posterior wall of the right atrium, albeit that the septum itself is not nearly as extensive as is often thought. This statement requires a degree of explanation. From the perspective of the anatomist, we take the stance that a septal structure is that part of the walls of the heart that can be removed without encroaching on extracardiac space. In this way, we distinguish true partitions between adjacent chambers from folds or sandwiches [15]. When considered in this way, as we have already shown (Plate 1.11), the so-called "septum secundum" is no more than the superior interatrial fold, representing for the most part the deep infolding between the connections of the caval veins to the right atrium, and the right pulmonary veins to the left atrium. The anterior and superior border of the oval fossa is related directly to the aortic root (Plate 1.10). This anatomic feature is also of major significance to the interventionist, since the wall in this area often has crevices that can be mistaken for the space between the flap valve and the rim of the fossa itself. The interventionist seeking to achieve septal puncture may sometimes locate the perforating device in one of the crevices rather than within the oval fossa. It is then easy, but regrettable, to puncture the aortic root rather than to pass into the left atrium (Plate 1.17).

The Eustachian ridge itself, running between the orifice of the coronary sinus and the inferior margin of the fossa, becomes continuous with the anteroinferior margin, then forming the other truly septal component of the posterior wall (Plate 1.11). In the past, we were of the opinion that the anterior continuation of this buttress formed part of an atrioventricular muscular septum. We now know that, although this muscular wall does indeed interpose between the cavities of the right atrium and the left atrium, it is a sandwich rather than a true septum. This is because an extension from the inferior atrioventricular groove runs between the right atrial and left ventricular musculatures in this area, carrying the artery to the atrioventricular node (Plate 1.18). The atrial part of this musculature, nonetheless, is crucially important to the arrhythmologist, since it contains on its inferior surface the compact atrioventricular node.

We have made no mention thus far of the location of a body within the right atrium. The part of the myocardium derived from the primary atrium is squeezed between the septum and the leftward margin of the systemic venous sinus. It is not possible in the postnatal heart, however, to recognize any anatomic boundaries in this area distinguishing the origin of the different myocardial components, as is possible at the rightward margin, which is marked by the terminal crest and the remnants of the right venous valve. As we will discuss later, it is possible to recognize such a boundary in the developing heart, which is formed by the left venous valve. It is the "septo-valvar space" between the left venous valve and the septum that represents the body of the right atrium, this being the part from which, during development, the appendage has ballooned prior to incorporation of the systemic venous sinus.

Positional relationships of the components of the left atrium

As with the right atrium, the left atrium is made up of the appendage, the vestibule, the pulmonary venous component, and the left aspect of the septum.

The left atrium also retains the larger part of the atrial body derived from the primary atrium, albeit that there are no anatomic boundaries that show the different parts of the smooth-walled atrium derived from the various developmental components. The left atrium also lacks a terminal crest, or "crista terminalis," so there is no groove between appendage and the smooth-walled part of the atrium such as seen on the right side. The appendage is readily recognized, nonetheless, because of its tubular shape, and its narrow junction with the remainder of the left atrium (Plate 1.19). It is positioned anterosuperiorly and leftward relative to the body of the atrium (Plate 1.20). The pulmonary venous component is shaped like a pillow, with the pulmonary veins entering the four corners of the superoposterior aspect. The left veins enter the atrium more superiorly than the right veins, albeit that this relationship is grossly distorted in Plate 1.15. The true relationship is shown by reconstructions made from computed tomographic or magnetic resonance images (Plate 1.21). Variation in the number of veins entering the human left atrium is not uncommon. Sometimes two veins of one, or both, sides unite prior to entering the atrium. In others, an additional vein is found, more frequently on the right side. In a recent description based on tomographic images, emphasis was placed on recognizing a so-called "roof" vein [18]. It should also be noted that five or six pulmonary venous orifices are described for the canine heart [1], although some veins become confluent just before entering the left atrium. There are two veins, one on each side, in the porcine heart. In the murine heart, in contrast, there is but a solitary vein entering the left atrium [19]. These differences between species need to be taken into account when judging the significance of experimental results to arrhythmias as seen in the human. In our limited experience in assessing variations in the human, it is more common to find the right upper veins joining to enter as one vein, with the orifice located slightly superiorly to the common left upper venous orifice. The septal aspect of the left atrium, forming the anterior wall of the chamber, is usually marked by shallow and irregular pits on the flap valve of the oval fossa. A crescent marks the free edge of the flap valve (Plate 1.19). It is through this margin that a probe or catheter can be pushed obliquely and anterosuperiorly along the fossal surface on the right side to enter the left atrium. Indeed, in up to one third of the normal population, there is no anatomic fusion between the flap valve and the left side of the margins of the oval fossa [20]. Such failure of fusion produces a probe-patent oval foramen, now known to be a harbinger for cryptogenic stroke [21], and perhaps even a cause of migraine [22]. As we have stressed when discussing the right atrium, the anterior rims of the oval fossa can themselves exhibit holes or crevices. The walls are also very thin close to this point, increasing the risk of exiting the heart during attempted septal puncture. As with the right atrium, the vestibular musculature inserts into the left atrioventricular junction around the margins of the annulus of the mitral valve. Unlike the right side, however, the left-sided vestibule is a complete ring of muscle.

An important structure related to the left atrium is the coronary sinus, albeit that this venous channel, as already discussed opens into the systemic venous sinus of the right atrium. In the past, we thought that the wall of the sinus was directly continuous with that of the posterior vestibular of the left atrium, the two representing a "party wall." We now know that this is not the case (Plate 1.20), the elegant study of Chauvin and colleagues [23] proving that the walls of the sinus are discrete entities, albeit with muscular bridges running from the wall of the sinus to the left atrial musculature. In the normal individual, the coronary sinus, representing the remnant of the left sinus horn, does no more than serve as a conduit to channel most of the coronary venous return to the right atrium. The remaining part of the initially symmetrical left cardinal vein is then seen as the oblique vein of the left atrium, the site of this venous channel being taken by some as marking the junction of the coronary sinus and the great cardiac vein (Plate 1.22). Others use the location of the prominent valve within the venous conduit, the valve of Vieussens, as the boundary between the great cardiac vein and the sinus. As can be seen from the cast shown in Plate 1.22, this junction is somewhat arbitrary, since the venous conduit continues as an uninterrupted channel throughout the left atrioventricular groove. In the adult heart, the walls of the funnel-shaped venous channel are located approximately 1–1.5 cm proximal to the internal plane corresponding to the mitral valvar orifice [24].

The muscular walls and muscular venous sleeves

The atrial mass is an integral muscular whole, albeit with walls of varying thickness and complexity, and with relatively limited connections between the two atriums. The varying thickness of the walls is particularly well seen in the right atrium. The most prominent bundles are the terminal crest, the Eustachian ridge, the rim of the oval fossa, the pectinate muscles, and the tricuspid vestibule. When attention is given to the epicardial aspect of the terminal crest at the crest of the right atrial appendage, then a prominent band of muscular aggregates can be traced from the superior cavoatrial junction leftward to become the superficial fibers of the left atrium. Best known as Bachmann's bundle, this band crosses the anterior interatrial groove (Plate 1.23). As initially emphasized by Bachmann himself [25], the bundle is not ensheathed by fibrous tissue, and is of varying widths and thicknesses in different hearts. It lacks distinct margins, and it is the parallel arrangement of myofibers that almost certainly confer upon it the state of the superhighway for interatrial conduction. There are then other important interatrial bundles that cross the superior or posterior parts of the interatrial groove, and still others that connect the wall of the coronary sinus to the left atrium (Plate 1.24). The floor of the oval fossa, however, is made up largely of fibrous tissue in the adult human heart, and is therefore electrically inert. The anteroinferior margin of the oval fossa, nonetheless, is a true septal structure, so this area also constitutes an electrical bridge between the atriums. In all these prominent muscle bundles, it is the alignment of the long axis of the myocytes that sets the scene for preferential conduction, since as we will emphasize shortly, there are no discrete insulated muscular tracts running through the atrial walls, either between the sinus and atrioventricular nodes, or between the atriums.

Being mainly smooth, the left atrial wall gives the impression of muscular homogeneity. Detailed dissections through its full thickness, however, reveal it to be composed of overlapping broad bands of myofibers. These run in different directions, but the layers again are not insulated one from the other by fibrous sheaths. The superficial myofibers are mostly orientated parallel to the atrioventricular junction, while the deeper fibers run obliquely or perpendicularly to the junction. The superior wall, however, is composed mainly of the perpendicular or oblique fibers of the septopulmonary bundle (Plate 1.24).

The recording of electrical activity in the thoracic veins, and the ablation technique developed by Haissaguerre and his colleagues for treating paroxysmal atrial fibrillation [11], have focused attention on the muscular sleeves surrounding the proximal parts of the both the systemic and the pulmonary veins. Encircling the veins to varying extents, the sleeves are continuations of atrial musculature along the epicardial aspect of the venous wall [6]. They tend to be thicker and more complete near the cavoatrial or pulmonary–atrial junctions, but taper and fragment as they move further away from the junction. When considering the pulmonary veins, the upper veins tend to have longer sleeves than the lower ones, which are often devoid of sleeves (Plate 1.25). It is no coincidence that ectopic focuses are most commonly found in the superior veins. Although claims have been made for the existence of "specialized" cells in the human heart [5], we have found no evidence demonstrating specialization of the cells (Plate 1.26) [6, 26]. It is almost certainly the nonuniform anisotropic pattern of the myocytes in their supporting fibrous matrix that sets the scene for focal activity (Plate 1.27). Muscular sleeves are seldom well-developed around the inferior caval vein. In contrast, the superior caval vein usually has a discernible cuff of atrial muscle extending some distance from the cavoatrial junction. The sleeves around the caval veins, irrespective of their length, when judged histologically are again made up exclusively of working myocardium. Some have suggested that the oblique vein of the left atrium might also be a site of arrhythmogenesis. We find this unlikely, since the vein is a small structure, representing no more than the remnant of the left cardinal vein.

The location of the specialized atrial myocardium

As we have already demonstrated and discussed, the larger parts of the atrial walls are made up of ordinary working myocytes. The myocytes themselves are aggregated within a supporting matrix of fibrous tissue, the parallel alignment of these aggregates favoring preferential conduction along the direction of their long axis, the overall arrangement being one of nonuniform anisotropy [27]. Within the overall structure of the atrial walls, nonetheless, certain parts of the myocardium show so-called histologically "specialized" characteristics. One of these areas, the sinus node, is known to be the generator of the cardiac impulse [28]. Another area, the atrioventricular node and its zones of transitional cells, is the atrial component of the solitary axis of muscular tissue, which joins the atrial and ventricular muscle masses [29]. At various times, and in various places, however, multiple investigators have suggested that other parts of the atrial myocardium are histologically specialized. For quite some time, these suggestions focused on the presence or absence of muscular "tracts" extending between the sinus and atrioventricular nodes [30]. More recently, the suggestions have centered on the possibility that additional areas of "specialized" tissue could form the focus for abnormal atrial rhythmicity [2, 3, 5]. All these potential controversies, however, could have been avoided had the protagonists for histological specialization followed the criteria suggested by the great German pathologists, Aschoff [31] and Mönckeberg [32]. The need for these criteria had appeared when Thorel, another German investigator, was the first to suggest that the atrial myocardium interposed between the newly discovered sinus and atrioventricular nodes was histologically specialized [33]. Aschoff [31], and Mönckeberg [32], in presentation to a meeting of the German Society of Pathology, held in Marburg in 1910, pointed out that the careful studies of Tawara [29] provided the basis for appreciating the histological essence of "specialization." In a truly epochal study, first published in 1906 as a monograph in German, but now available in an excellent English translation [29], Tawara had shown that the axis for atrioventricular conduction took its origin from the "knoten," or atrioventricular node. The axis then penetrated the insulating tissues separating the atrial and ventricular muscle masses, and then continued to be insulated from the ventricular myocardium as the branches of the atrioventricular bundle, enclosed in fibrous sheaths, coursed on either side of the muscular ventricular septum, merging with the ventricular myocardial mass only when they had reached the ventricular apexes. Taking this account as their example, Aschoff and Mönckeberg suggested that specialized tracts within the walls of the heart should, first, be composed of cells which are histologically distinct from their neighboring walls of working myocardium, second, should be enclosed by fibrous sheaths, and third, should be followed from section to section in blocks of myocardium prepared using the technique of serial sectioning. The paradigm for such a tract is the right bundle branch (Plate 1.28). When examining the atrial myocardium histologically, then no structures are to be found which satisfy all three of the criteria suggested by Mönckeberg [32] and Aschoff [31], criteria which still retain their currency, and have yet to be superceded by better "rules" for recognition of histologically specialized tissue. Thus, when examined in the light of the existing rules, it is now established beyond any doubt that insulated tracts of atrial myocardium do not exist within the atrial walls. As we will see, there are areas of the walls that show differences one from the other, but none which satisfy the criteria for existence as tracts comparable to the ventricular bundle branches.

When we examine the histological arrangement of the sinus and atrioventricular nodes, structures of which the functions are no longer in doubt, then we find that they satisfy only two of the three criteria established by Aschoff [31] and Mönckeberg [32]. These nodes are histologically discrete from the adjacent working myocardium, and can be followed from section to section in serially sectioned histological blocks. The cells of the nodes, however, are not insulated from the adjacent myocardium. Indeed, it would destroy their purpose where they thus insulated. The purpose of the sinus node (Plate 1.29) is to generate the cardiac impulse. The pacemaking cells, therefore, need to be in electrical contact with the adjacent working myocardial cells. This transition from the nodal tissue to working atrial myocardium occurs at all borders of the node where there is contact with the atrial walls. But there are no "tracts" emanating from the node other than the tail extending for variable distance down the terminal groove. Similarly, the atrial myocardial cells adjacent to the atrioven-

tricular node change their histological structure, becoming isolated and elongated, and recognizable as transitional cells (Plate 1.30). These transitional cells themselves then undergo further transitions, grouping themselves together to become the compact node, which is then engulfed by the fibrous tissue of the central fibrous body to become the bundle of His (Plate 1.30). When we apply these two criteria, histological differentiation and the ability to follow structures through serial sections, we then find other areas of atrial myocardium that are histologically specialized (Plate 1.31). These are the node-like structures found at various points within the vestibule of the tricuspid valve. Originally discovered by Kent in 1893 [34], and illustrated in 1913 [35], Kent wrongly assumed that the nodes extended across the insulating fibrofatty groove between the right atrium and the right ventricle. As we showed subsequently [36], the structures, which truly resemble a miniature atrioventricular node (Plate 1.31), are located within the insertions of the right atrial vestibular into the orifice of the tricuspid valve. As we will show below, they are the remnants of a more extensive ring of primary myocardium that initially surrounds the atrioventricular junction and embryonic interventricular foramen, and which also becomes incorporated into the developing right atrial vestibule. In the normal heart, the nodal remnants make no contact with the ventricular myocardium. It has been suggested that the part of the original ring in the septal isthmus forms the slow pathway into the atrioventricular node [37], albeit that not all patients with atrioventricular nodal tachycardia possess such histologically identifiable structures [38]. The node-like structures, nonetheless, can function as part of electrical atrioventricular connections, either in the so-called "Mahaim" type of preexcitation [39], or in congenitally malformed hearts such as congenitally corrected transposition [40]. Other than the sinus and atrioventricular nodes, and the remnants of specialized tissue known as the atrioventricular ring tissue [36], and despite claims to the contrary [2, 3, 5], there are no other areas of the walls of the right or left atrium, including the pulmonary venous sleeves, which are histologically specialized when set against the criteria established by Aschoff [31] and Mönckeberg [32] in 1910.

The location of the cardiac nodes

It is important for the clinician, and particularly the electrophysiologist, to be able to identify with accuracy the locations of the sinus and atrioventricular nodes within the walls of the right atrium. The sinus node is a small, cigar-shaped, structure set immediately subepicardially within the terminal groove, its body being wedged between the wall of the superior caval vein and the musculature of the terminal crest. In an earlier study [41], we found that, in addition to a tail extending for various distances down the terminal groove toward the orifice of the inferior caval vein, in one tenth of the specimens studied, the node also extended in horseshoe fashion across the crest of the right atrial appendage. In a subsequent study of adult human hearts [42], however, we did not encounter any horseshoe nodes, all examples lying laterally within the terminal groove (Plate 1.15). The nodal cells themselves are immediately subepicardial, and make short transitions with the atrial myocardium throughout the boundary between the node and the terminal crest (Plate 1.29). It is noteworthy that, in most individuals, a prominent artery courses through the middle of the node, although the specific arrangement varies from heart to heart [43]. This artery to the sinus node is an early branch of the right coronary artery in just over half individuals, taking origin from the initial course of the circumflex artery in just under half, with rare individuals exhibiting lateral origin from more distal parts of the right or circumflex arteries. This variation in arterial supply is likely to be of greater significance to the cardiac surgeon than to the electrophysiologist [43].

As we have emphasized, there are no insulated tracts emanating from the sinus node and coursing either into the left atrium, or toward the atrioventricular node [44]. As was shown by Bachmann himself [25], it is the parallel arrangement of the aggregates of myocytes that is responsible for preferential conduction along the prominent thick atrial muscular bundles. Amongst these, the most important are Bachmann's bundle itself (Plate 1.23), the margins of the oval foramen, and the vestibule of the tricuspid valve (Plate 1.14). It is the latter muscular structures, which make up the approaches to

the atrioventricular node, but not forgetting that, as an interatrial structure, the node is also in electrical contact with the left atrial side of the septum (Plate 1.30). The anatomical landmark to the location of the atrioventricular node is the triangle of Koch. This triangular area is delineated on the atrial side by the course of the tendon of Todaro through the Eustachian ridge to the central fibrous body, and on the ventricular side by the hingeline of the septal leaflet of the tricuspid valve (Plate 1.14). These sloping borders meet superiorly at the apex of the triangle, formed by the central fibrous body. The base of the triangle, containing the mouth of the coronary sinus, is the cavo-tricuspid isthmus. The atrial wall of this triangle is a thin layer of myocardium that is separated from the underlying ventricular myocardium by an extension from the fibrofatty atrioventricular groove. This groove is traversed by the artery to the atrioventricular node, which takes its origin from the dominant coronary artery, this being the right coronary artery in nine tenths of the population. The artery courses superiorly, entering the compact node, which is located in the union of the right and left atrial walls at the apex of the triangle (Plate 1.30). When traced further superiorly, the compact node itself then becomes engulfed by the tissues of the central fibrous body. This body, the strongest part of the cardiac skeleton, is formed from the union of the right fibrous trigone, the rightward end of the region of continuity between the leaflets of the aortic and mitral valves, and the membranous part of the ventricular septum. This arrangement is best appreciated from the aspect of the left ventricular outflow tract (Plate 1.32). In the setting of atrial fibrillation, the interventionist is likely to wish to know the site of penetration of the conduction axis so as to ablate it. As can be appreciated from Plate 1.14, 1.30, and 1.32, this can best be achieved from either the right side, or through the subaortic outflow tract. From the right side, the landmark to penetration of the bundle of His is the apex of the triangle of Koch. In the subaortic outflow tract, the bundle emerges onto the crest of the muscular ventricular septum immediately beneath the zone of apposition between the right coronary and noncoronary leaflets of the aortic valve. The node can also be approached from the left atrium, but is then much deeper within the atrial septum (Plate 1.30). The landmark from the left atrial side is the atrial vestibule immediately adjacent to the septal end of the zone of apposition between the two leaflets of the mitral valve [43]. Although of less immediate significance to the treatment of atrial fibrillation, the interventionist also needs to be aware of the sites of the so-called "slow" and "fast" pathways into the atrioventricular node. As we have already discussed, the slow pathway is located within the septal isthmus (Plate 1.11), albeit that the anatomical substrate has still to be determined with certainty [37, 38]. The fast pathway is located in the anterosuperior rim of the oval fossa, immediately superior to the location of the tendon of Todaro. Again, the anatomic substrate of this structure has yet to be established, but our bias remains that conduction through both pathways into the node is conditioned by the variability in alignment of the myocardial aggregates within the atrial walls [37].

Substrates for abnormal atrial rhythmogenicity

We have emphasized in the preceding paragraphs that there are no insulated tracts of atrial myocardium extending between the sinus and atrioventricular nodes, with preferential conduction between the nodes achieved because of the morphologic arrangement of the working myocardial cells [27]. This does not mean, however, that the cells in these areas have never shown differences from the remainder of the atrial walls. Recognition of this fact is the more significant because, although not recognizable anatomically in the postnatal heart as conduction tissues, the cells forming the internodal atrial area are known to be the substrate for focal atrial tachycardias [45]. The features of these cells that differentiate them from the remainder of the atrial walls cannot be determined on the basis of classical histology. The features, nonetheless, have been clarified by recent findings in the fields of molecular biology and immunohistochemistry, which also impact on the nature of the myocardial sleeves surrounding the pulmonary veins. Taken together, the findings show the need to broaden our recognition of the conduction system based exclusively on histological criteria, considering also the potential substrates for abnormal electrical events as seen within the heart as it develops.

In the postnatal human heart, each heartbeat is generated by a wave of depolarizing impulses originating from the sinus node. Having traversed the working atrial myocardium, and activating it to contract, the impulse is collected in the atrioventricular node, where it is slowed, before being conducted rapidly through the histologically specialized and insulated fibers of the ventricular conduction axis to the ramifications of the peripheral ventricular conduction system, where it finally activates the ventricular working myocardium to contract. This sequence of electrical myocardial activation is registered in the electrocardiogram. The working myocardium of the cardiac chambers themselves, in addition to the anatomic components of the conduction system, is necessary to produce a normal electrocardiogram, as is the insulation found at the atrioventricular junctions at all points other than the penetration of the bundle of His. Although essential components of the overall system, neither the working myocardial elements, nor the fibrofatty elements providing electrical insulation, are considered traditionally as parts of the anatomic conduction system.

This distinction between "specialized" and "working" elements is the more pertinent to the arrangements of the hearts found in lower vertebrates, and to the morphology seen in the hearts of mammals and birds during their development. In lower vertebrates, and in mammalian and avian embryos early in their development, it is possible to record normal electrocardiograms. Yet neither in the hearts of fishes, nor early in the developing heart of birds and mammals, is it possible to recognize the morphologically discrete elements that we subsequently identify as conduction tissues using the definitions of Aschoff [31] and Mönckeberg [32]. The consecutive recordings of depolarizations of atrial and ventricular working myocardium, along with a period of atrioventricular delay, nonetheless, are a fundamental element of electrical patterning of the vertebrate heart. And the basis for development of this electrical design is the key to understanding the function of the components that generate and disseminate the impulse, irrespective of whether or not the components themselves are anatomically distinct.

In all species, the heart tube, when first formed, is simply a myocardial mantle enfolding a ventrally located endocardial tube. Within the walls of the tube at this stage, each myocyte is potentially a pacemaking cell, being inherently rhythmical, and poorly coupled to its neighbors because of a scarcity of gap junctions containing connexin45. Myocardium of this type can be dubbed "primary" myocardium [4, 46]. An electrocardiogram comparable to that seen in the postnatal heart, however, is not recorded until the larger part of the myocardium forming the walls of the atriums and ventricles is ballooned from this primary heart tube (Plate 1.33). This ballooning myocardium, therefore, can be considered secondary, or chamber, myocardium [4]. It is characterized electrically by its ability to conduct rapidly, containing gap junctions rich in both connexin40 and connexin43. The chamber myocardium also stains positively for atrial natriuretic factor. This permits its immunocytochemical distinction from the primary myocardium, which does not contain either atrial natriuretic factor, or connexin40 (Plate 1.34). As these secondary parts of the chambers are ballooned from the primary tube, the interposing areas of myocardium retain their primary characteristics, having high automaticity and conducting slowly. Indeed, small parts of the primary myocardium will retain these initial characteristics throughout development, eventually becoming the sinus and atrioventricular nodes, as will the other parts of the atrioventricular canal which persist as components of atrioventricular ring tissue [36] recognized using the criteria of Aschoff [31] and Mönckeberg [32]. We must ask, therefore, why all this primary myocardium does not persist and become histologically recognizable conduction tissues? This can be answered by recent findings concerning the role of transcription factors of the T-box family.

Transcription factors of the T-box family are essential to many of the processes needed for patterning of the vertebrate embryo [47]. Tbx5, for example, is known to be expressed in a caudocranial gradient along the heart tube. It is able to condition the appropriate development of the cardiac chambers, as well as the individual components of the anatomic conduction system. Haploinsufficiency of the gene produces not only septal defects, but also problems with conduction [48].

This particular transcription factor is also needed to activate the gene that encodes both atrial natriuretic factor and connexin40 [48, 49]. These are some of the proteins expressed in the chamber myocardium that balloons from the primary tube, but they are lacking from the areas of primary myocardium (Plate 1.34). Establishing the pattern of expression of Tbx5 itself, however, does not explain why the genes for atrial natriuretic factor and connexin40 are activated only in the chamber myocardium.

We now know that, concomitant with formation of the myocardium of the chambers, other genes of the Tbx family, initially Tbx2, and slightly later Tbx3, become expressed in the walls of the systemic venous tributaries, the atrioventricular canal, and the developing outflow tract [49], all these areas composed initially of primary myocardium. These latter genes are repressors of transcription [50]. In cooperation with Nkx2-5, they are able to repress the expression of the genes producing atrial natriuretic factor and connexin40. In this way, they permit the primary myocardium to persist in parts of the developing atriums, where it forms a corridor between the atrioventricular canal and the systemic venous tributaries (Plate 1.35). And it is at either end of this area that, eventually, we find the nodes of the anatomic conduction system.

In this respect, it is noteworthy that the original anatomic descriptions of Keith and Flack [28], as well as those subsequently made by Benninghoff [51], match almost seamlessly the patterns of expression for the T-box transcription factors and connexin40. The reconstruction shown in Plate 1.35, from a mouse heart at 9.5 days gestation, shows how the roof of the atrium, at this stage, consists of the rapidly expanding chamber myocardium. Its floor, in contrast, is primary myocardium, interposing between the eventual sites of formation of the cardiac nodes. With ongoing development, the entrances of the systemic venous tributaries, and part of septating atrioventricular canal, become incorporated within the developing right atrium, as does the intervening corridor of primary myocardium, from which the sinus node will be formed at one of its extremities, and the atrioventricular node at the other (Plate 1.35).

In this respect, Rentschler and coworkers [52], using as a molecular marker the reporter gene engrailed-LacZ, have shown that, in the mouse, all the components of the anatomically recognized cardiac conduction system, but in addition the internodal area along with the entire atrioventricular junctional area, are initially under the same transcriptional control. The mechanism of regulation, however, as yet remains undefined. The patterns noted during development for the expression of connexin45, nonetheless, display a remarkable similarity to those seen for Tbx2 and Tbx3, with all being expressed in the regions initially composed of primary myocardium.

Connexin45 is the first connexin to be detected in the embryonic heart tube, being first seen at 8.5 days of development in the mouse. It can subsequently be found in all the individually recognized components of the conduction system, and also in the terminal crest and the atrioventricular region, as well as in the myocardium of the developing outflow tract [53]. The presence of connexin45, therefore, serves to identify the initial location of the primary myocardium, its subsequent location in the anatomical conduction system, and its persistence in a number of associated areas.

If we combine this evidence that has emerged from the findings concerning the T-box transcription factors, engrailed-LacZ, and connexin45, it seems that parts of the walls of the developing atrial chambers are shielded from formation of secondary myocardium. In the postnatal heart, it is parts of these shielded areas that persist as the anatomically recognizable parts of the atrial portion of the conduction system. Other parts remain in vestigial form (Plate 1.36). Although we have been at pains to emphasize that atrial tracts analogous to the ventricular pathways for conduction do not exist, we do not seek to deny that a prominent region of the developing heart can be found along the terminal crest that expresses Tbx3, and which also runs between the definitive nodes. The markers used identify this area of the developing heart as being primary myocardium. In the postnatal human heart, it has become indistinguishable morphologically and histologically from the remainder of the right atrial myocardium.

All the molecular studies discussed above also show the atrioventricular region to be a distinct component of the atrial chambers, lacking as it does expression of connexin40, connexin43, and atrial natriuretic factor, but being positive for Tbx3. It is this atrioventricular region that forms the right and left atrial vestibules. In terms of their gross histology, these vestibules are indistinguishable, in their greater part, from the working myocardium of the remainder of the atrial chambers. A small part of the initially dorsal aspect of the region, of course, persists as the atrioventricular node. The remaining parts have reverted anatomically to a working phenotype, even though McGuire and coworkers showed that, when studied electrophysiologically, the entire region had nodal characteristics [54]. It is surely more than coincidence, therefore, that ectopic nodes are found in these areas in congenitally malformed hearts [40], and the specialized atrioventricular ring tissue is to be found in the right atrial vestibule even in the normal heart (Plate 1.31).

It is then also surely more than coincidence that focal tachycardias arising from the right atrium are far from randomly distributed, originating primarily along the long axis of the terminal crest, around the atrioventricular bundle, around the orifice of the coronary sinus, and around the vestibules of the mitral and tricuspid valves [45]. These are the precise areas identified anatomically and molecularly as representing the residue of the primary myocardium. We speculate, therefore, that these regions maintain their embryonic phenotype relatively long during development. Despite achieving a working anatomic phenotype in postnatal life, it is likely that their developmental heritage renders them prone to the generation of arrhythmias.

Finally, these molecular considerations can be extended to the sleeves of myocardium surrounding the pulmonary veins. We have already discussed the lack of evidence for histologic specialization of the myocytes making up the sleeves. From the stance of development, both the pulmonary and the systemic tributaries of the venous pole of the developing heart constitute a dynamic region, which is rapidly growing and remodeling [52]. The rapid changes occurring within the region are reflected in the expression of markers such as HNK1 [2, 3]. When considered in terms of the pattern of expression of atrial natriuretic factor and connexin40, however, the pulmonary myocardium is negative for the first, and positive for the second, indicating that it is not primary myocardium. The myocardium surrounding the systemic tributaries, in contrast, is negative for both atrial natriuretic factor and connexin40, showing that it is primary in its origin. The pulmonary myocardium, therefore, is a new development not only in evolutionary, but also in embryonic terms [10]. There is no convincing evidence to support its anatomically specialized nature.

Etiological factors relating to atrial fibrillation

Although the focus of our chapter has been anatomic features pertinent to the treatment of patients with atrial fibrillation, thus far we have not discussed any morphologic features specific to such patients. This is because, to the best of our knowledge, studies comparing the atrial morphology of groups of patients with and without fibrillation are largely lacking. Studies have demonstrated an increase in fibrous tissue in the sinus nodes [55], and overall increase in the content of fibrous tissue within the dilated walls of the left atriums [56], albeit not always from patients with fibrillating hearts. We do not know with certainty, therefore, whether these changes cause the atriums to fibrillate, or whether, in the hearts that are fibrillating, the changes are the cause or the effect of the fibrillation. Similarly, studies of the pulmonary venous sleeves have largely been carried out on samples removed from patients with normal rather than fibrillating hearts. Thus, we now know much more about how fibrillation can be stopped by focal ablation in the pulmonary veins, or by compartmentation of the atriums using maze procedures, either surgically or by means of interventional catheterization, but we have yet to identify specific morphologic features precipitating the onset of fibrillation. There is much still to be learnt with regard to the structure and histology of the fibrillating heart.

Acknowledgment

Many thanks to Pfizer Ireland for sponsoring this chapter.

References

1 Ho SY, Anderson RH, Sánchez-Quintana D. Gross structure of the atriums: more than an anatomical curiosity. *PACE* 2002; **25**: 342–350.

2 Blom NA, Gittenberger-de Groot AC, deRuiter MC, Poelmann RE, Mentink MM, Ottenkamp J. Development of the cardiac conduction tissue in human embryos using HNK-1 antigen expression: possible relevance for understanding of abnormal atrial automaticity. *Circulation* 1999; **99**: 800–806.

3 Jongbloed MRM, Schalij MJ, Poelmann RE *et al.* Embryonic conduction tissue: a spatial correlation with adult arrhythmogenic areas. *J Cardiovasc Electrophysiol* 2004; **15**: 349–355.

4 Moorman AFM, Christoffels VM, Anderson RH. Anatomic substrates for cardiac conduction. *Heart Rhythm* 2005; **2**: 875–886.

5 Perez-Lugones A, McMahon JT, Ratliff NB *et al.* Evidence of specialized conduction cells in human pulmonary veins of patients with atrial fibrillation. *J Cardiovasc Electrophysiol* 2003; **14**: 803–809.

6 Ho SY, Cabrera JA, Tran VH, Farre J, Anderson RH, Sanchez-Quintana D. Architecture of the pulmonary veins: relevance to radiofrequency ablation. *Heart* 2001; **86**: 265–270.

7 Cury RC, Abbara S, Schmidt S *et al.* Relationship of the esophagus and aorta to the left atrium and pulmonary veins: implications for catheter ablation of atrial fibrillation. *Heart Rhythm* 2005; **2**: 1317–1323.

8 Cosio FC, Anderson RH, Kuck K *et al.* Living anatomy of the atrioventricular junctions. A guide to electrophysiological mapping. A consensus statement from the Cardiac Nomenclature Study Group, Working Group of Arrhythmias, European Society of Cardiology, and the Task Force on Cardiac Nomenclature from NASPE. *Circulation* 1999; **100**: e31–e37. *Eur Heart J* 1999; **20**: 1068–1075. *J Cardiovasc Electrophysiol* 1999; **10**; 1162–1170.

9 Cook AC, Anderson RH. Attitudinally correct nomenclature [Editorial]. *Heart* 2002; **87**: 503–506.

10 Anderson RH, Brown NA, Moorman AFM. Development and structures of the venous pole of the heart. *Dev Dyn* 2006; **235**: 2–9.

11 Haissaguerre M, Jais P, Shah DC *et al.* Electrophysiological end point for catheter ablation of atrial fibrillation initiated from multiple pulmonary venous foci. *Circulation* 2000; **101**: 1409–1417.

12 Anderson RH, Razavi R, Taylor AM. Cardiac anatomy revisited. *J Anat* 2004; **205**: 159–177.

13 Sanchez-Quintana D, Cabrera JA, Climent V, Farre J, Weiglein A, Ho SY. How close are the phrenic nerves to cardiac structures? Implications for cardiac interventionalists. *J Cardiovasc Electrophysiol* 2005; **16**: 309–313.

14 Chevalier P, Tabib A, Meyronnet D *et al.* Quantitative study of nerves of the human left atrium. *Heart Rhythm* 2005; 2: 518–522.

15 Anderson RH, Webb S, Brown NA. Clinical anatomy of the atrial septum with reference to its developmental components. *Clin Anat* 1999; 12: 362–374.

16 Uemura H, Ho SY, Devine WA *et al.* Analysis of visceral heterotaxy according to splenic status, appendage morphology, or both. *Am J Cardiol* 1995; 76: 846–849.

17 Trento A, Zuberbuhler JR, Anderson RH, Park SC, Siewers RD. Divided right atrium (prominence of the Eustachian and Thebesian valves). *J Thorac Cardiovasc Surg* 1988; 96: 457–463.

18 Lickfett L, Kato R, Tandri H *et al.* Characterization of a new pulmonary vein variant using magnetic resonance angiography. *J Cardiovasc Electrophysiol* 2004; 15: 538–543.

19 Webb S, Brown NA, Wessels A, Anderson RH. Development of the murine pulmonary vein and its relationship to the embryonic venous sinus. *Anat Rec* 1998; 250: 325–334.

20 Hagen P, Scholz DG, Edwards WD. Incidence and size of patent foramen ovale during the first decades of life: an autopsy study of 965 normal hearts. *Mayo Clin Proc* 1984; 59: 1489–1494.

21 Wilmshurst PT, Nightingale S, Walsh KP, Morrison WL. Effect on migraine of closure of cardiac right-to-left shunts to prevent recurrence of decompression illness or stroke for haemodynamic reasons. *Lancet* 2000; 356: 1648–1651.

22 Wilmshurst PT, Nightingale S, Walsh KP, Morrison WL. Clopidogrel reduces migraine with aura after transcatheter closure of persistent foramen ovale and atrial septal defects. *Heart* 2005; 91: 1173–1175.

23 Chauvin M, Shah DC, Haissaguerre M, Marcellin L, Brechenmacher C. The anatomic basis of connections between the coronary sinus musculature and the left atrium in humans. *Circulation* 2000; 101: 647–652.

24 Ho SY, Sanchez-Quintana D, Becker AE. A review of the coronary venous system: a road less travelled. *Heart Rhythm* 2004; 1: 107–112.

25 Bachmann G. The inter-auricular time interval. *Am J Physiol* 1916; 41: 309–320.

26 Ho SY, Anderson RH, Sanchez-Quintana D. Atrial structure and fibres: morphological basis of atrial conduction. *Cardiovasc Res* 2002; 54: 325–336.

27 Spach MS, Kootsey JM. The nature of electrical propagation in cardiac muscle. *Am J Physiol* 1983; 244: H3–H22.

28 Keith A, Flack M. The form and nature of the muscular connections between the primary divisions of the vertebrate heart. *J Anat Physiol* 1907; 41: 172–189.

29 Tawara S. *The Conduction System of the Mammalian Heart: An Anatomico-histological Study of the Atrioventricular Bundle and the Purkinje Fibers.* Imperial College Press, London, 2000.

30 James TN. The internodal pathways of the human heart. *Prog Cardiovasc Dis* 2001; 43: 495–535.

31 Aschoff L. Referat uber die Herzstorungen in ihren Beziehungen zu den Spezifischen Muskelsystem des Herzens. *Verh Dtsch Ges Pathol* 1910; 14: 3–35.

32 Mönckeberg JG. Beitrage zur normalen und pathologischen Anatomie des Herzens. *Verh Dtsch Ges Pathol* 1910; 14: 64–71.

33 Thorel C. Vorläufige Mitteulungen über eine besondere Muskelverbindung zwischen der Cava superior und dem Hisschen bündel. *Munch Med Woch* 1909; 56: 2159–2161.

34 Kent AFS. Researches on the structure and function of the mammalian heart. *J Physiol* 1893; 14: 233–254.

35 Kent AFS. The structure of the cardiac tissues at the auricular–ventricular junction. *J Physiol* 1913; 47: xvii–xviii.

36 Anderson RH, Davies MJ, Becker AE. Atrioventricular ring specialised tissues in the normal heart. *Eur J Cardiol* 1974; 2: 219–230.

37 Inoue S, Becker AE, Riccardi R, Gaita F. Interruption of the inferior extension of the compact atrioventricular node underlies successful radio frequency ablation of atrioventricular nodal reentrant tachycardia. *J Interv Card Electrophysiol* 1999; 3: 273–277.

38 Sanchez-Quintana D, Davies DW, Ho SY, Oslizlok P, Anderson RH. Architecture of the atrial musculature in and around the Triangle of Koch: its potential relevance to atrioventricular nodal reentry. *J Cardiovasc Electrophysiol* 1997; 8: 1396–1407.

39 Anderson RH, Ho SY, Gillette PC, Becker AE. Mahaim, Kent and abnormal atrioventricular conduction. *Cardiovasc Res* 1996; 31: 480–491.

40 Anderson RH, Becker AE, Arnold R, Wilkinson JL. The conducting tissues in congenitally corrected transposition. *Circulation* 1974; 50: 911–923.

41 Anderson KR, Ho SY, Anderson RH. Location and vascular supply of sinus node in human heart. *Br Heart J* 1979; 41: 28–32.

42 Sánchez-Quintana D, Cabrera JA, Farré J, Climant V, Anderson RH, Ho SY. Sinus node revisited in the era of electroanatomical mapping and catheter ablation. *Heart* 2005; 91: 189–194.

43 Wilcox BR, Cook AC, Anderson RH. *Surgical Anatomy of the Heart*, 3rd edn. Cambridge University Press, Cambridge, 2004: 12–44.

44 Janse MJ, Anderson RH. Specialized internodal atrial pathways—fact or fiction? *Eur J Cardiol* 1974; 2: 117–136.

45 Kalman JM, Olgin JE, Karch MR, Hamdan M, Lee RJ, Lesh MD. "Cristal tachycardias": origin of right atrial tachycardias from the crista terminalis identified by intracardiac echocardiography. *J Am Coll Cardiol* 1998; **31**: 451–459.

46 Moorman AFM, Lamers WH. Molecular anatomy of the developing heart. *Trends Cardiovasc Med* 1994; **4**: 257–264.

47 Papaioannou VE, Silver LM. The T-box gene family. *Bioessays* 1998; **20**: 9–19.

48 Bruneau BG, Nemer G, Schmitt JP *et al*. A murine model of Holt-Oram syndrome defines roles of the T-box transcription factor Tbx5 in cardiogenesis and disease. *Cell* 2001; **106**: 709–721.

49 Habets PEMH, Moorman AFM, Clout DEW *et al*. Cooperative action of Tbx2 and Nkx2.5 inhibits ANF expression in the atrioventricular canal: implications for cardiac chamber formation. *Genes Dev* 2002; **16**: 1234–1246.

50 Paxton C, Zhao H, Chin Y, Langner K, Reecy J. Murine Tbx2 contains domains that activate and repress gene transcription. *Gene* 2002; **283**: 117–124.

51 Benninghoff A. Über die Beziehungen des Reizleitungssystems und der papillarmuskeln zu den Konturfasern des Herzschlauches. *Verh Anat Gesellsch* 1923; **57**: 185–208.

52 Rentschler S, Vaidya DM, Tamaddon H *et al*. Visualization and functional characterization of the developing murine cardiac conduction system. *Development* 2001; **128**: 1785–1792.

53 Coppen SR, Severs NJ, Gourdie RG. Connexin45 (alpha 6) expression delineates an extended conduction system in the embryonic and mature rodent heart. *Dev Genet* 1999; **24**: 82–90.

54 McGuire MA, De Bakker JMT, Vermeulen JT *et al*. Atrioventricular junctional tissue. Discrepancy between histological and electrophysiological characteristics. *Circulation* 1996; **94**: 571–577.

55 Sims BA. Pathogenesis of arrhythmias. *Br Heart J* 1972; **34**: 346–350.

56 Davies MJ, Pomerance A. A quantitative study of ageing in the human sinuatrial node and internodal tracts. *Br Heart J* 1972; **34**: 150–152.

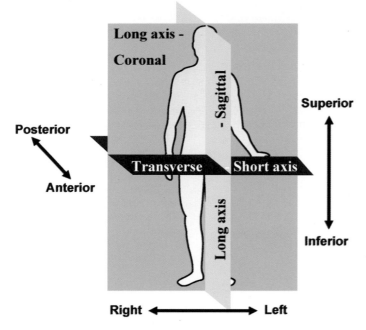

Plate 1.1 The cartoon shows the so-called anatomical position. The subject is standing upright and facing the observer. All structures within the body, by convention, are then described relative to the three orthogonal planes of the body, two in the long axis, the coronal and sagittal planes, and the third in the short axis. As shown, structures are described as being right or left relative to the coronal plane, anterior and posterior relative to the sagittal plane, and superior or inferior according to their position within the short axis series of planes.

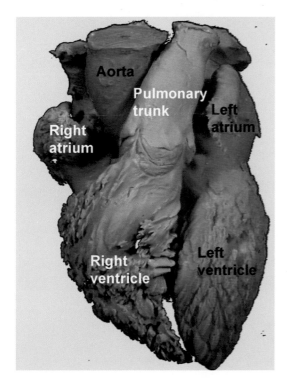

Plate 1.2 The casts of the right and left sides of the heart have been positioned with the heart itself on its apex—the current convention of describing cardiac structures. With this "Valentine" orientation, then the so-called "right-" and "left-sided" structures are appropriately described relative to their counterparts. This situation, however, does not pertain when the heart is in its usual position within the thorax (see Plate 1.3). It is wrong to describe cardiac structures using these coordinates.

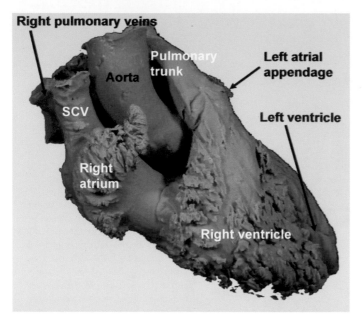

Plate 1.3 The casts of the heart as shown in Plate 1.2 have been reorientated to match the position the heart usually occupies within the thorax. As can be seen, the so-called "right" chambers, in reality, are positioned anteriorly relative to their purported "left-sided" counterparts. All that is seen of the left atrium with the heart in attitudinally appropriate location is the tip of the left atrial appendage. And only a small strip of the left ventricle is seen extending to the cardiac apex. Note the relationship of the superior caval vein (SCV) relative to the right pulmonary veins.

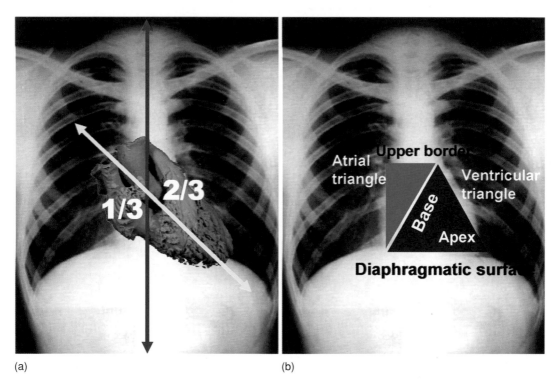

(a) (b)

Plate 1.4 The casts of the heart shown in Plate 1.3 have been superimposed on the chest radiograph, emphasizing the importance of attitudinally appropriate description. As shown in (a), in the usual situation there is a marked discrepancy between the long axis of the body (red arrow) and that of the heart itself (yellow arrow). The heart is typically positioned with one third of its bulk to the right of the midline. As shown in (b), the silhouette projected to the anterior surface of the chest is trapezoidal, but this can be analyzed in terms of atrial and ventricular triangles. Note that the arterial trunks emerge from the base of the ventricular mass through the upper surface of the cardiac silhouette, with the aorta to the right of the pulmonary trunk.

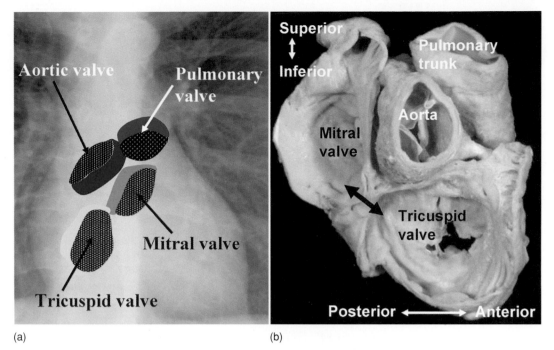

(a)　　　　　　　　　　　　　　　　　　　(b)

Plate 1.5 The montage as shown in (a) was created by reconstructing the locations of the cardiac valves from a dataset obtained using magnetic resonance imaging from the subject whose chest radiograph is shown in the figure. The anatomic relationships of the valves is shown from a different subject in (b), as viewed having removed most of the atrial myocardium and the arterial trunks, and looking at the ventricular base from posteriorly and the right side. Note the "wedged" location of the aorta relative to the site of the atrial septum (double-headed arrow).

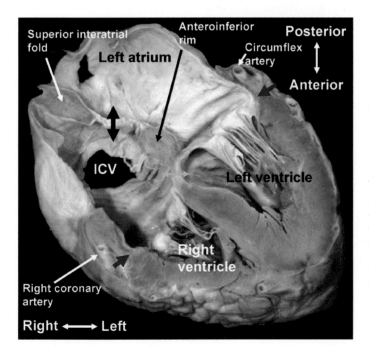

Plate 1.6 The heart has been sectioned to replicate the echocardiographic "four chamber" projection. The section shows how the atrial myocardium is insulated from the ventricular muscle mass by the fibrofatty atrioventricular junctions (red arrows), apart from at the site of penetration of the bundle of His from the apex of the triangle of Koch to the crest of the ventricular septum in the subaortic outflow tract of the left ventricle (double-headed yellow arrow). Note the orientation of the atrial septum (double-headed black arrow), with the so-called "septum secundum" being no more than the superior interatrial fold, but the anteroinferior rim formed by a prominent muscular buttress. ICV, inferior caval vein.

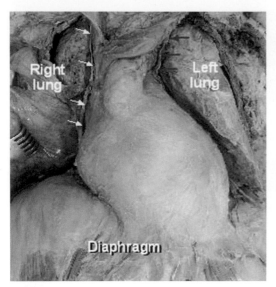

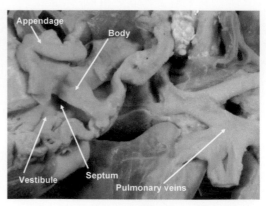

Plate 1.8 The specimen comes from a patient who had totally anomalous pulmonary venous connection. As can be seen, in addition to the appendage, vestibule, and septum, the left atrium possesses a significant body despite the fact that all the pulmonary veins are connected to an extracardiac site, in this instance the portal venous system.

Plate 1.7 This dissection, made by Damian Sanchez-Quintana, of the University of Badajoz, Spain, and reproduced with his permission, shows the relationships of the phrenic nerves to the heart contained within its pericardial sac.

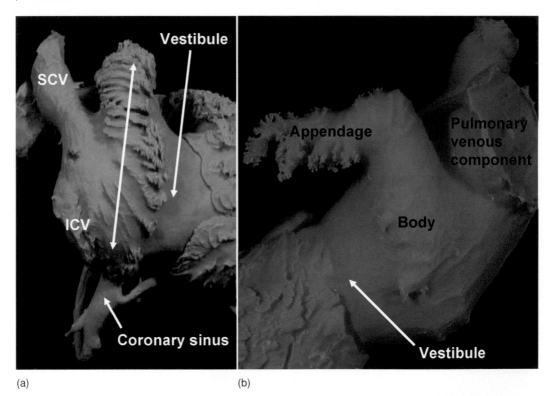

(a)   (b)

Plate 1.9 The casts of the atrial chambers from the heart shown in Plate 1.2 and 1.3 are shown in greater detail. The cast of the right atrium (a) is photographed from the right and posteriorly. Note the extent of the pectinate muscles of the appendage (white double-headed arrow), which makes up the entirety of the anterior wall of the chamber. The pectinated appendage interposes between the smooth-walled systemic venous sinus and the vestibular, the venous sinus receiving the superior and inferior caval veins (SCV, ICV), as well as the coronary sinus. The cast of the left atrium (b) is photographed from the left and laterally. The pectinate muscles are confined within the tubular appendage, with the remainder of the chamber, made up of vestibule, body, and venous component, having smooth walls. Neither the septum nor the body of the right atrium is visible in these photographs.

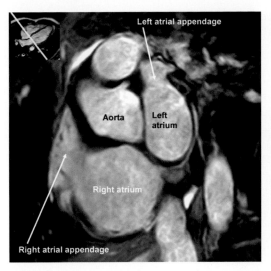

Plate 1.10 This magnetic resonance image, taken in the plane shown in the inset, shows the relationships of the atrial appendages to their respective chambers.

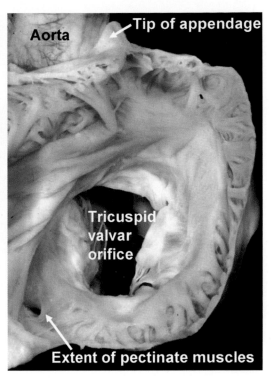

Plate 1.12 The right atrium has been opened through a cut in the appendage parallel to the vestibular, and is photographed from above and behind. Note the extent of the pectinate muscles round the vestibular. Note also the triangular tip of the appendage, which abuts against the aorta.

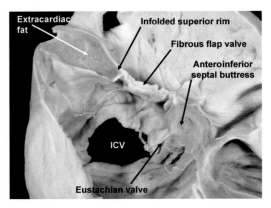

Plate 1.11 This close-up of the specimen shown in Plate 1.6 reveals the salient features of septal morphology. The floor of the oval fossa is formed by the fibrous flap valve of the septum, which closes against the infolded superior rim, often described as the "septum secundum." As can be seen, in reality this structure is a deep fold, containing extracardiac fat. The flap valve is hinged from the extensive anteroinferior septal buttress, into which inserts the fibrous remnant of the Eustachian valve, which becomes the tendon of Todaro.

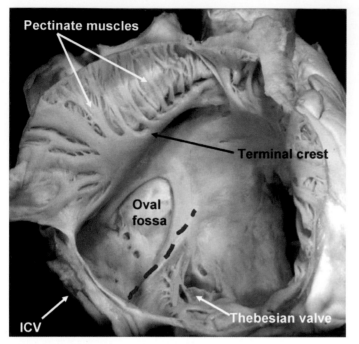

Plate 1.13 The right atrium has again been opened through a cut parallel to the atrioventricular junction, but in this heart, the appendage has been reflected superiorly, and the chamber is photographed from the front. Note the extent of the terminal crest, and the pectinate muscles that radiate from the crest into the appendage. The green arrow shows the inferior extent of the pectinate muscles, while the dotted red line marks the Eustachian ridge. ICV, inferior caval vein.

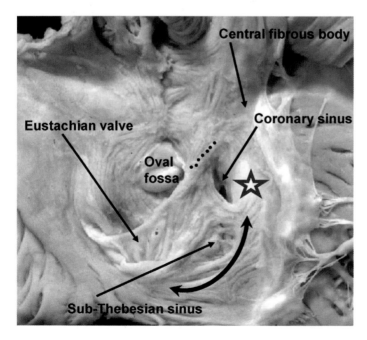

Plate 1.14 In this heart, the parietal wall of the right atrium has been opened, and the endocardial lining dissected away from the posterior wall to reveal the orientation of the myocardial aggregates forming the atrial walls. The dotted black line shows the continuation of the Eustachian valve as the tendon of Todaro, while the double-headed black arrow shows the location of the cavo-tricuspid isthmus, with the red star showing the location of the septal isthmus.

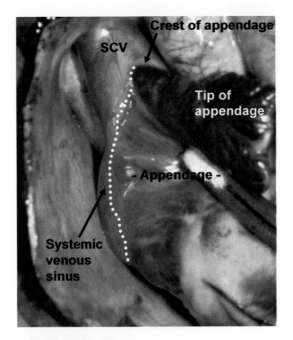

Plate 1.15 This picture, taken in the operating room by Dr Ben Wilcox, University of North Carolina, and reproduced with his permission, shows the relationship of the right atrial appendage to the systemic venous sinus. The white dotted line shows the location of the terminal groove, with the usual position of the sinus node outlined by the green dashed line. Note the triangular tip of the appendage lying adjacent to the aorta, but note also the extent of the appendage inferiorly. SCV, superior caval vein.

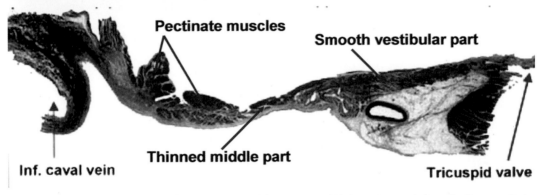

Plate 1.16 This histological section shows the structure of the cavo-tricuspid isthmus. It extends from the fibrous wall of the inferior caval vein to the hinge of the tricuspid valve. Note the varying thickness of its muscular walls in its posterior, middle, and anterior components.

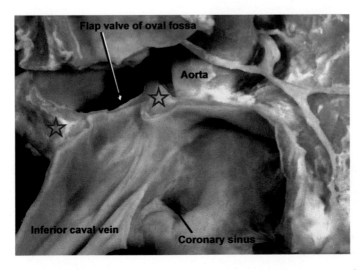

Plate 1.17 This heart from an infant has been transacted across the middle of the oval fossa. This shows how the anterior and posterior margins of the fossa are infoldings in the walls of the atrium. Significantly, the anterior infolding overlies the aortic root. As can be appreciated, it would be feasible, albeit unwanted, to pass a device across this wall, rather than through the floor of the oval fossa itself, unless taking care when attempting septal puncture.

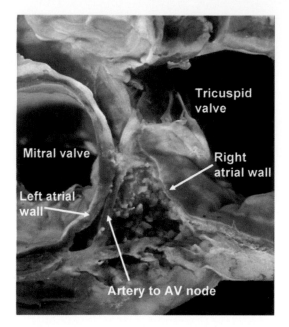

Plate 1.18 In this heart, the inferoanterior continuation of the margin of the oval fossa has been dissected away to show how the walls of the right atrium diverge to overlay the wall of the left ventricle. The artery to the atrioventricular node extends superiorly through this extension of the inferior atrioventricular groove, arising in this heart from a dominant circumflex artery.

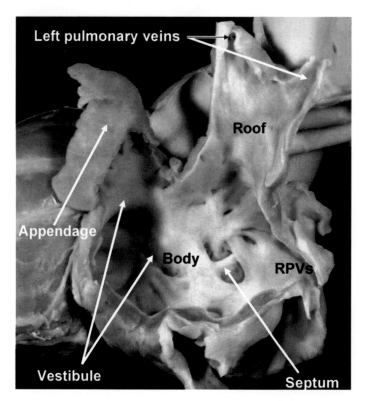

Plate 1.19 The left atrium has been dissected to show its component parts, and is photographed from the left side. Note that almost all the walls are smooth on the internal aspect, the pectinate muscle, not well seen in this photograph, being confined within the tubular appendage (see Illustration 1.2b). The atrial roof, formed by the pulmonary veins, is reflected upward, with the right pulmonary veins (RPVs) seen inferiorly, whereas in reality one vein is found at each corner of the atrial roof.

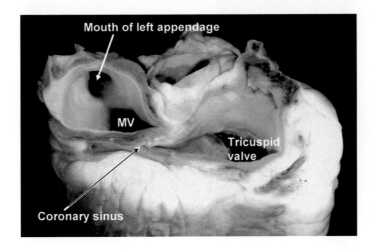

Plate 1.20 The heart has been sectioned through its diaphragmatic surface, showing the course of the coronary sinus through the left atrioventricular groove. Note that the wall of the sinus is discrete and separate from the wall of the left atrium, albeit that muscular bridges run between the two muscular components. Note also the site of the opening to the left atrial appendage. MV, orifice of mitral valve.

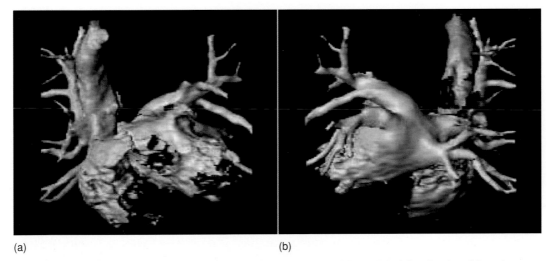

(a) (b)

Plate 1.21 These reconstructions of the atrial chambers, the right atrium in blue and the left atrium in red, have been made from a dataset acquired using magnetic resonance imaging. They show the chambers seen from the front (a) and the back (b). Note the relationships of the pulmonary veins.

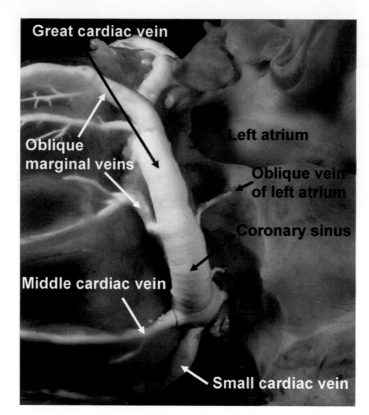

Great cardiac vein

Oblique marginal veins

Middle cardiac vein

Left atrium

Oblique vein of left atrium

Coronary sinus

Small cardiac vein

Plate 1.22 The cast shows the usual pattern of venous drainage to the coronary sinus. The junction of the oblique vein of the left atrium with the venous conduit within the left atrioventricular junction is often taken as the site of origin of the coronary sinus, although others place the boundary between sinus and the great cardiac vein as the location of the valve of Vieussens.

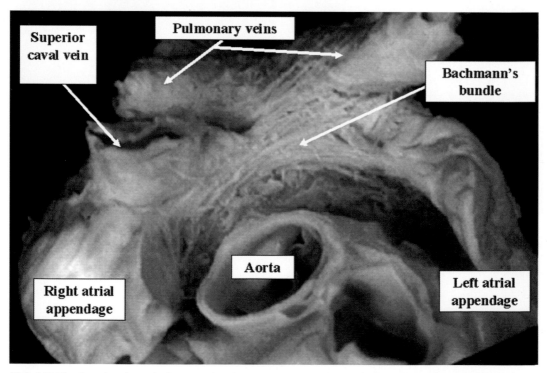

Superior caval vein

Pulmonary veins

Bachmann's bundle

Aorta

Right atrial appendage

Left atrial appendage

Plate 1.23 The dissection shows the location of Bachmann's bundle, which extends from the superior and leftward aspect of the terminal crest, crosses the interatrial groove, and ramifies within the wall of the left atrium. It is the parallel alignment of the myocytes within the bundle that confers upon it the facility to perform as a "superhighway" for interatrial conduction.

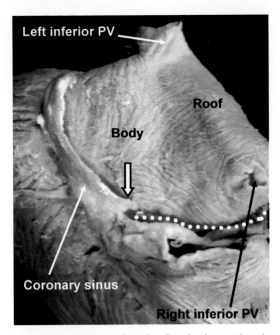

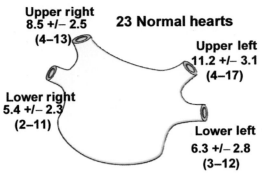

Measurements in millimeters – Ho *et al.*, *JCE*, 1999: 10: 1525–1533

Plate 1.25 The dimensions of the myocardial sleeves extending along the pulmonary veins in a series of 23 human hearts. Reproduced with permission.

Plate 1.24 In this heart, the epicardium has been stripped away to show the orientation of the aggregates of myocytes within the atrial walls. Note that the coronary sinus possesses its own wall, and note also the bridge (arrow) between the walls of the sinus and the left atrium. The white dotted line marks the deep superior interatrial fold. The posterior aspect of the heart is photographed from above and from the right side.

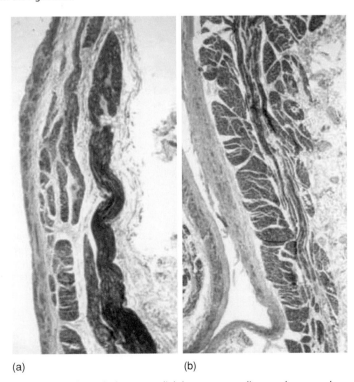

(a)   (b)

Plate 1.26 These sections are taken through the myocardial sleeves surrounding one human pulmonary vein, with the sections taken close to the venoatrial junction (a) and more distally (b). The sleeves are composed exclusively of working myocardium.

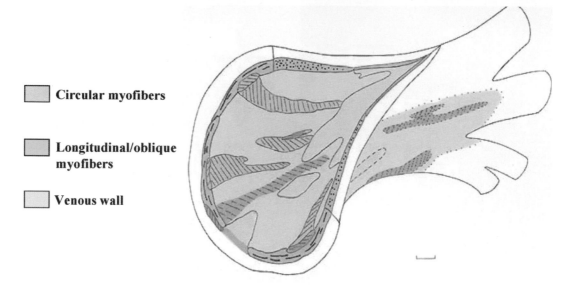

Circular myofibers

Longitudinal/oblique myofibers

Venous wall

Plate 1.27 A reconstruction of the myocardial sleeve surrounding an upper left pulmonary vein from a normal heart. Note the intermingling of the circumferential and longitudinal fibers. It is probably this nonuniform anisotropy, perhaps coupled with an increase of the fibrous matrix, that sets the scene for abnormal focal activity.

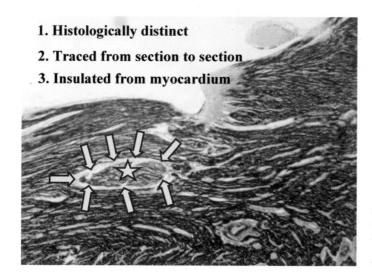

1. **Histologically distinct**
2. **Traced from section to section**
3. **Insulated from myocardium**

Plate 1.28 The histological section shows how the right bundle branch satisfies all three criteria suggested by Aschoff [31], and Mönckeberg [32], for recognition of tracts of conduction tissue.

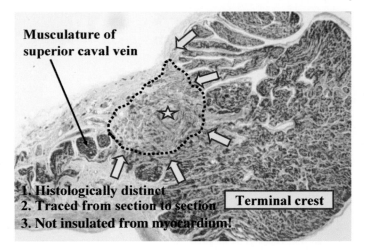

Musculature of superior caval vein

1. **Histologically distinct**
2. **Traced from section to section**
3. **Not insulated from myocardium!**

Terminal crest

Plate 1.29 This section is through the junction of the terminal crest with the lateral wall of the superior caval vein. It shows that the cells of the sinus node satisfy only two of the three criteria for histological specialization, not being insulated from the atrial myocardium.

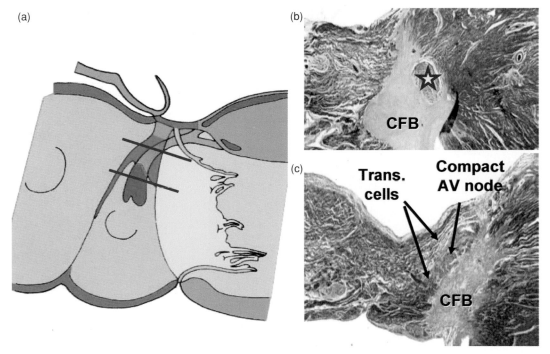

(a)

(b)

CFB

(c)

Trans. cells

Compact AV node

CFB

Plate 1.30 The cartoon (a) shows a diagrammatic representation of the triangle of Koch. The two blue lines show the level of the histological sections seen in the right hand panels. (c) shows the compact node and its transitional cells, again satisfying only two of the three German criteria for specialization. (b) shows how the axis becomes engulfed within the central fibrous body to become the bundle of His (star).

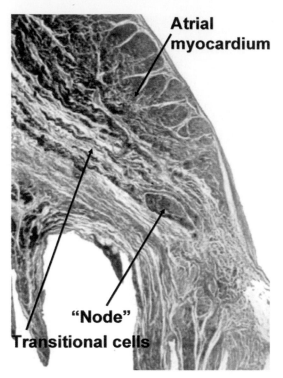

Plate 1.31 This histological section is through the right atrial vestibule. It shows how a component of the terminal insertion of the myocardium is recognized as specialized using the German criteria. This is the atrioventricular ring tissue.

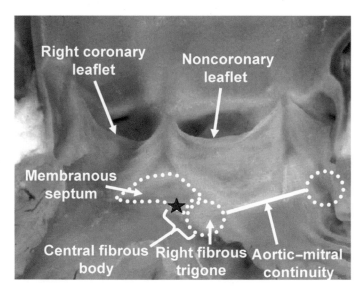

Plate 1.32 The subaortic outflow tract has been opened through its anterior wall and photographed from the front and from the left side. Note how the membranous septum and right fibrous trigone fuse to form the so-called central fibrous body. The point of penetration of the conduction axis is shown by the star.

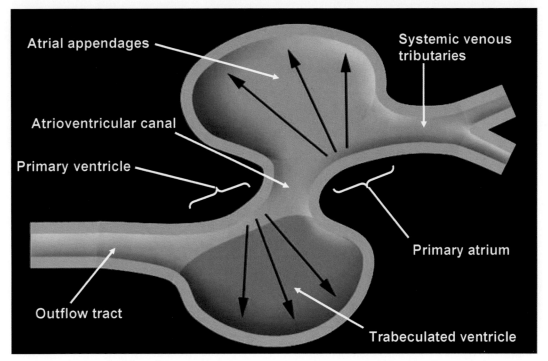

Plate 1.33 The cartoon illustrates the general architectural plan for formation of the vertebrate heart. The primary heart tube, shown in grey, buds ventrally and dorsally to produce chamber myocardium. The ventral buds, two in the human heart, form the atrial appendages. The dorsal bud forms the trabeculated part of the left ventricle, with the right ventricle budding from an additional component of the primary tube added at a later stage.

Connexin 40 (Cx 40)

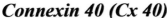

Molecular phenotype

Cx40– / ANF– myocardium
Cx 40+/ANF + myocardium
Cx40+/ ANF– myocardium

Atrial natriuretic factor (ANF)

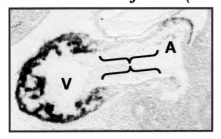

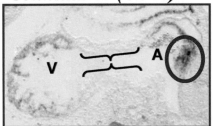

Components

Primary myocardium
Chamber myocardium
Pulmonary myocardium

Plate 1.34 The sections of the heart from an embryonic mouse of 9.5 days gestation have been processed to demonstrate either connexin40 or atrial natriuretic factor. The differential patterns of expression permit the distinction of primary, chamber, and pulmonary myocardium.

(a)

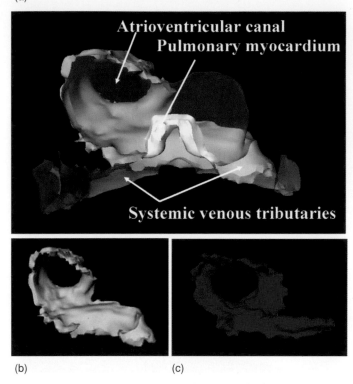

Atrioventricular canal
Pulmonary myocardium

Systemic venous tributaries

(b)   (c)

Plate 1.35 These reconstructions are from a mouse heart at 9.5 days gestation. (a) shows the atrial component viewed from behind, with the systemic venous tributaries seen inferiorly. (b) shows the corridor of primary myocardium extending from the atrioventricular canal to the openings of the systemic venous tributaries. It is identical in location to the area delineated by expression of the transcription factor Tbx3, shown in red in (c).

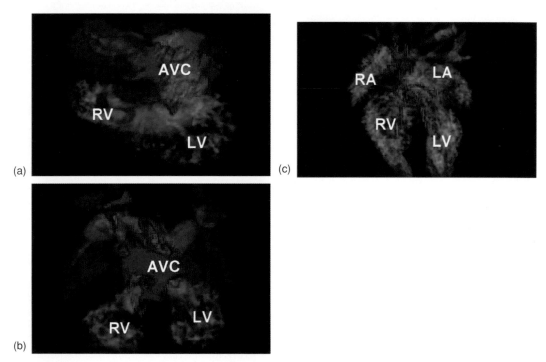

Plate 1.36 These reconstructions, all shown from the front, show the extent of the areas expressing Tbx3 at 9.5 days (a), 13.5 days (b), and 17.5 days (c) gestation. The areas are much more extensive at the earlier than the later stages. See text for further discussion.

CHAPTER 2

Pathophysiology of atrial fibrillation

Robert A. Byrne & Kieran Daly

Introduction

Although the first electrocardiographic recording of atrial fibrillation (AF) was made by Einthoven in 1906, it was not until Sir Thomas Lewis described the presence of irregular f waves in a patient with "arrhythmia perpetua" and ascribed these as originating from continual fibrillatory activity of the auricle, that the atrial basis of the arrhythmia was recognized [1]. Ever since, the precise electrical mechanisms underlying the pathophysiology of AF have remained elusive. It may be argued that our current inability to adequately manage or prevent AF is a direct result of our poor understanding of the mechanics of AF. In fact, in recent years, there has been a noticeable clinical shift downstream in our management strategies with concentration on the prevention of the consequences of AF rather than clinical attempts at effective rhythm modification. Almost simultaneously, however, there has been a very significant expansion in our understanding of the electrophysiological basis of the arrhythmia at a basic science level. This provides hope for clinical interventions aimed at the underlying disease process and a reversion in our management drift of an evolving cardiovascular epidemic.

Writing in a recent Insight review paper for *Nature*, Stanley Nattel notes that much of our conceptual framework for understanding AF mechanisms is grounded in the work of early twentieth century research [2]. As early as 1907, Winberg surmised that rapidly firing ectopic atrial foci were the primary driving forces behind the arrhythmia. Mines first advanced the circus movement of reentry (i.e. multiple-circuit reentry) in 1914, and in the same year, Lewis proposed a flutter-like single-circuit reentry underlying AF. In multiple reentry excitation, irregular atrial activity is inherent, whereas in ectopic foci and single-circuit reentry, irregularity is consequent on interactions between wavefronts from the primary generator and the spatial variance in the refractory properties of atrial tissue. After the publication of the seminal research work of Moe and Abildskov in 1959 [3], there was general acceptance of the primacy of the multiple wavelet hypothesis and this remained the case until advances in high-resolution mapping, which began in the 1970s, allowed more precise delineation of electrophysiological mechanisms and improved catheter-based technology offered opportunity for potential curative intervention. Before exploring the electrophysiological basis of the arrhythmia we will briefly discuss AF in its clinical context.

Clinicopathological considerations

In the normal resting individual, heart rate is controlled by the opposing forces of the two discrete limbs of the autonomic nervous system. At rest, vagal tone predominates over sympathetic innervation and heart rate is typically maintained between 60 and 100 beats/min. Pharmacological blockade of the autonomic nervous system or denervation of the heart, for example, following cardiac transplantation, results in unregulated sinoatrial automaticity and resting heart rates of approximately 100 beats/min. AF results in loss of physiological autonomic control of chronotropy with

Manual of Surgical Treatment of Atrial Fibrillation.
Edited by Hauw T. Sie *et al.* © 2008 Blackwell Publishing,
ISBN: 978-1-4051-4032-4.

resultant rapid ventricular response rates which are hallmarks of the clinical condition. Loss of autonomic chronotropic control is typically associated with rapid acceleration of ventricular rates with exercise, reduced functional capacity, and exertional dyspnea. Incessant atrial tachycardia may lead to the development of systolic cardiac dysfunction and clinical manifestations of heart failure, in patients with otherwise structurally normal hearts [4, 5].

During AF, atrial cells fire at rates in the order of 400–600/min. As a result, functional mechanical synchronicity of atrial tissue is lost, resulting in incoordinated fibrillatory activity or quivering of the atria. Atrial contraction in late ventricular diastole typically accounts for approximately 10% of ventricular filling volumes and loss of "atrial kick" appreciably compromises cardiac output. Patients with LV systolic dysfunction or impaired relaxation, for example, hypertrophic cardiomyopathy, are particularly dependent on the atrial component of ventricular filling as this may comprise in excess of 25% of end-diastolic volumes, and consequently this subset tends to tolerate AF particularly poorly with a high potential for clinical decompensation.

In clinicopathological terms, two distinct clinical pictures exist. The majority of cases of AF (approximately 85%) occur secondary to predisposing clinical cardiac conditions [6]. These include hypertension, coronary artery disease, heart failure, valvular dysfunction, pericardial disease, and cardiac surgery. Arrhythmogenesis is postulated to be mediated by altered vascular compliance, impaired ventricular relaxation, elevated filling pressures, and left atrial (LA) stretch. This disease entity tends to be associated with a dysfunctional cardiovascular substrate and is associated with a higher incidence of complications, such as systemic thromboembolism. A smaller proportion of cases (approximately 15%) occur in patients without structural cardiac or vascular diseases. The term "lone AF" has been coined to refer to this clinical picture and systemic complications, such as thromboembolism, are rare. Although there are many similarities in the electrical mechanisms underlying the generation and propagation of AF in both categories, there is an increasing consensus that the clinical manifestations and risks associated with AF when coupled with cardiovascular disease, across the spectrum from endothelial dysfunction through impaired relaxation to structural heart disease, are very significantly different from AF occurring in the absence of cardiac disease. This has important implications in terms of risk management strategies.

Novel risk factors predictive of AF have been described. In particular, an association of AF with sleep apnea, obesity, and metabolic syndrome, and C-reactive protein (CRP) has been seen. Obstructive sleep apnea rates have been shown to be significantly higher in a cohort of patients with AF compared with those without AF [7]. Obesity also appears to be an independent predictor of AF with one study finding a relative risk of $1.39/10 \text{ kg/m}^2$ for developing AF after multivariate analysis [8]. An association between CRP and AF is also noted. It would seem that the central mechanism underlying these newer risk factors might be endothelial dysfunction and abnormalities of diastolic function with CRP being a surrogate marker for the presence, albeit subclinically, of atherosclerotic endothelial dysfunction.

Diastolic dysfunction and electromechanical coupling

Evidence supporting the central pathophysiological association between diastolic dysfunction AF was described recently in a cohort of 840 consecutive patients over the age of 65 who underwent routine echocardiographic examination [9]. Patients with known atrial arrhythmia, valvular heart disease, or stroke were excluded and eligible subjects were followed in their medical record for documentation of first episode of AF. Abnormal relaxation, pseudonormal, and restrictive left ventricular diastolic filling were associated with hazard ratios for developing AF of 3.33, 4.84, and 5.26, when compared with normal diastolic function. The subsequent development of AF over a 5-year period was only 1% in patients who did not have diastolic dysfunction compared with approximately 12% of patients with moderate dysfunction and 20% of those with restrictive physiology. The investigators concluded that the presence and severity of diastolic dysfunction were independent predictors of incident nonvalvular AF.

Atrial histology shows marked variation in the concentration of myocyte packing within their connective tissue sheaths in different locations throughout the atrium. Mechanical stretch is therefore distributed differently to myocytes in different regions of the atria. Uneven distribution of stretch within myocyte groups will generate differences in electrical contraction coupling and may promote dispersion of refractoriness. These variations may be more marked in conditions predisposing to increased atrial interstitial fibrosis, such as senescence, infarction, and heart failure. Conversely, however, in certain situations, interstitial collagenization may promote structural coherence and more even distribution of load, depending on preexisting geometrical arrangements.

One central tenet critical to the understanding of the pathophysiology of AF is the recognition that increased hemodynamic load on the atria promotes electrophysiological changes which confer predisposition to arrhythmogenesis. Using a model of increased LA pressure in isolated sheep hearts, Kalifa and investigators were the first to demonstrate that rising LA pressure elicits rapid atrial electrical activity [at the junction of the left atrium with the superior pulmonary veins (PVs)]. The sources were further identified as rotors, the frequency and spatial organization of which increased, at higher atrial pressures [10]. Below 10 cm H_2O, artificially induced AF terminated due to slow and unstable atrial reentry. The mechanism underlying this transduction remains to be fully elucidated. Stretch-induced nonselective cation current (I_{nsl}) can carry Na^+ into the cell and K^+ out, and is involved in depolarization from resting membrane potential (during phase 4) and initial very early repolarization after the termination of phase 0. The former favors spontaneous ectopic activity while opening in the latter circumstance favors earlier repolarization and reduced refractory periods. Interestingly, blockade of these stretch-activated channels by a tarantula toxin is associated with a suppression of stretch-induced AF and may represent a potential therapeutic target [11].

In a chronically instrumented human model, alterations in hemodynamic load on the atrium has been shown to directly affect myocyte depolarization duration independent of changes in rate or autonomic tone [12]. Acute reductions in resting membrane potential, action potential amplitude and duration, and the presence of after depolarizations causing extrasystoles have been demonstrated. These changes appear more pronounced in areas of greatest mechanical stretch [13].

Mechanical force transduction likely affects cellular electrophysiological activity via a number of different mechanisms. Firstly, stretch-activated ionic channels (SACs) may be opened as a direct result of transmembrane pressure effects or indirectly via cytoskeletal strain on membrane-bound integrins that are electrically coupled to SACs. Alterations in force–length relationships at a cellular level also impact on actin–myosin interaction at a sarcomeric level, which alters sarcoplasmic Ca^{2+} release and consequently affects transmembrane potentials. Finally, strain at a cellular level may have direct impacts on secondary signal transduction systems involved in transmembrane ionic channel opening. In addition to strain effects on mechanosensitive SACs, alteration in concentrations of L-type I_{Ca} channels has also been shown in response to cytoskeletal stretch. The central importance of this ion channel in regulating the duration of the atrial effective refractory period (ERP) and hence the dispersion of electrical signal propagation is discussed in detail at a later stage.

The central role of angiotensin-II

Increased cellular stress is also associated with catecholamine release and upregulation of angiotensin-II (Ang-II). Whether these changes are markers of the underlying cardiovascular disease process or effects of atrial stretch are unclear. Acetylcholine (via muscarinic receptors) and adrenaline (via beta-agonist effects) tend to oppose each other in the generation of adenylcyclase, which favors protein kinase A generation via cyclic AMP. Protein kinase A modulates intracellular Ca^{2+} via I_{Ca} opening and the release of sarcoplasmic reticular Ca^{2+} stores. Alpha-adrenergic receptor and angiotensin-II type 1 receptor (AT1) effects modulate calcium homeostasis via phosphatidylinositol second messenger systems. Activation of these latter two receptors also enhances protein kinase C generation that upregulates mitogen-activated protein kinase (MAPK) activity, which has a central role in hypertrophy and fibrosis [14].

Alterations in the activity of Ang-II alluded to above, seems to have an important role in explaining the inextricable link between AF and heart failure [15]. Maladaptive activation of the renal-angiotensin system (RAAS) is a hallmark of the congestive heart failure syndrome. Increased atrial Ang-II concentrations have clearly been demonstrated in AF associated with structural heart disease and RAAS activation has been shown to be associated with cardiac fibrosis in a variety of clinical settings. Exposure of fibroblasts to Ang-II in vitro promotes collagen synthesis while impairing collagenase activity. This correlates with analysis of atrial tissue samples removed at surgery in patients with AF, which have shown increased levels of ACE activity which is necessary for Ang-II generation and increased levels of extracellular signal-related kinase (ERK) which is a downstream product of Ang-II involved in fibrosis and hypertrophy at a cellular level [16]. The expression of AT1 receptors, which mediate these mitogenic effects, is downregulated in structural heart disease associated with AF. This is a manifestation of a classical receptor-kinetic response to the presence of increased levels of its agonist compound and likely represents a physiological compensatory response to atrial fibrosis [17].

Programmed cell death (apoptosis) has an important role in regulation of cellular expression under normal physiological circumstances. However, recent consensus suggests a pathological role for apoptosis in heart failure and cellular remodeling associated with myocardial infarction. Atrial apoptosis, evidenced by increased levels of proapoptotic caspace-3, has been demonstrated in chronically fibrillating human atria and replacement fibrosis appears to be the ultimate consequence [18].

Further support for the important role of Ang-II, and promise for intervention by its blockade, in causing substrate modification in AF comes from experimental canine model by Li *et al.* [19]. They induced LV dysfunction by rapid ventricular pacing in the presence and absence of enalapril therapy and measured Ang-II levels, MAPK activity, atrial collagenization, and mean duration of burst pacing induced AF. They found that ventricular tachycardic pacing successfully induced heart failure, raised levels of Ang-II and MAPK, and promoted atrial fibrosis. Enalapril significantly attenuated the increase in

Ang-II and MAPK (specifically ERK) activity (while hydralazine and nitrate therapy did not). Electrophysiological studies showed that enalapril reduced the higher conduction heterogeneity index seen in CHF and reduced the duration of burst pacing induced AF. They conclude that ACE inhibition interferes with the signal transduction mechanisms, which favor the development of an AF-promoting substrate, and offers potential as a therapeutic target for prevention of AF.

It is encouraging that this basic science experimental data has been borne out in a number of large-scale clinical trials. A systematic review of 11 studies, which recruited 56,308 patients, found that ACE inhibitors and angiotensin receptor blockers reduced the relative risk of AF by 28% [20]. There was no significant difference observed between the two classes in terms of efficacy, though benefit appeared to be limited to patients with heart failure or those hypertensives who had documented left ventricular hypertrophy. There appeared to be a large effect in patients postelectrical cardioversion (relative risk reduction of 48%) but the confidence limits were wide.

Electropathophysiological concepts

The role of the PVs

The electropathophysiology of AF is complex and involves the integration of framework models from across the spectrum of arrhythmology. Historical stand-alone models have been inadequate in explaining the mechanism of AF but recent developments are leading toward a more pervasive understanding of the underlying electropathophysiology. In common with other cardiac arrhythmia there are two processes necessary for arrhythmogenesis of AF, namely, an abnormal mechanism responsible for initiating the arrhythmia and the presence of an abnormal substrate that allows perpetuation of the abnormal rhythm.

For the best part of the last century, Moe's multiple wavelet reentry hypothesis was the dominant prevailing theory in our understanding of AF [3]. However, while this theory may play a role in explaining the propagation of the arrhythmia, it does not address the triggers responsible for its initiation in the first instance. Much of the work in elucidating the mechanisms of AF over the last century ignored arrhythmia-initiation because most studies focused on AF that had been iatrogenically induced in the electrophysiology lab. In addition, spontaneous initiation of AF in animal models is rare. However, a group of French electrophysiologists revived the original concept of Rothberger that a single focus may initiate AF. Haissaguerre et al. studied 45 consecutive patients with documented daily or alternate day episodes of AF [21]. Spontaneous ectopy was mapped using multielectrode catheters in the right and left atria and the earliest electrical activity immediately preceding the onset of AF was recorded. Sixty-nine foci were discovered, 3 in the right atrium, 1 in the left atrium, and 65 (94%) in the PVs. Radiofrequency (RF) catheter ablation was then performed in an attempt to isolate the initiating focus and the accuracy of their mapping was confirmed by the abrupt disappearance of triggering beats after catheter ablation. Their seminal paper concluded that PV foci played a vital role in the initiation of AF and that RF catheter ablation could successfully eliminate paroxysms of AF in a majority of patients.

Subsequent studies have confirmed that although the majority of early electrical activity foci are located in the PVs, other atrial locations such as the ligament of Marshall (a venous remnant in the left atrium) and the superior vena cava have also demonstrated important early electrical activation [22, 23].

The reasons why PVs play such an important role in the initiation of AF is not well understood. Triggering ectopic activity appears to be localized to "sleeves" of atrial myocardial tissue that extend into the distal PVs. This tissue likely resembles the islets of atrial myocardium and vascular smooth muscle cells found within the coronary sinus and the AV valves that appear to exhibit focal triggering activity in response to rapid electrical stimulation or increased mechanical stretch. Multiple electrophysiologic mechanisms have been proposed as the basis for focal PV firing, including abnormal automaticity, triggered activity, and micro-reentry; however, the exact mechanism for conversion of the focal PV activity into AF is still unknown.

There is increasing evidence that local autonomic innervation of the PVs plays an important role in the modulation of PV foci output and the transduc-

tion of these impulses into a propagated arrhythmia. Recent animal work by Scherlag et al. showed that stimulation of local autonomic ganglia in epicardial fat pads produced a vagal response which was associated with a reduction in the number of PV premature depolarizations required to induce AF [24]. Conversely, vagal denervation, via localized lignocaine injection, abolished transduction of PV stimuli into propagated AF. RF ablation around PV ostia frequently induces vagal responses and a recent study of patients undergoing RFA showed that 34% exhibited vagal responses [25]. The most common sites of parasympathetic innervation were the roof junction of the left superior PV and the posteroinferior junction of the left and right inferior PVs. Successful vagal denervation by continued RF application at the site of the evoked response was achieved in the vast majority of patients. Patients in whom vagal responses were elicited and abolished were significantly more likely to remain in sinus rhythm. The conclusion is that parasympathetic attenuation by PV denervation confers added benefit in patients undergoing circumferential PV isolation for paroxysmal AF.

Many commentators have recognized the importance of fluctuation in autonomic tone preceding the onset of paroxysms of AF. The main tool used to evaluate autonomic tone in clinical cardiology is the analysis of heart rate variance on Holter monitoring. Analysis of Holter monitor recordings in unselected AF patients has demonstrated significant changes in autonomic tone prior to the onset of sustained AF. Bettoni and Zimmermann studied time–domain and frequency–domain data from six antecedent time periods: the 24-hour period, the hour preceding AF, and four consecutive 5-minute periods in the 20 minutes immediately before the onset of AF [26, 27]. Their data suggested a primary increase in adrenergic drive occurring over at least 20 minutes before the onset of AF followed by an abrupt shift toward vagal predominance immediately before onset. Increased vagal tone is frequently involved in the onset of AF in patients with structurally normal hearts. Parasympathetic stimulation shortens the atrial effective refractory period, increases its dispersion, and decreases the wavelength of reentrant circuits that facilitate initiation and perpetuation of AF. In addition to reducing the critical mass necessary to sustain multiple reentry circuits, the maze procedure causes partial parasympathetic denervation, which dual mechanism of action may account for its high clinical success rates [28]. Long-term vagal denervation of the atria renders AF less easily inducible, presumably because of increased electrophysiological homogeneity. Conversely, however, increased adrenergic drive seems to predominate in AF due to secondary causes.

Opposing models of propagation

Historically, the majority of our conceptual basis for understanding the pathophysiology of AF is derived from competing theories explaining the mechanisms of perpetuation of an artificially initiated arrhythmia. In 1959, using a cholinergic canine model of AF, Moe and Abildskov attempted to elucidate the critical frequency at which macro-reentrant atrial flutter would degenerate into AF [3]. Their observation that electrically induced atrial flutter could be terminated by injection of aconitine, when the initiating stimulus was removed, but that AF could not, resulted in the conclusion that AF could exist as a stable self-sustaining arrhythmia independent of its initiating trigger. They explained this by proposing that differences in atrial refractory periods resulted in advancing wavefronts encountering atrial tissue in variously advanced stages of refractoriness. This resulted in fractionating of wavefronts about islets of refractory tissue and the generation of independent daughter wavelets that became subjected to this same process. "Fully developed fibrillation would then be a state in which many of such randomly wandering wavelets coexist."

In a subsequent computer-generated model, the same group showed that AF was most likely perpetuated by multiple chaotic circuits, widely scattered in the myocardium, varying constantly in size, location, and number, and exhibiting mutual reinitiation and extinguishment .[29]. They further observed that continued perpetuation of the rhythm seemed critically dependent on the number of coexistent reentrant wavelets, which itself was a function of the atrial mass available for arrhythmogenesis. "Large mass, short wavelength and slow conduction will all favour perpetuation of the arrhythmia by permitting the coexistence of many independent, randomly wandering wavelets." This concept of a "critical mass" was supported by their

observations that application of a clamp across the base of the fibrillating atrium to disconnect the atrial appendage from the remainder of the atrium, resulted in the persistence of fibrillatory activity in the atrium and termination in the appendage. These theories have obvious clinical implications both in terms of surgical- or catheter-based techniques for division of atrial mass [28] and pharmacotherapy involving drugs that lengthen refractory periods.

Moe's multiple wavelet theory was further refined by Allessie and colleagues [30]. They introduced the concept of "wavelength of reentry" which is defined as the shortest pathway length that can sustain reentry in a given reentrant pathway. The wavelength of an impulse is described as the distance traveled over the course of a single action potential refractory period and is equal to the product of the conduction velocity times the duration of the refractory period. It follows that any impulse with a wavelength which is greater than the pathway length of its reentrant circuit will encounter refractory tissue on completion of the circuit and therefore become extinguished. Thus, the wavelength of reentry is the shortest path length that can sustain reentry. Furthermore, the authors claimed, functional reentry tends to naturally establish itself in a path length which is equal to its wavelength. Consequently, the number of reentrant circuits that can be accommodated is a simple function of atrial mass and wavelength. This mechanism they termed the "leading circle" hypothesis. Pharmacological manipulation of the ERP increases the wavelength of reentry and therefore reduces the number of reentrant circuits that can be maintained which in turn favors termination of the arrhythmia. On the other hand, physical division of the atrial chambers by surgical- or catheter-based techniques reduce the critical mass necessary to sustain the arrhythmia.

An alternative hypothesis of arrhythmia propagation based on single-circuit reentry has evolved since the late 1970s. It is proposed that the maintenance of AF, whether paroxysmal or persistent, may depend on the periodic activity of a small number of rotors located in the posterior left atrium and PV region [31]. A "rotor" is defined as a stably rotating pattern of reaction and diffusion about a pivot point, also known as a "phase singularity." These engines activate the atria at exceedingly high rates giving rise to curved spiraling wavefronts and fibrillatory conduction throughout the atria. Combining newer optical mapping and electrographic techniques, a number of investigators have shown strong evidence for significant spatiotemporal periodicity activity during AF in isolated heart and animal models. Although both RA (right atrial) and LA are capable of harboring such rotors, it is proposed that those rotors whose rotating periods are shorter acted as dominant frequency sources responsible for sustaining the arrhythmia, and these appear to arise in the main from the posterior wall of the left atrium at the PV–LA junction. Demonstration of a hierarchy of distribution of cycle lengths across the atria from the PV–LA junction to the LA to the RA further supports this hypothesis. The method of transmission of this highly periodic rotor activity via fibrillatory conduction to the rest of the LA and RA is complex. These changes appear to be frequency dependent and somewhat surprisingly are independent of refractory period but rather seem to be related to structural dispersion by the crista terminalis and pectinate muscle network of the right atrium which increase the complexity of the fibrillatory conduction.

AF begets AF—electrical remodeling

Clinical experience attests to the fact that paroxysmal AF is a recurrent disorder. Over 90% of patients suffering an episode of paroxysmal AF will have a recurrent episode and even in the absence of concomitant cardiovascular disease the natural history is of progression to permanent AF over time. An important breakthrough into the understanding of the electrophysiological mechanism behind this was made by Alessie's group in 1995. In an elegant model in awake chronically instrumented goats, an atrial fibrillator device maintained the animals in AF continuously over a specified time period, and a series of experiments were performed at baseline, after 24 hours and after approximately 3 weeks of sustained AF [32]. In normal goat atria, electrically induced AF lasted only a few seconds and terminated spontaneously. In animals maintained in AF for greater than 24 hours, both duration of induced AF increased significantly and fibrillatory rates increased significantly. The inducibility of AF by a single pre-

mature stimulus increased from 24 to 76%. The electrophysiological basis of these findings seemed to stem from a shortening of atrial ERPs by one third, and the loss of normal adaptation of the atrial action potential to rapid atrial rates (i.e. a lesser degree of shortening of atrial ERPs at higher rates). All electrophysiological changes reverted to normal 1 week following restoration of sinus rhythm. This process, termed "electrical remodeling" is believed to arise, at least in part, from altered expression of ionic channel proteins as outlined below.

The role of transcellular ionic currents

The duration of the plateau phase of the myocardial action potential is determined by the relative contributions of the inward L-type Ca^{2+} current (I_{Ca}) and the outward so-called "delayed rectifier" potassium currents (I_{Kur}, I_{Kr}, I_{Ks}). At atrial rates of roughly 10 times normal, that are observed during AF, the inward transfer of Ca^{2+} with each action potential results in the accumulation of potentially toxic intracellular Ca^{2+}. As a result, in the long term, there is compensatory downregulation of expression of the pore-forming I_{Ca} alpha-subunit and in turn a reduction in I_{Ca} magnitude. This has the effect of limiting further excessive inward Ca^{2+} transfer but as a consequence the "delayed rectifier" potassium currents predominate in the plateau phase of the action potential with earlier return to resting membrane potential and shortening of the atrial ERP.

In addition to a reduction in atrial ERP observed in steady state atrial tachycardia, there is altered restitution of action potential duration in response to abrupt changes in rate. The normal response to an abrupt decrease in cycle length (i.e. an acceleration in rate of depolarization) is a reduction in ERP but in studies on the atria of chronically fibrillating dogs, significant rate adaptation of action potential duration did not occur in response to abrupt cycle length changes. Administration of a calcium blocker, ryanodine, appeared to restore rate adaptation, demonstrating the importance of calcium release mechanics in rate adaptation of fibrillating atria [33]. Subsequent work in humans has shown that action potential duration restitution (APDR) kinetics has a characteristic appearance in patients with AF when compared with controls. Furthermore, patients with persistent AF show greater regional variation in APDR kinetics across a range of sampled atrial areas than do patients with paroxysmal AF [34].

Thus, reduced action potential duration as a response to potential intracellular calcium toxicity and "failure of restitution" play a central role in the electrical remodeling by increasing the potential number of reentry circuits and by promoting electrical dispersion of refractoriness. Regardless of the mechanism of initiation of AF then, promotion of maintenance of AF by enhanced multiple-circuit reentry, in the setting of shorter atrial ERPs, is a postulated "final common pathway" of sustained AF.

Genetics of AF

While AF is generally not considered a heritable condition, seemingly rare familial cases have long been recognized. These families have aroused considerable interest in the hope that identification of the abnormal gene and its product would shed some light on the poorly understood molecular basis of the arrhythmia. Several researchers have identified families with autosomal dominant patterns of transmission and in a novel analysis of pooled DNA from affected and unaffected members of one proband in Spain, Brugada and coworkers identified a genetic locus for the disease at 10q22-24. They subsequently confirmed this in two further families [35]. However, further work in this field has revealed that familial atrial fibrillation (FAF) may not be as uncommon as previously thought and that its genetics may be more heterogeneous than initial studies suggested. A group from Rochester examined 914 consecutive patients with AF referred to a specialist arrhythmia clinic. Even allowing for referral bias they surprisingly identified 50 probands (5% of all AF; 15% of lone AF) with AF and a significant family history. None of these four multigenerational families showed linkage to the 10q22-24 locus, suggesting that, at the very least, two distinct gene abnormalities are involved in the disorder [36].

Several studies have described families with AF and indeed linkage analysis has identified a number of disparate chromosome loci containing candidate causative genes. In general, individuals affected in FAF present at a younger age than the typical patients who compromise the bulk of the clinical disease burden. Whether such putative candidate genes are involved in the formation of a predisposing atrial substrate, acted upon by environmental factors such as endothelial dysfunction, resulting in the genesis of senescence-related AF remains an intriguing question [37].

Conclusion

This is an exciting time in the development of our knowledge of the pathophysiology of AF. The past 10 years has seen an explosion in research into the mechanisms underlying this seemingly pervasive arrhythmia. The primacy of the multiple wavelet hypothesis has been challenged by newer scientific endeavors, and the repercussions have spawned new belief in the old theories of single-circuit reentry and enhanced automaticity that were first mooted 100 years ago. Effervescing strands of research encompass such diverse fields as catheter-based electrophysiological mapping, electrical action potential delineation, structural and molecular atrial remodeling, cellular ionic transport, and genetic linkage analysis. Enhanced scientific understanding of the pathogenesis of AF already shows promise in furthering our ultimate goal of moving away from the palliative therapeutics of rate control and thromboprophylaxis, to interventions aimed at the restoration and maintenance of sinus rhythm.

References

1 Lewis T. Auricular fibrillation and its relationship to clinical irregularity of the heart. *Br Heart J* 1910; **1**: 306–372.

2 Nattel S. New ideas about atrial fibrillation 50 years on. *Nature* 2002; **415**(6868): 219–226.

3 Moe GK, Abildskov JA. Atrial fibrillation as a self-sustaining arrhythmia independent of focal discharge. *Am Heart J* 1959; **58**(1): 59–70.

4 Phillips E, Levine SA. Auricular fibrillation without other evidence of heart disease: a cause of reversible heart failure. *Am J Med* 1949; **7**: 478–489.

5 Fenelon G *et al.* Tachycardiomyopathy: mechanisms and clinical implications. *Pacing Clin Electrophysiol* 1996; **19**(1): 95–106.

6 Kannel WB *et al.* Epidemiologic features of chronic atrial fibrillation: the Framingham study. *N Engl J Med* 1982; **306**(17): 1018–1022.

7 Gami AS *et al.* Association of atrial fibrillation and obstructive sleep apnea. *Circulation* 2004; **110**(4): 364–367.

8 Barnes ME. Obesity as an independent predictor of first atrial fibrillation in adults aged greater than or equal to 65 years [Abstract 885]. *J Am Coll Cardiol* 2004; **43**: 240A.

9 Tsang TS *et al.* Left ventricular diastolic dysfunction as a predictor of the first diagnosed nonvalvular atrial fibrillation in 840 elderly men and women. *J Am Coll Cardiol* 2002; **40**(9): 1636–1644.

10 Kalifa J *et al.* Intra-atrial pressure increases rate and organization of waves emanating from the superior pulmonary veins during atrial fibrillation. *Circulation* 2003; **108**(6): 668–671.

11 Bode F, Sachs F, Franz MR. Tarantula peptide inhibits atrial fibrillation. *Nature* 2001; **409**(6816): 35–36.

12 Nanthakumar K *et al.* Effect of physiological mechanical perturbations on intact human myocardial repolarization. *Cardiovasc Res* 2000; **45**(2): 303–309.

13 Franz MR. Mechano-electrical feedback. *Cardiovasc Res* 2000; **45**(2): 263–266.

14 Allessie MA *et al.* Pathophysiology and prevention of atrial fibrillation. *Circulation* 2001; **103**(5): 769–777.

15 Maisel WH, Stevenson LW. Atrial fibrillation in heart failure: epidemiology, pathophysiology, and rationale for therapy. *Am J Cardiol* 2003; **91**(6A): 2D–8D.

16 Goette A *et al.* Increased expression of extracellular signal-regulated kinase and angiotensin-converting enzyme in human atria during atrial fibrillation. *J Am Coll Cardiol* 2000; **35**(6): 1669–1677.

17 Goette A *et al.* Regulation of angiotensin II receptor subtypes during atrial fibrillation in humans. *Circulation* 2000; **101**(23): 2678–2681.

18 Aime-Sempe C *et al.* Myocardial cell death in fibrillating and dilated human right atria. *J Am Coll Cardiol* 1999; **34**(5): 1577–1586.

19 Li D *et al.* Effects of angiotensin-converting enzyme inhibition on the development of the atrial fibrillation substrate in dogs with ventricular tachypacing-induced congestive heart failure. *Circulation* 2001; **104**(21): 2608–2614.

20 Healey JS *et al.* Prevention of atrial fibrillation with angiotensin-converting enzyme inhibitors and angiotensin receptor blockers: a meta-analysis. *J Am Coll Cardiol* 2005; **45**(11): 1832–1839.

21 Haissaguerre M *et al.* Spontaneous initiation of atrial fibrillation by ectopic beats originating in the pulmonary veins. *N Engl J Med* 1998; **339**(10): 659–666.

22 Wu TJ *et al.* Pulmonary veins and ligament of Marshall as sources of rapid activations in a canine model of sustained atrial fibrillation. *Circulation* 2001; **103**(8): 1157–1163.

23 Tsai CF *et al.* Initiation of atrial fibrillation by ectopic beats originating from the superior vena cava: electrophysiological characteristics and results of radiofrequency ablation. *Circulation* 2000; **102**(1): 67–74.

24 Scherlag BJ *et al.* Autonomically induced conversion of pulmonary vein focal firing into atrial fibrillation. *J Am Coll Cardiol* 2005; **45**(11): 1878–1886.

25 Pappone C *et al.* Pulmonary vein denervation enhances long-term benefit after circumferential ablation for paroxysmal atrial fibrillation. *Circulation* 2004; **109**(3): 327–334.

26 Bettoni M, Zimmermann M. Autonomic tone variations before the onset of paroxysmal atrial fibrillation. *Circulation* 2002; **105**(23): 2753–2759.

27 Zimmermann M, Kalusche D. Fluctuation in autonomic tone is a major determinant of sustained atrial arrhythmias in patients with focal ectopy originating from the pulmonary veins. *J Cardiovasc Electrophysiol* 2001; **12**(3): 285–291.

28 Cox JL, Ad N. New surgical and catheter-based modifications of the maze procedure. *Semin Thorac Cardiovasc Surg* 2000; **12**(1): 68–73.

29 Moe G, Rheinboldt W, Abildskov J. A computer model of atrial fibrillation. *Am Heart J* 1964; **67**: 200–220.

30 Allessie MA, Bonke FI, Schopman FJ. Circus movement in rabbit atrial muscle as a mechanism of tachycardia. III. The "leading circle" concept: a new model of circus movement in cardiac tissue without the involvement of an anatomical obstacle. *Circ Res* 1977; **41**(1): 9–18.

31 Jalife J. Rotors and spiral waves in atrial fibrillation. *J Cardiovasc Electrophysiol* 2003; **14**(7): 776–780.

32 Wijffels MC *et al.* Atrial fibrillation begets atrial fibrillation. A study in awake chronically instrumented goats. *Circulation* 1995; **92**(7): 1954–1968.

33 Hara M *et al.* Steady-state and nonsteady-state action potentials in fibrillating canine atrium: abnormal rate adaptation and its possible mechanisms. *Cardiovasc Res* 1999; **42**(2): 455–469.

34 Kim BS *et al.* Action potential duration restitution kinetics in human atrial fibrillation. *J Am Coll Cardiol* 2002; **39**(8): 1329–1336.

35 Brugada R *et al.* Identification of a genetic locus for familial atrial fibrillation. *N Engl J Med* 1997; **336**(13): 905–911.

36 Darbar D *et al.* Familial atrial fibrillation is a genetically heterogeneous disorder. *J Am Coll Cardiol* 2003; **41**(12): 2185–2192.

37 Mestroni L. Genomic medicine and atrial fibrillation. *J Am Coll Cardiol* 2003; **41**(12): 2193–2196.

CHAPTER 3

Genetics of atrial fibrillation

Ramon Brugada

Overview

Atrial fibrillation (AF) remains one of the most challenging arrhythmias for the clinician and basic researcher. Different approaches have been undertaken from the basic standpoint to improve its understanding, from the development of animal models to the analysis of genetic backgrounds in individuals with familial and acquired forms of the disease. In the last years, a large body of evidence has shown that alterations in ionic currents are involved in the disease. But it has not been until recently, with the genetic link between mutations in proteins responsible for these ionic currents and the familial disease, that we have been given the final evidence that AF can also be primarily an ion channelopathy. Despite the limited prevalence of the inherited diseases, it has been shown before that the knowledge gained in their study will be helpful in dealing with the most common acquired forms of the disease. Therefore, as data keep unraveling, clinicians can expect that soon better therapeutic and preventive options for this arrhythmia will emerge from basic science.

Introduction

A balance between structural and ionic components is required for the electromechanical impulse to propagate orderly across the myocardial cells. When structural heart disease or genetic or iatrogenic factors modify this interaction, the result can be the formation of a chaotic electrical activity or fibrillation that can affect either chamber of the heart,

atria, or ventricles. The atrial chaos or AF is defined as an erratic activation of the atria, causing an irregular heart rhythm at the ventricular level. AF is the most common sustained arrhythmia encountered in clinical practice. It affects over 3 million Americans and its prevalence increases with age to about 6% in people over the age of 65 [1]. The disease doubles the mortality and it accounts for over one third of all cardioembolic episodes [2]. AF is usually associated with cardiac pathology including hypertensive heart disease, cardiomyopathy, valvular disease, or atherosclerotic cardiovascular disease. AF can be transient (paroxysmal) or persistent. Paroxysmal AF accounts for 35–40% of all cases seen by physicians and is not a benign entity in individuals with underlying cardiac pathology. The disease carries a high mortality and high incidence of stroke, and despite being a self-terminating arrhythmia, there is a 30–50% chance of converting to a chronic state depending on the underlying pathology. In some instances, especially in the young, the disease has no apparent etiology, and is called "lone" AF. Lone AF accounts for 2–16% of all cases and in the absence of risk factors like hypertension, diabetes, or previous stroke, has a low risk of embolism and does not require the use of anticoagulation before the age of 65. Among the "lone" AF group falls the familial forms of the disease, in which a genetic basis and no cardiac pathology are the main characteristics. Limited studies have shown that the familial form has also a higher risk of embolism after the age of 65, data that support the use of anticoagulation in these individuals.

There are three main goals in the therapy of AF: control of heart rate, prevention of thromboembolism, and restoration of sinus rhythm. The first two are successfully achieved in the majority of cases with the use of medications. The latter remains a

Manual of Surgical Treatment of Atrial Fibrillation.
Edited by Hauw T. Sie *et al.* © 2008 Blackwell Publishing,
ISBN: 978-1-4051-4032-4.

challenge. While the pharmacological approach to restore sinus rhythm can be helpful in some cases, it carries a high recurrence rate and a potential proarrhythmic effect, especially in individuals with underlying cardiac pathology. Surgery and ablation have emerged in the last decade as promising techniques to terminate the arrhythmia, but to date they are very time consuming and few selected patients can benefit from these procedures.

Molecular mechanisms in AF

The limited success in the therapy of AF is in part due to our poor understanding of its molecular pathophysiology. Advances in genetics and molecular biology will likely give new insights into the development of the disease. In the human, research efforts to elucidate the molecular basis of AF are focused into two main areas: genetics in the human and alterations in genetic expression of ion channels. The study in alterations in expression is usually performed in animal models of the disease but can also be performed, in a more limited scale, in the human (because of tissue availability). These experiments will mainly provide information on the molecular changes triggered by the disease and may explain some of the mechanisms that perpetuate the arrhythmia into a chronic form. However, it will be very difficult to prove whether the molecular changes that occur in the atria are the etiology of the disease, a maladaptation or a compensating mechanism [3].

These doubts could in part be clarified by the identification of genetic defects in the human that play a role in the disease. Study in genetics of AF can also be attained from different perspectives: (1) the analysis of AF as a monogenic disease, in which different members of a family have the arrhythmia as a primary electrical disease, (2) the analysis of the arrhythmia presenting in the setting of another familial disease, and (3) the analysis genetic backgrounds that may predispose to the disease without it segregating in the family. The first two, analysis of familial forms of the disease, provide a definitive insight into the etiology of the disease and require the analysis of families with the disease segregating in several members, with or without another pathology. The last one is achieved by comparing cases of nonfamilial AF to age- and gender-matched con-

trols. The analysis is performed as an association study, aimed at identifying differences in segregation of genetic backgrounds between both groups which may explain the development of the disease.

AF as a monogenic disease

It is not generally appreciated that AF may be inherited. It was first reported as a familial form in 1943 [4]. Recent analysis of the Framingham data has shown that there is a genetic susceptibility to AF, shown by the fact that parental AF increased the risk of AF in the offspring [5]. A study by Darbar *et al.* [6] indicates that 5% of the patients with AF and up to 15% of the individuals with lone AF may have a familial form. This study indicates that the familial form of the disease may have a higher prevalence than previously suspected. In 1996, we identified three families in Catalonia, Spain, with AF inherited with an autosomal dominant pattern. These families were later expanded to six with a total of 132 individuals. Fifty of them presented with AF, with an age of diagnosis of the arrhythmia from 0 to 45 years (two patients were diagnosed in utero). The echocardiograms were within the normal range when the patients were diagnosed. Some of them have subsequently developed dilatation of the left atrium on follow-up. Two patients have mild left ventricular dysfunction, one of them probably related to her advanced age and the other due to tachycardiomyopathy secondary to poorly controlled heart rate. In six patients, electrical cardioversion was unsuccessful despite a structurally normal heart. The majority of the individuals in these six families are asymptomatic, and only six patients presently suffer from palpitations, but otherwise have a normal life. The disease is chronic in all but two individuals, one has been progressively having more and longer episodes of paroxysmal AF suggesting that she will probably become chronic. The second patient died suddenly, while being treated with antiarrhythmic drugs. With techniques of linkage analysis the locus was identified in 10q22, which was segregating with the affected individuals [7]. The gene has not been identified yet.

The first genes for AF have been identified in these last years, providing the first links of ion channelopathies to the disease. A four-generation family from China was segregating the disease with a locus on chromosome 11 [8]. The analysis of KVLQT1 (KCNQ1) identified a missense mutation resulting in the amino acid change S140G. Electrophysiological studies revealed a gain of function in I_{Ks} current when the mutated channel was expressed with the β-subunits minK and MirP1. This gain of function explains well the shortening of the action potential duration and effective refractory period, which are thought to be the culprits of the disease. Mutations in KCNQ1 causing a loss of function had been described before as responsible for long QT syndrome type 1. Interestingly, despite the gain of function 9 out of 16 individuals presented QT prolongation of the electrocardiogram [8]. Just recently, also from the same group in China, a link between KCNE2 and AF has been provided with the identification of a same mutation in two families with AF [9]. The mutation R27C caused a gain of function when coexpressed with KCNQ1 but had no effect when expressed with HERG. This confirms the role of mutations in channels responsible for potassium currents in the development of AF. New loci, 6q14-16 [10] and 5p13 [11], have been identified in this last year.

AF associated with other monogenic diseases

AF has been described in other cardiac monogenic diseases as a concomitant disease. It has been identified in families with hypertrophic cardiomyopathy [12], skeletal myopathies [13], familial amyloidosis [14], and in monogenic diseases predisposing to atrial abnormalities. In these cases, the disease is probably related to morphological changes in the atria caused by the underlying cardiac pathology. The disease can also be present in other ion channelopathies like Long QT 4 [15], Brugada syndrome [16], and Short QT syndrome [17]. In the latter, the mutations described in HERG cause a gain of function of I_{Kr}, responsible for sudden cardiac death. The high incidence of atrial arrhythmias in patients with Short QT syndrome and the data on gain of function mutations in I_{Ks} currents point to an important role for the shortening of the action potential in the development of AF. A mutation in KCNQ1 (V141M) has been identified this last year as responsible for AF and Short QT syndrome in utero, showing also a gain of function in I_{Ks} current [18].

Genetic predisposition to acquired AF

The familial form of AF is uncommon. The majority of the cases are acquired and related to structural abnormalities. However, not all individuals with the same cardiac pathology develop AF, indicating that there are probably genetic factors that predispose some of them to the arrhythmia. Few centers have been trying to unravel some of these genetic backgrounds with the use of association studies. One report from Japan [19] tested the hypothesis that genetic factors that increase cardiac fibrosis would be a determinant for the development of lone AF. These investigators analyzed a polymorphism in the ACE gene, an enzyme that interacts with angiotensin II and affects cardiac remodeling. ACE gene can be inherited with an intronic deletion, which has been linked to higher circulating levels of enzyme and higher degree of hypertrophy and myocardial fibrosis [20]. While this cardiac fibrosis has been described at the ventricular level, they hypothesized that it would also affect the atria and cause the arrhythmia. They compared the genotypes of 77 patients with lone AF to 83 controls. They did not find any difference in the distribution of the ACE genotypes between the affected individuals and controls. There was no correlation with the type of AF, namely, paroxysmal or chronic and the genotype. However, a larger study in the last months has shown that there may be a relation between non-familial structural AF and polymorphisms in the renin–angiotensin system [21].

A second study has looked at a polymorphism in minK and relation with the disease. There was an association with the 38G allele and AF. It is still a matter of debate regarding the functional significance of the polymorphism. Further studies will be required to confirm this association [22].

In this last year, a study has addressed the relationship between inflammation and the risk of developing postoperative AF. In this study, they investigated the role of the -174G/C Interleukin-6 polymorphism in 110 patients undergoing coronary artery bypass surgery [23]. This polymorphism had been previously associated to postoperative Interleukin-6 levels. Twenty-six patients developed AF in the postoperative period. Analysis of the polymorphism revealed a significant prevalence of the GG genotype (34% versus 10%) in patients with AF. Likewise, the levels of interleukin and fibrinogen were higher in patients with GG phenotype. Therefore, this study has shown a possible role of inflammatory component in the development of AF. As in all association studies, larger patient population will be required to confirm the relationship.

Genetic studies: implications for the future

The discovery of the structure of the ion channels, their function, and pathophysiology have helped unravel in part the role played by the different ionic currents in both the electrical activity, electromechanical coupling, and arrhythmogenecity. With the advances in genetics and the discovery of mutations causing familial diseases we have been able to jump from the most basic level to the clinical arena. Cardiac arrhythmias predisposing to sudden death, like Long QT, Brugada syndrome, and Short QT syndrome, have benefited tremendously from the advances in genetics and molecular biology. The information gained in genetics, biophysics, and experimental models have opened new insights into preventive and therapeutic options.

Arrhythmias like AF will therefore undoubtedly benefit from the discovery of the genes that cause the familial forms of the disease and from the knowledge of the alterations in gene expression as a consequence of it. The interaction of all these genes with the structural cardiac abnormalities will probably shed light not only on the factors that induce the first episode but also on the determinants that prolong this episode into a chronic form. The largest benefit that will be drawn from all these data is the much better understanding of the disease, how it is initiated, how it is chronified. Like it has happened in the previously mentioned diseases, once this preliminary data is obtained, the development of better therapeutic and preventive measures will be a possibility.

References

1 Feinberg WM, Blackshear JL, Laupacis A, Kronmal R, Hart RG. Prevalence, age distribution, and gender of patients with atrial fibrillation. Analysis and implications. *Arch Intern Med* March 13, 1995; **155**(5): 469–473.

2 Wolf PA, Singer DE. Preventing stroke in atrial fibrillation. *Am Fam Phys* December 1997; **56**(9): 2242–2250.

3 Brugada R. Molecular biology of atrial fibrillation. *Minerva Cardioangiol* April 2004; **52**(2): 65–72.

4 Wolff L. Familiar auricular fibrillation. *New Engl J Med* 1943; **229**: 396.

5 Fox CS, Parise H, D'Agostino RB, Sr *et al.* Parental atrial fibrillation as a risk factor for atrial fibrillation in offspring. *JAMA* June 16, 2004; **291**(23): 2851–2855.

6 Darbar D, Herron KJ, Ballew JD *et al.* Familial atrial fibrillation is a genetically heterogeneous disorder. *J Am Coll Cardiol* June 18, 2003; **41**(12): 2185–2192.

7 Brugada R, Tapscott T, Czernuszewicz GZ *et al.* Identification of a genetic locus for familial atrial fibrillation. *N Engl J Med* March 27, 1997; **336**(13): 905–911.

8 Chen YH, Xu SJ, Bendahhou S *et al.* KCNQ1 gain-of-function mutation in familial atrial fibrillation. *Science* January 10, 2003; **299**(5604): 251–254.

9 Yang Y, Xia M, Jin Q *et al.* Identification of a KCNE2 gain-of-function mutation in patients with familial atrial fibrillation. *Am J Hum Genet* November 2004; **75**(5): 899–905.

10 Ellinor PT, Shin JT, Moore RK, Yoerger DM, MacRae CA. Locus for atrial fibrillation maps to chromosome 6q14-16. *Circulation* June 17, 2003; **107**(23): 2880–2883.

11 Oberti C, Wang L, Li L *et al.* Genome-wide linkage scan identifies a novel genetic locus on chromosome 5p13 for neonatal atrial fibrillation associated with sudden death and variable cardiomyopathy. *Circulation* 2005; **110**(25): 3753–3759.

12 Gruver EJ, Fatkin D, Dodds GA *et al.* Familial hypertrophic cardiomyopathy and atrial fibrillation caused by Arg663His beta-cardiac myosin heavy chain mutation. *Am J Cardiol* June 17, 1999; **83**(12A): 13H–18H.

13 Ohkubo R, Nakagawa M, Higuchi I *et al.* Familial skeletal myopathy with atrioventricular block. *Intern Med* November 1999; **38**(11): 856–860.

14 Gillmore JD, Booth DR, Pepys MB, Hawkins PN. Hereditary cardiac amyloidosis associated with the transthyretin Ile122 mutation in a white man. *Heart* September 1999; **82**(3): e2.

15 Schott JJ, Charpentier F, Peltier S *et al.* Mapping of a gene for long QT syndrome to chromosome 4q25-27. *Am J Hum Genet* November 1995; **57**(5): 1114–1122.

16 Morita H, Kusano-Fukushima K, Nagase S *et al.* Atrial fibrillation and atrial vulnerability in patients with Brugada syndrome. *J Am Coll Cardiol* October 16, 2002; **40**(8): 1437–1444.

17 Brugada R, Hong K, Dumaine R *et al.* Sudden death associated with short-QT syndrome linked to mutations in HERG. *Circulation* January 6, 2004; **109**(1): 30–35.

18 Hong K, Piper DR, az-Valdecantos A *et al.* De novo KCNQ1 mutation responsible for atrial fibrillation and

short QT syndrome in utero. *Cardiovasc Res* August 16, 2005; **3**: 433-440.

19 Yamashita T, Hayami N, Ajiki K *et al.* Is ACE gene polymorphism associated with lone atrial fibrillation? *Jpn Heart J* September 1997; **38**(5): 637–641.

20 Nakai K, Itoh C, Miura Y *et al.* Deletion polymorphism of the angiotensin I-converting enzyme gene is associated with serum ACE concentration and increased risk for CAD in the Japanese. *Circulation* November 1994; **90**(5): 2199–2202.

21 Tsai CT, Lai LP, Lin JL *et al.* Renin–angiotensin system gene polymorphisms and atrial fibrillation. *Circulation* April 6, 2004; **109**(13): 1640–1646.

22 Lai LP, Lin JL, Huang SK. Molecular genetic studies in atrial fibrillation. *Cardiology* 2003; **100**(3): 109–113.

23 Gaudino M, Andreotti F, Zamparelli R *et al.* The −174G/C interleukin-6 polymorphism influences postoperative interleukin-6 levels and postoperative atrial fibrillation. Is atrial fibrillation an inflammatory complication? *Circulation* September 9, 2003; **108**(suppl 1): II195–II199.

CHAPTER 4

Pharmacological management of atrial fibrillation

Yvonne Smyth & Kieran Daly

Introduction

Atrial fibrillation (AF) is the most common sustained arrhythmia, the arrhythmia most commonly encountered in clinical practice and with the aging population in the Western world, one which is becoming increasingly prevalent. The prevalence of AF increases with age, affecting more than 10% of those over 80. It is estimated that 2.2 million people in the United States have AF. This number is expected to double by 2035. AF is associated with significant mortality and morbidity, particularly from thromboembolic stroke. It is thought to account for one sixth of all ischemic strokes in patients over 60 [1–3].

Significant advances in recent years in the understanding of the pathophysiology of AF have led to the development of new treatment modalities. Despite this, the vast majority of patients with AF are still managed with medication; 99.4% of all patients with AF are treated with some form of drug therapy, compared with 0.6% who are currently treated with catheter ablation, antitachycardia pacing and/or surgical techniques [4]. Medical management is aimed at reducing thromboembolic risk and controlling symptoms. The latter can be achieved by either control of ventricular response rate or restoration and maintenance of sinus rhythm.

Manual of Surgical Treatment of Atrial Fibrillation.
Edited by Hauw T. Sie *et al.* © 2008 Blackwell Publishing, ISBN: 978-1-4051-4032-4.

Treatment strategies for AF

Essentially there are two ways to manage patients with persistent AF, either to restore and maintain sinus rhythm (rhythm control) or allow the patient to remain in AF and ensure the ventricular response rate is controlled with atrioventricular (AV) nodal blocking drugs (rate control) [5]. Each approach has advantages and disadvantages. The most appropriate approach for an individual patient is determined by a number of factors including the duration of the AF, how symptomatic the patient is, the age of the patient and patient preference.

Rhythm control

Rhythm control has the potential advantages of fewer symptoms, better exercise tolerance, a lower incidence of stroke and the possibility that warfarin could be stopped if sinus rhythm was maintained. However, the major drawback of this approach is the lack of efficacy of and the side effect profile of the currently available antiarrhythmic drugs that have significant risks of proarrhythmia.

There are two standard approaches to converting AF to sinus rhythm: synchronized external DC cardioversion and pharmacologic cardioversion. The timing of attempted cardioversion is influenced by the duration of AF. For patients with AF for more than 48 hours or those with AF of unknown duration, cardioversion should be delayed until the patient has been anticoagulated at appropriate levels (INR 2.0–3.0) for 3–4 weeks. Anticoagulation should be continued for at least 1 month after successful cardioversion to prevent thrombus formation that may result from a transient period of atrial stunning postcardioversion. Where immediate cardioversion is required and the duration of AF is unknown or greater than 48 hours, a transesophageal echocardiogram should be performed to out rule left appendage thrombus prior to cardioversion [6].

DC cardioversion is indicated in patients who are hemodynamically unstable; in stable patients in whom spontaneous reversion due to correction of an underlying disease is not likely either DC or pharmacologic cardioversion can be performed. Electrical cardioversion is often preferred because of greater efficiency and a low risk of proarrhythmia. The overall success rate of electrical cardioversion for AF is 75–93% and is related inversely both to the duration of AF and to left atrial size. Where the duration of AF exceeds 6 months, success rates for DC cardioversion can be as low as 50%. Direct current cardioversion requires sedation or general anesthetic whereas chemical cardioversion does not. There is no difference in the risk of stroke or systemic embolization with either method so the anticoagulation guidelines are the same for both [7].

A number of antiarrhythmic drugs are more effective than placebo, converting 30–60% of patients to sinus rhythm. Antiarrhythmic drugs are classified according to the phase of the action potential they directly affect and which ion channel of the cardiac myocyte they interact with. There are four main classes (Vaughan Williams classification) of antiarrhythmic agents:

Class I agents interfere with the sodium channel. They are subdivided into Ia, Ib, and Ic according to their mechanism of action.

Class II agents are antisympathetic agents. All agents in this class are beta-blockers.

Class III agents affect potassium influx and prolong repolarization.

Class IV agents affect the AV node. They are slow calcium channel blockers [8].

Evidence of efficacy from randomized trials is best established for dofetilide, flecainide, ibutilide, propafenone, amiodarone, and quinine. The ACC/AHA/ESC guidelines concluded that evidence for benefit from specific antiarrhythmic drugs varies with the duration of AF: dofetilide, flecainide, ibutilide, propafenone, or to a lesser degree, amiodarone (unless the patient has left ventricular dysfunction or heart failure) if it is less than 7 days duration; and dofetilide or, to a lesser degree, amiodarone or ibutilide if AF is more prolonged [1].

Dofetilide is a class III antiarrhythmic agent that blocks the delayed rectifier cardiac potassium channel and prolongs repolarization. The United States Food and Drug Administration (FDA) has approved the use of dofetilide for the conversion of AF and atrial flutter to normal sinus rhythm and for maintenance of normal sinus rhythm. Because of the risk of torsades de pointes, patients must be hospitalized for a minimum of 3 days for dofetilide initiation at a facility that can provide measurement of creatinine clearance, cardiac monitoring, and cardiac resuscitation. The majority of episodes of torsades de pointes occur within this 3-day period, the time of peak increase in the QT interval.

Several studies have evaluated the efficacy of intravenous and oral dofetilide for the termination of supraventricular arrhythmias and the use of oral dofetilide for the prevention of recurrent paroxysmal supraventricular tachycardia or AF after reversion to sinus rhythm [9]. Results from the SAPPHIRE-D trial suggest that dofetilide is more effective for the cardioversion of atrial flutter than AF [10]. Dofetilide is more effective than placebo for the pharmacological cardioversion of AF that has persisted for more than 1 week. When given orally dofetilide may take days or even weeks to produce a response.

Flecainide is a class Ic antiarrhythmic agent and it has a similar mechanism of action to dofetilide. It has been shown to be effective for the cardioversion of recent onset AF in placebo-controlled trials. It can be administered orally or intravenously. When given orally it usually produces a response within 3 hours and when given intravenously usually within 1 hour. Not infrequently it causes atrial flutter and bradycardia. Hypertension and neurological side effects are less common [7, 11].

The Cardiac Arrhythmia Suppression Trial sought to evaluate the efficacy and safety of arrhythmia suppression therapy in patients with asymptomatic or mildly symptomatic ventricular arrhythmia after myocardial infarction. After less than 1 year of follow-up the encainide and flecainide arms of the trial were stopped due to increased mortality and nonfatal cardiac arrests compared to placebo [12]. For this reason it is recommended that flecainide be given with caution or avoided completely in patients with underlying organic heart disease involving abnormal LV function.

Ibutilide is a class III antiarrhythmic drug available only for intravenous use for the termination of certain arrhythmias. An oral form is not available because of extensive first-pass metabolism. Ibutilide is effective for the termination of AF and atrial flutter of recent onset. An effect should be seen within 1 hour of administration. Since there is no oral preparation of ibutilide, it has no role in the long-term prevention of these arrhythmias. Ibutilide is not approved or the treatment of ventricular arrhythmias and its efficacy for these arrhythmias is unknown. The most frequent and serious side effects are those involving the cardiovascular system. There is a small but definite risk or torsades de pointes. For this reason it is recommended that serum magnesium and potassium concentrations should be measured prior to administration and that patients have at least 4 hours of continuous ECG monitoring after receiving ibutilide.

Propafenone is a class Ic antiarrhythmic drug that also has some beta-blocking activity. It can be given orally or intravenously for cardioversion of recent onset AF. A response is usually 2–6 hours after oral administration and earlier if it is administered intravenously. The most common side effects are cardiovascular. It has a negative inotropic effect at higher doses and for this reason should be avoided in patients with LV dysfunction (EF < 40%). It is not recommended for use in patients with obstructive lung disease because of its beta-blocking activity.

Quinidine is a class 1a antiarrhythmic agent. It can be given orally or intravenously. It successfully terminates AF in 20–60% of patients. The shorter the duration of AF, the more effective it is. A clinical response may be expected 3–4 hours after administration. It is usually given after digoxin or verapamil has been given to control the ventricular response rate. Side effects include torsades de pointes, nausea,

diarrhea, fever, hepatic dysfunction, and thrombocytopenia.

Amiodarone is a very effective antiarrhythmic drug and is widely used. In addition to its efficacy, it has very little negative inotropic activity and a very low rate of proarrhythmia compared to other antiarrhythmic drugs. However, the use of amiodarone is associated with a relatively high incidence of noncardiac side effects, making it a complicated drug to use safely. Amiodarone can be given both orally and intravenously. Oral amiodarone has a delayed onset of action that varies with the dosing regimen but usually takes at least 2–3 days, while intravenous amiodarone begins to act within hours. The delayed effect with the oral therapy is largely related to the fact that amiodarone is highly lipophilic.

Amiodarone is one of the more commonly used drugs to maintain sinus rhythm in patients with AF. If the arrhythmia recurs after successful cardioversion, amiodarone can slow the ventricular response at rest and with exercise. Amiodarone is the preferred drug to maintain sinus rhythm in patients with heart failure because a very low risk or proarrhythmia and lack of negative inotropic activity. Amiodarone can convert some patients with AF to sinus rhythm. However, it acts less rapidly and less effectively than other agents, so amiodarone is generally not a first-line therapy for pharmacologic cardioversion except in patients with heart failure. Amiodarone provides effective rate control and can improve hemodynamics in critically ill patients with AF or flutter that is refractory to conventional therapy. A recent meta-analysis has shown that amiodarone lowers the incidence of postoperative AF by 36% in patients undergoing cardiac surgery. It also reduces major cardiovascular morbidity and length of stay [13].

In some situations it is appropriate to commence antiarrhythmic drugs outside hospital to increase the chances of successful DC cardioversion by lowering the defibrillation threshold. The ESC guidelines recommend amiodarone, flecainide, ibutilide, propafenone, quinidine, and sotalol to enhance cardioversion and prevent the immediate recurrence of AF. This approach should be avoided for patients with LV dysfunction, SA, or AV node dysfunction, or a prolonged QT interval on safety grounds.

Drugs used for pharmacological cardioversion of AF.

Drug	Route of administration	Dosage	Potential adverse effects
Dofetilide	Oral	500 mcg BD (reduce in renal impairment)	Torsades de pointes, QT prolongation
Flecainide	Oral or intravenous	200–300 mg PO; 1.5–3.0 mg/kg over 10–20 min	Hypotension, rapidly conducting atrial flutter
Ibutilide	Intravenous	1 mg over 10 min; repeat if necessary	Torsades de pointes, QT prolongation
Propafenone	Oral or intravenous	450–600 mg PO; 1.5–2 mg/kg over 10–20 min	Hypotension, rapidly conducting atrial flutter
Amiodarone	Oral or intravenous	PO: 1.2–1.8 g/day in divided dose until 10 g given then 200–400 mg/day maintenance IV: 5–7 mg/kg over 30–60 min then 1.2–1.8 g/day until 10 g given then 200–400 mg maintenance	Hypotension, bradycardia, QT prolongation, torsades de pointes, GI upset, constipation, phlebitis
Quinidine	Oral	0.75–1.5 g in divided doses over 6–12 h	Torsades de pointes, QT prolongation, GI upset, hypotension

One year after successful cardioversion, only 20–30% of patients will remain in sinus rhythm without antiarrhythmic drug treatment. The drugs with efficacy for the maintenance of sinus rhythm are amiodarone, flecainide, sotalol, quinidine, disopyramide, and propafenone. The most appropriate choice varies from patient to patient. Typically flecainide is used in patients with no significant heart disease, amiodarone for those with LV dysfunction and sotalol in those with coronary artery disease.

Sotalol has both beta-blocking and class III antiarrhythmic actions. It has not been shown to be particularly effective for cardioversion of AF, but can be used to prevent its recurrence at doses of 80–160 mg twice daily. At lower doses sotalol has only a beta-blocking effect. Sotalol is completely renally excreted and doses must be adjusted to reflect renal function. It should be avoided completely in those with significant renal impairment. The need for QT monitoring after commencing sotalol usually necessitates inpatient initiation of the drug.

There is increasing evidence that amiodarone may be more effective than sotalol for maintenance of sinus rhythm. In the Canadian Trial of Atrial Fibrillation (CTAF) amiodarone was more effective than either sotalol or propafenone [14]. The SAFE-T trial randomized 655 patients with persistent AF on anticoagulants to receive amiodarone, sotalol or placebo [15]. The median times to recurrence of AF were 487 days in the amiodarone group, 74 days in the sotalol group, and 6 days in the placebo group. Amiodarone was superior to sotalol ($p < 0.001$) and placebo ($p < 0.001$) and sotalol was superior to placebo ($p < 0.001$). The number of adverse events was surprisingly few—one case of torsades de pointes in the sotalol group and three cases of adverse pulmonary effects, two in the amiodarone group, one in the placebo group. Restoration of sinus rhythm improved quality of life and exercise capacity. Despite this evidence caution is still advised in the use of amiodarone given its side effect profile.

Disopyramide is a class Ia antiarrhythmic agent and is quite similar to quinidine. It prolongs the QT interval and thus involves the risk of torsades de pointes. It improves AV conduction because of its anticholinergic action but this also causes significant side effects the most common of which is urinary retention. Another disadvantage of disopyramide is its negatively inotropic effect [1, 8, 16].

Although it would seem reasonable after cardioversion to continue antiarrhythmic therapy to maintain sinus rhythm in all patients, this would not be in keeping with the current guidelines and that is due to concerns regarding the proarrhythmic potential of these agents. According to the ESC/AHA/ACC guidelines the only class I indication for pharmacologic therapy to maintain sinus rhythm is for patients with disabling or otherwise troublesome symptoms during AF [1]. The choice of therapy in that case should be made primarily on safety. Reducing the frequency of recurrence of AF and preventing tachycardia-mediated cardiomyopathy are deemed class IIa indications for ongoing antiarrhythmic treatment.

Drugs used to maintain sinus rhythm in patients with AF.

Amiodarone	100–400 mg	Photosensitivity, pulmonary fibrosis, neuropathy, GI upset, thyroid dysfunction, hepatic toxicity, bradycardia, torsades de pointes
Disopyramide	400–750 mg	Torsades de pointes, glaucoma, dry mouth, urinary retention
Dofetilide	500–1000 mcg	Torsades de pointes
Flecainide	200–300 mg	VT, congestive heart failure
Propafenone	450–900 mg	VT, congestive heart failure, conversion to atrial flutter
Sotalol	240–320 mg	Bradycardia, bronchospasm, torsades de pointes, congestive heart failure

Rate control

The rationale behind a rate control strategy is avoidance of symptoms and hemodynamic instability and the prevention of tachycardia-mediated cardiomyopathy. Beta-blockers, calcium channel blockers and digoxin either alone or in combination are the mainstay of rate control. They all act by slowing AV nodal conduction. The adequacy of rate control is determined by both symptoms and ECG monitoring. It should be assessed both at rest and during exercise. Ambulatory monitoring or ex-ercise stress testing can be useful in this regard. It is usually advised that the resting heart rate be 60–80 beats/min and the heart rate during mild exercise should not exceed 100 beats/min [17]. Without treatment and in the absence of AV nodal disease, the ventricular rate usually varies between 90 and 170 beats/min.

In general, beta-blockers are the most effective agents for controlling ventricular response rates during exercise. Calcium channel blockers are effective both at rest and during exercise and are useful for patients with contraindications to beta-blockers. Digoxin, although not particularly useful for rate control in acute AF, is effective for rate control in persistent AF at rest, but not during exercise. For this reason it is frequently combined with a beta-blocker or calcium channel blocker. Digoxin alone rarely achieves adequate control unless the patient has underlying conduction system disease.

Beta-blockers

Beta-blockers are available in both intravenous and oral form. Intravenous beta-blockers are particularly useful for rate control of acute AF. The most commonly used agents are esmolol and metoprolol. Esmolol is a rapidly acting intravenous beta-blocker which has a very short duration of action. This can be useful for a therapeutic trial if it uncertain whether a beta-blocker will be tolerated. It is usually given as a bolus of 0.5 mg/kg infused over 1 minute followed by 50 mcg/min. If this fails to produce an adequate response, the dose is gradually up titrated. Metoprolol is given as an intravenous bolus of 2.5–5 mg over 2 minutes. It can be repeated at 5-minute intervals up to a total of 15 mg if necessary to achieve rate control.

Oral blockers are recommended as first-line therapy for rate control of AF. In a review of 17 beta-blockers all were shown to be effective for controlling ventricular rate during exercise, but some provided better rate control at rest including metoprolol and atenolol [6]. While they effectively reduce heart rate both at rest and during exercise, they may also reduce exercise tolerance. They can be used in combination with either digoxin or diltiazem. They have a number of side effects including hypotension, heart block, bronchospasm, worsening heart failure, cold extremities, and impotence.

Calcium channel blockers

The nondihydropyridine calcium channel blockers, diltiazem and verapamil, can be used either orally or intravenously for rate control.

Verapamil acts by inhibiting the calcium-mediated depolarization of the upper and middle regions of the AV node. Given intravenously in doses of 5–10 mg it acts within 2–3 minutes, oral verapamil takes 2 hours to act and its effect peaks at 3 hours [18]. The starting dose of oral verapamil is 40 mg three times a day, which can be increased to a maximum of 360 mg/day in divided doses. The equivalent dose of a sustained release preparation can be used once a day. Verapamil has a negative inotropic effect and should be avoided in those with LV dysfunction or hypotension. Intravenous verapamil should also be avoided in those with pre-existing beta-blockade and those with second- or third-degree AV block. As with all calcium channel blockers, verapamil can cause headaches, facial flushing, and dizziness. Constipation is a common side effect of verapamil that can be particularly troublesome for older patients.

Diltiazem is similar to verapamil, having similar indications and contraindications. It is also available in intravenous and oral form. The oral dose is 120–360 mg given in divided doses of a short-acting formulation or once or twice a day with slow release preparations. Although its negatively inotropic effect is less than that of verapamil, diltiazem is contraindicated in those with an ejection fraction <40%. Side effects include headaches, dizziness, and ankle edema although these are infrequent.

Digoxin

Digoxin has a vagolytic effect on the AV node and at higher doses also slows AV conduction. It can be given intravenously or orally. Intravenous digoxin begins to act within 15–30 minutes with a peak effect at 5 hours. The typical starting dose of oral digoxin is 0.25 mg, but a lower dose of 0.125 mg or even 0.0625 mg may be appropriate for older patients or patients with renal dysfunction. Serum digoxin levels should be measured periodically. Digoxin toxicity can manifest itself as nausea, vomiting, diarrhea, confusion, vertigo, colored vision, or arrhythmias. It is important to remember the interaction of digoxin and verapamil, which causes serum digoxin levels to rise by 50–75%. Amiodarone also increases serum digoxin levels. Diuretics can cause hypokalemia that sensitize the heart to digoxin [19].

Digoxin is less effective than beta-blockers and calcium channel blockers for rate control during exercise. It is not useful for cardioversion of AF and it has no impact on the heart rate in those with paroxysmal AF. For this reason it should not be used as a first-line agent for rate control of AF except for patients with heart failure. Despite this it is still very widely used for rate control in AF [5].

Rate control versus rhythm control

Until recently there was very little data comparing these two approaches.

Intuitively rhythm control would seem to be the first-line approach and this was the approach favored by most physicians prior to the publication of some recent major randomized trials. The largest of these was the AFFIRM trial [17]. In total 4060 patients with predominantly persistent AF and a mean age of 70 years were enrolled. They were randomly allocated to rate control using digoxin, beta-blocker and/or calcium channel blocker or rhythm control. The most frequently used drugs in the rhythm control arm were amiodarone (38%) and sotalol (31%). Propafenone, procainamide, quinidine, flecainide, and disopyramide were used to a lesser extent. All patients were anticoagulated with warfarin, but those in the rhythm control group who maintained sinus rhythm could be withdrawn from it at the treating physician's discretion.

After a mean of 3.5 years follow-up in the AFFIRM trial, 60% of patients in the rhythm control arm were in sinus rhythm. Satisfactory rate control was achieved in 80% in the rate control arm. Crossover from rhythm control to rate control occurred in 17 and 38% at 1 and 5 years due to inability to maintain sinus rhythm and drug intolerance. Crossover from rate control to rhythm control was 8 and 15% primarily due to symptoms and heart failure. All-cause mortality was not significantly different between the two groups although there was a trend favoring rate control. There was no difference in the secondary endpoints including stroke rate, quality of life, and functional status. Most of the strokes occurred in those patients whose warfarin had been stopped or who had subtherapeutic INRs. The number of patients requiring hospitalization was greater in the rhythm control group. In patients under the age of 65 in this trial a trend favoring rhythm control was noted.

The RACE trial randomized 522 patients with a mean age of 68 years to a rate control strategy or a rhythm control strategy [20]. These patients had persistent AF or atrial flutter and had previously been cardioverted. Rate control was achieved with beta-blockers, calcium channel blockers, and digoxin. Initial therapy for rhythm control was sotalol, this was changed to flecainide or propafenone if AF recurred. If it recurred again within 6 months, amiodarone was commenced. Late recurrence was treated with DC cardioversion. All patients received warfarin at least until they were in sinus rhythm for 1 month.

The primary endpoint was a composite of cardiovascular death, heart failure, thromboembolic event, severe bleeding, pacemaker implantation, or severe side effects from antiarrhythmic agents. After a mean of 2.3 years follow-up 39% of patients were in sinus rhythm in the rhythm control group compared to 10% in the rate control group. There was an almost significant trend toward lower incidence of primary endpoint with rate control (17% versus 23%). There were no significant differences in quality of life between the two groups.

The AFFIRM and RACE trials demonstrated that embolic events occurred as frequently in the rhythm control groups as in the rate control groups. Most embolic events (113 of 157 strokes in AFFIRM and 29 of 35 strokes in RACE) occurred when warfarin had been stopped or the INR was subtherapeutic. These findings suggest that chronic warfarin anticoagulation is necessary in high-risk patients even if it seems that sinus rhythm has been restored.

A recent meta-analysis of the five randomized trials comparing rate and rhythm control strategies included the AFFIRM, RACE, HOT CAFÉ, PIAF, and STAF trials [21]. In total these five trials included 5239 patients with persistent or recurrent AF. No significant difference was found between the two strategies regarding all-cause mortality although a strong trend in favor of the rate control approach was found. They concluded that in ap-propriate patients a strategy of rate control with anticoagulation was at least equivalent to rhythm control using currently available antiarrhythmic agents.

These trials have shown that rate control is an acceptable approach and should probably be the primary approach for the type of patients included in these trials. None of the presumed benefits of rhythm control was borne out. AFFIRM and RACE demonstrated the need for chronic anticoagulation with both strategies. However, it is important to recognize the limitations of these trials. The majority of the patients in these trials had persistent AF, had a high risk of thromboembolic events, were older and they were not particularly symptomatic. These results should not be extrapolated to patients with paroxysmal AF at a low risk of recurrence or at low risk of thromboembolic events.

One of the possible explanations for the lack of benefit in the rhythm control group is the lack of efficacy and the high frequency of cardiac and non-cardiac side effects of the currently available antiarrhythmic agents. If safer, more effective agents become available this may have an impact on the rate versus rhythm control debate.

Dronedarone is a noniodinated amiodarone derivative which is currently in the late stages of development. Unlike amiodarone it has little effect on thyroid receptors. Results from two recent phase III trials EURIDIS and ADONIS were promising, but unfortunately the ANDROMEDA study was terminated prematurely due to possible increased mortality in the dronedarone group [22].

Azimilide is a new class III antiarrhythmic agent which is also in the late stages of development. The ALIVE study examined its effects on mortality in patients with impaired LV function [23]. Although it did not affect mortality, it significantly reduced the incidence of AF compared to placebo and had a low incidence of adverse effects.

RSD 1235 is a novel antiarrhythmic agent which is atrial selective. It blocks several ion channels known to be active in AF. It exists in both intravenous and oral preparations. Results from phase III trials ACT 1 and ACT 3 have been promising. ACT 2 which is examining the role of RSD 1235 in postoperative AF is ongoing. All these trials relate to the intravenous preparation of this agent, but trials on the oral form are planned [24].

Thromboembolic risk and AF

These are the current AHA/ACC/ESC recommendations for antithrombotic therapy in patients with AF:

1 Administer antithrombotic therapy (oral anticoagulation or aspirin) to all patients with AF to prevent thromboembolism.

2 Individualize the selection of the antithrombotic agent based upon assessment of the absolute risks of stroke and bleeding and the relative risk and benefit for a particular patient.

3 Chronic oral anticoagulation therapy should be given in a dose adjusted to achieve target intensity INR of 2–3 in patients at high risk of stroke, unless contraindicated.

4 Aspirin 325 mg daily is an alternative in low-risk patients or those with certain contraindications to oral anticoagulation [1].

AF is a powerful independent risk factor for stroke, conferring approximately a fivefold increase in risk for those with nonvalvular AF, although risk varies significantly from patient to patient. The risk of thromboembolic phenomenon occurs as early as 72 hours after the onset of AF [25]. For this reason, current guidelines recommend that patients who have been in AF for longer than 48 hours should be anticoagulated.

Warfarin is the single most effective agent for the prevention of stroke in AF and the mainstay of thromboprophylaxis. Risk factors associated with stroke in patients with nonvalvular AF include previous stroke or TIA, diabetes, hypertension, CHF, increased age, coronary artery disease, and increased left atrial size [2].

A number of trials have compared the benefits of warfarin and aspirin for stroke prevention in patients with AF including five randomized trials—AFASAK [26], BAATAF [27], CAFA [28], SPAF [29], and SPINAF [30]. Together these trials included 2313 patients with AF with no previous stroke or TIA. The mean follow-up was 1.5 years. A similar reduction in stroke in patients taking warfarin was seen in all five trials with the overall OR of 0.39 or a relative risk reduction of 61% and an OR of 0.34 for ischemic stroke. In terms of the number needed to treat (NNT), 25 strokes were prevented per 100 patients treated with warfarin. The rate of intracranial and extracranial hemorrhage was not significantly increased in these trials although this was most certainly influenced to a certain extent by the close monitoring of anticoagulation in the setting of a clinical trial [31–33].

Oral anticoagulation with warfarin is approximately twice as effective as aspirin for the prevention of ischemic stroke in patients with AF. Patients aged under 65 years who have a structurally normal heart on echocardiography and no risk factors have a very low risk of stroke. Aspirin may be an acceptable alternative to warfarin anticoagulation for these patients and for those patients who have contraindications to warfarin [31].

The CHADS2 score attempts to estimate the risk of ischemic stroke or peripheral embolization in patients with AF [34].

Clinical parameter	Points
Congestive heart failure (any history)	1
Hypertension (prior history)	1
Age >75	1
Diabetes mellitus	1
Secondary prevention in patients with Ischemic stroke or TIA	2

Patients with a score of 0 are at low risk and can be managed with aspirin. Patients with a score of 3 or more are high risk and in the absence of contraindications should be anticoagulated with warfarin. The difficulty arises in choosing between aspirin and warfarin in intermediate risk patients. This decision must be based on the physician's estimate of risk, availability of INR monitoring, bleeding risk, and patient preference.

Despite compelling evidence for warfarin anticoagulation in the majority of patients with AF, it continues to be underutilized. The magnitude of this problem in the United States was demonstrated in the ATRIA trial, which was designed to look at the prevalence of and the risk factors for AF [3]. Among patients with no known contraindications to anticoagulation, only 53% were receiving warfarin; among patients without a contraindication to anticoagulation who had one or more risk factors for stroke, only 59% were receiving warfarin. The use of warfarin is hampered by a number of inherent difficulties including slow onset and offset of antithrombotic action, significant patient inter-variability, numerous food and drug interactions, and a narrow therapeutic window that necessitates regular monitoring with blood tests.

The limitations of warfarin have provided the impetus for the new treatment strategies and new antithrombotic agents. The combination of the antiplatelet agents, aspirin and clopidogrel, have been shown to be effective in both STEMI and NSTEMI and in the prevention of subacute stent thrombosis [35, 36]. Aspirin and clopidogrel target different pathways in platelet activation and aggregation. The use of this combination in AF is being examined in the Atrial Fibrillation Clopidogrel Trial with Irbesartan for prevention of Vascular Events (AC-TIVE) trial which is ongoing [37]. The trial aims to determine whether aspirin in combination with clopidogrel is noninferior to warfarin and superior to aspirin alone for preventing vascular events in patients with AF.

Unfortunately, the MATCH trial (Management of Atherosclerosis with Clopidogrel in High Risk Patients with Recent Transient Attack or Ischemic Stroke) which examined this combination in 7599 patients who had previously had a stroke or TIA showed no significant benefits in reducing vascular events but a significantly increased risk of major bleeding [38]. One arm of the ACTIVE was stopped prematurely in September 2005, because of a lower event rate in the warfarin group than in those taking a combination of clopidogrel and aspirin [39]. However, the ACTIVE trial has two other arms that are continuing to enroll patients. These are evaluating clopidogrel plus aspirin versus aspirin alone in AF in patients who cannot or will not take warfarin and the role of blood-pressure lowering with irbesartan in AF.

Idraparinux is a synthetic pentasaccharide that specifically targets factor Xa. Like heparin, it must be administered parentally. As it has a very long half-life it can be given subcutaneously once weekly. Like low-molecular-weight heparin, it produces a predictable anticoagulant response obviating the need for blood test monitoring. AMADEUS is an ongoing phase III trial comparing idraparinux with warfarin in patients with AF and at least one other risk factor for stroke. It is a noninferiority trial with a primary efficacy outcome of all strokes and systemic embolic events [40]. The primary safety endpoint is bleeding. One potential disadvantage of idraparinux is the lack of an antidote particularly when it has such a long half-life. Reversal in patients who develop major bleeding or who require urgent surgery may be problematic.

Ximelagatran is a new antithrombotic agent that acts by indirectly inhibiting thrombin. It is administered orally. Its efficacy in stroke prevention in patients with AF has been assessed in the SPORTIF III and V trials [41]. The results of these trials were promising. Ximelagatran, 36 mg twice daily, was compared to warfarin (target INR 2–3) in moderate to high-risk patients. Both trials demonstrated the noninferiority of ximelagatran compared to warfarin in this patient population. However, there were elevations in liver enzymes specifically alanine aminotransferase (ALT) greater than three times the upper limit of normal in 6.2% of those receiving ximelagatran compared to 0.8% of those receiving warfarin.

Ximelagatran was turned down for approval by the FDA panel in September 2004, because of concerns about hepatotoxicity. Whether it will ever be marketed in the United States is in doubt. The oral DTI ximelagatran has received regulatory approval in various European countries for the prevention of thromboembolic events in patients undergoing elective total hip—or total knee replacement surgery, but the compound has not gained regulatory approval for thromboprophylaxis in AF patients [41, 42].

Conclusion

AF is a common problem and one which is becoming increasingly more frequent. Medical management is the most common approach to this problem at present, but this may change in the future as advances in catheter ablation and surgical techniques offer the prospect of a permanent cure. All patients with AF whether it is persistent or paroxysmal are at risk of thromboembolic events, the most devastating of which is stroke. Until new agents become available or new combinations of existing agents are proven to be effective, patients at high risk should receive warfarin anticoagulation. For patients under the age of 65 years with structurally normal hearts and no risk factors, aspirin is probably sufficient although evidence for this is somewhat limited.

The optimum treatment strategy for managing patients with AF remains controversial. Ultimately, treatment needs to be individualized. A rate control strategy may be reasonable one for older patients or for those who are not particularly symptomatic. Beta-blockers and calcium channel blockers are much more effective than digoxin alone in achieving rate control. Younger patients and symptomatic patients may benefit from restoration and maintenance of sinus rhythm. This can be achieved with DC cardioversion or chemical cardioversion with antiarrhythmic drugs all of which have a proarrhythmic potential. As new agents with fewer side effects become available rhythm control may become a more attractive option.

References

1 Fuster V, Ryden LE, Asinger RW *et al.* ACC/AHA/ESC guidelines for the management of patients with atrial fibrillation: executive summary. A Report of the American College of Cardiology/American Heart Association Task Force on Practice Guidelines and the European Society of Cardiology Committee for Practice Guidelines and Policy Conferences (Committee to Develop Guidelines for the Management of Patients with Atrial Fibrillation): developed in Collaboration with the North American Society of Pacing and Electrophysiology. *J Am Coll Cardiol* October 2001; **38**(4): 1231–1266.

2 Feinberg WM, Blackshear JL, Laupacis A, Kronmal R, Hart RG. Prevalence, age distribution, and gender of patients with atrial fibrillation. Analysis and implications. *Arch Intern Med* March 13, 1995; **155**(5): 469–473.

3 Go AS, Hylek EM, Borowsky LH, Phillips KA, Selby JV, Singer DE. Warfarin use among ambulatory patients with nonvalvular atrial fibrillation: the anticoagulation and risk factors in atrial fibrillation (ATRIA) study. *Ann Intern Med* December 21, 1999; **131**(12): 927–934.

4 Cox JL. Surgical management of atrial fibrillation. *Medscape Cardiol* 2005. Available at www.medscape.com/viewarticele/512480_2. Accessed October 10, 2005.

5 Markides V, Schilling RJ. Atrial fibrillation: classification, pathophysiology, mechanisms and drug treatment. *Heart* August 2003; **89**(8): 939–943.

6 McNamara RL, Tamariz LJ, Segal JB, Bass EB. Management of atrial fibrillation: review of the evidence for the role of pharmacologic therapy, electrical cardioversion, and echocardiography. *Ann Intern Med* December 16, 2003; **139**(12): 1018–1033.

7 Gallagher MM, Guo XH, Poloniecki JD, Guan YY, Ward D, Camm AJ. Initial energy setting, outcome and efficiency in direct current cardioversion of atrial fibrillation and flutter. *J Am Coll Cardiol* November 1, 2001; **38**(5): 1498–1504.

8 Miller JM. Therapy for cardiac arrhythmias. In: Zipes DP, Libby P, Bonow RO & Braunwald E, eds. *Braunwald's Heart Disease*, 7th edn. Elselvier, Philadelphia, 2005: 713–766.

9 Pedersen OD, Bagger H, Keller N, Marchant B, Kober L, Torp-Pedersen C. Efficacy of dofetilide in the treatment of atrial fibrillation–flutter in patients with reduced left ventricular function: a Danish investigations of arrhythmia and mortality on dofetilide (diamond) substudy. *Circulation* July 17, 2001; **104**(3): 292–296.

10 Singh SN. Role of dofetilide in patients with atrial fibrillation. Insights from the Symptomatic Atrial Fibrillation Investigative Research on Dofetilide (SAFIRE-D) study. *Card Electrophysiol Rev* September 2003; **7**(3): 225–228.

11 Falk RH, Fogel RI. Flecainide. *J Cardiovasc Electrophysiol* November 1994; **5**(11): 964–981.

12 Pratt CM, Moye LA. The cardiac arrhythmia suppression trial: background, interim results and implications. *Am J Cardiol* January 16, 1990; **65**(4): 20B–29B.

13 Aasbo JD, Lawrence AT, Krishnan K, Kim MH, Trohman RG. Amiodarone prophylaxis reduces major cardiovascular morbidity and length of stay after cardiac surgery: a meta-analysis. *Ann Intern Med* September 6, 2005; **143**(5): 327–336.

14 Roy D, Talajic M, Dorian P *et al.*, for Canadian Trial of Atrial Fibrillation Investigators. Amiodarone to prevent recurrence of atrial fibrillation. *N Engl J Med* March 30, 2000; **342**(13): 913–920.

15 Singh BN, Singh SN, Reda DJ *et al.* Amiodarone versus sotalol for atrial fibrillation. *N Engl J Med* May 5, 2005; **352**(18): 1861–1872.

16 Camm AJ, Al-Saaady NM, Opie LH. Antiarrhythmic drugs. In: Opie LH & Gersh BJ, eds. *Drugs for the Heart*, 5th edn. WB Saunders, Philadelphia, 2001.

17 Wyse DG, Waldo AL, DiMarco JP *et al.* A comparison of rate control and rhythm control in patients with atrial fibrillation. *N Engl J Med* December 5, 2002; **347**(23): 1825–1833.

18 Opie LH. Calcium channel blockers. In: Opie LH & Gersh BJ, eds. *Drugs for the Heart*, 5th edn. WB Saunders, Philadelphia, 2001: 53–83.

19 Opie LH, Gersh BJ, eds. Digitalis, acute inotropes and inotropic dilators. In: *Drugs for the Heart*, 5th edn. WB Saunders, Philadelphia, 2001: 154–186.

20 van Gelder I, Hagens VE, Bosker HA *et al.* A comparison of rate control and rhythm control in patients with recurrent persistent atrial fibrillation. *N Engl J Med* December 5, 2002; **347**(23): 1834–1840.

21 Testa L, Biondi-Zoccai GG, Russo AD, Bellocci F, Andreotti F, Crea F. Rate-control vs. rhythm-control in patients with atrial fibrillation: a meta-analysis. *Eur Heart J* October 2005; **26**(19): 2000–2006.

22 Kathofer S, Thomas D, Karle CA. The novel antiarrhythmic drug dronedarone: comparison with amiodarone. *Cardiovasc Drug Rev* 2005; **23**(3): 217–230.

23 Pratt CM, Singh SN, Al-Khalidi HR *et al.* The efficacy of azimilide in the treatment of atrial fibrillation in the presence of left ventricular systolic dysfunction: results from the azimilide postinfarct survival evaluation (ALIVE) trial. *J Am Coll Cardiol* April 7, 2004; **43**(7): 1211–1216.

24 Roy D, Rowe BH, Stiell IG *et al.* A randomized, controlled trial of RSD1235, a novel anti-arrhythmic agent, in the treatment of recent onset atrial fibrillation. *J Am Coll Cardiol* December 21, 2004; **44**(12): 2355–2361.

25 Stoddard MF, Dawkins PR, Prince CR, Ammash NM. Left atrial appendage thrombus is not uncommon in patients with acute atrial fibrillation and a recent embolic event: a transesophageal echocardiographic study. *J Am Coll Cardiol* February 1995; **25**(2): 452–459.

26 Petersen P, Boysen G, Godtfredsen J, Andersen ED, Andersen B. Placebo-controlled, randomised trial of warfarin and aspirin for prevention of thromboembolic complications in chronic atrial fibrillation. The Copenhagen AFASAK study. *Lancet* January 28, 1989; **1**(8631): 175–179.

27 Singer DE, Hughes RA, Gress DR *et al.* The effect of aspirin on the risk of stroke in patients with nonrheumatic atrial fibrillation: The BAATAF Study. *Am Heart J* December 1992; **124**(6): 1567–1573.

28 Connolly SJ, Laupacis A, Gent M, Roberts RS, Cairns JA, Joyner C. Canadian atrial fibrillation anticoagulation (CAFA) study. *J Am Coll Cardiol* August 1991; **18**(2): 349–355.

29 Hart RG, Halperin JL, Pearce LA *et al.* Lessons from the stroke prevention in atrial fibrillation trials. *Ann Intern Med* May 20, 2003; **138**(10): 831–838.

30 Ezekowitz MD, Bridgers SL, James KE *et al.* Warfarin in the prevention of stroke associated with nonrheumatic atrial fibrillation. Veterans affairs stroke prevention in nonrheumatic atrial fibrillation investigators. *N Engl J Med* November 12, 1992; **327**(20): 1406–1412.

31 Hart RG, Feinberg WM, Halperin JL. Stroke prevention guidelines. *Ann Intern Med* February 1, 1995; **122**(3): 235–236.

32 Morley J, Marinchak R, Rials SJ, Kowey P. Atrial fibrillation, anticoagulation, and stroke. *Am J Cardiol* January 25, 1996; **77**(3): 38A–44A.

33 Aguilar M, Hart R. Oral anticoagulants for preventing stroke in patients with non-valvular atrial fibrillation and no previous history of stroke or transient ischemic attacks. *Cochrane Database Syst Rev* 2005; (3): CD001927.

34 Gage BF, Waterman AD, Shannon W, Boechler M, Rich MW, Radford MJ. Validation of clinical classification schemes for predicting stroke: results from the National Registry of Atrial Fibrillation. *JAMA* Junuary 13, 2001; **285**(22): 2864–2870.

35 Yusuf S, Zhao F, Mehta SR, Chrolavicius S, Tognoni G, Fox KK. Effects of clopidogrel in addition to aspirin in patients with acute coronary syndromes without ST-segment elevation. *N Engl J Med* August 16, 2001; **345**(7): 494–502.

36 Sabatine MS, Cannon CP, Gibson CM *et al.* Addition of clopidogrel to aspirin and fibrinolytic therapy for myocardial infarction with ST-segment elevation. *N Engl J Med* March 24, 2005; **352**(12): 1179–1189.

37 Donnan GA, Dewey HM, Chambers BR. Warfarin for atrial fibrillation: the end of an era? *Lancet Neurol* May 2004; **3**(5): 305–308.

38 Weinberger J. Management of Atherothrombosis in High-risk Patients with Recent Transient Ischemic Attack or Ischemic Stroke: the MATCH Trial. *Curr Cardiol Rep* January 2005; **7**(1): 8–9.

39 Cleland JG, Coletta AP, Lammiman M *et al.* Clinical trials update from the European Society of Cardiology meeting 2005: CARE-HF extension study, ESSENTIAL, CIBIS-III, S-ICD, ISSUE-2, STRIDE-2, SOFA, IMAGINE, PREAMI, SIRIUS-II and ACTIVE. *Eur J Heart Fail* October 2005; **7**(6): 1070–1075.

40 O'Donnell M, Weitz JI. Novel antithrombotic therapies for the prevention of stroke in patients with atrial fibrillation. *Am J Manag Care* April 2004; **10**(suppl 3): S72–S82.

41 Olsson SB. Stroke prevention with the oral direct thrombin inhibitor ximelagatran compared with warfarin in patients with non-valvular atrial fibrillation (SPORTIF III): randomised controlled trial. *Lancet* November 22, 2003; **362**(9397): 1691–1698.

42 Gurewich V. Ximelagatran—promises and concerns. *JAMA* February 9, 2005; **293**(6): 736–739.

5

Electrophysiological basis of atrial fibrillation

Sander Verheule, Thomas van Brakel, Erik Harks,
Maura Greiser, & Maurits Allessie

Introduction

Atrial fibrillation (AF) is characterized by a rapid, irregular atrial rhythm with a variable atrial activation pattern. Both experimental and clinical studies have shown that various etiologies are associated with an increased risk of AF and it is becoming increasingly clear that the underlying mechanisms responsible for initiation and maintenance of AF can also be diverse. In this chapter, we will first describe the theory of various electrophysiological mechanisms that have been proposed to explain AF. Subsequently, we will present some seminal results from animal studies, illustrating the variability in the mechanism underlying AF. Finally, we will present an overview of studies into human AF and discuss to what extent insights from animal models are applicable to humans, and how therapeutic strategies have contributed to our understanding of AF.

Theory of AF mechanisms

Broadly, perpetuation of AF can be divided into "hierarchical" and "anarchical" mechanisms. In the case of "hierarchical" AF, a rapid source is responsible for "driving" AF. Because of the high rate of this source, the rest of the atria cannot follow one-to-one and fibrillatory conduction ensues (Figure 5.1a). Theoretically, ablation of the source

Manual of Surgical Treatment of Atrial Fibrillation.
Edited by Hauw T. Sie *et al.* © 2008 Blackwell Publishing, ISBN: 978-1-4051-4032-4.

would stop AF. In the case of "anarchical" AF, multiple sources act "anarchically" to sustain AF and as long as a sufficient number of sources is present simultaneously, AF will be maintained (Figure 5.1b).

What constitutes a "source" in this view of AF? Two main types of sources have been proposed: an "ectopic focus" and a "reentrant wave." In the first case, an area of tissue exhibits automaticity due to its intrinsic cellular membrane properties. Either spontaneously or when triggered, this tissue area, or "focus," begins firing autonomously and becomes the driver for AF in the rest of the atrium. An early demonstration that such a rapidly firing focus can indeed produce AF was provided by Scherf [1]. A rapidly firing focus was created by injection of the sodium channel opener aconitine in the epicardium of the atrial appendage, causing fibrillatory conduction to the rest of the atrium. When the aconitine-treated area was clamped or cooled, AF stopped, indicating that this area served as a "driver" for AF.

The second type of source for AF is a reentrant wave. The first description of a reentrant mechanism was provided by Mayer in his classic experiments on rings of muscle tissue from the jellyfish *Cassiopeia xamachana* [2]. In this preparation, illustrated in Figure 5.1c, Mayer showed that an activation wavefront can travel around the ring in one direction and "reenter" (i.e. reexcite) previously excited tissue, leading to sustained circus movement of activation. To allow reentry in this preparation, the wavefront has to continuously encounter tissue that has recovered from the previous excitation. Several factors increase the likelihood that this condition is

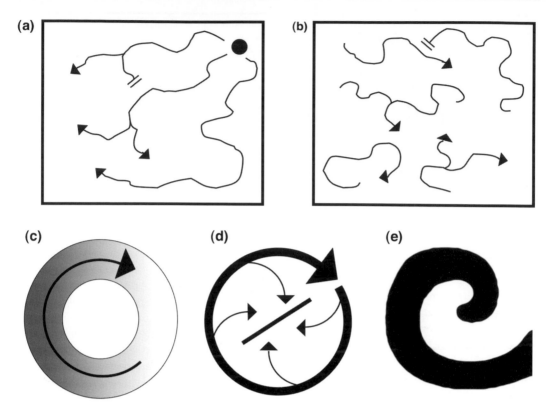

Figure 5.1 Mechanisms of atrial fibrillation. (a) "Hierarchical AF": a localized source (a focus, (micro)-reentrant circuit or rotor) driving fibrillatory conduction in the rest of the tissue. If the substrate itself supports sustained AF, it is sufficient that the source merely acts as a trigger; if not, the continued activity of the source is necessary to maintain AF. (b) "Anarchical AF": multiple wavelet reentry: several wavelets wander simultaneously over the atrium, displaying block (upper left wavelets), fusion (middle two wavelets), and a wavelet splitting up (lower left). (c, d, e) Reentrant sources for tachycardia; (c) An anatomically defined circuit: Mayer's classic experiment on anatomically determined reentry in a ring of Jellyfish muscle. The wavelength (WL) of the reentrant wave is the product of conduction velocity (CV) and effective refractory period (ERP). The time span in which the tissue is excitable but not excited is the "excitable gap." (d) Leading circle reentry: a reentrant wave with a circumference equal to the WL circles around a line of functional block. (e) Spiral wave or rotor.

met: a larger ring size, a slower conduction velocity (CV) of the wave around the ring, and a faster recovery time of the tissue (i.e. a shorter effective refractory period, ERP). The wavelength (WL) of the reentrant wave can be calculated simply as the product of CV and ERP [3]. The minimal ring size able to sustain reentry is equal to the WL of the reentrant wave. If the ring size is larger than this minimum, there is a delay between the recovery of the tissue from a previous excitation and its reexcitation that is referred to as the "excitable gap."

The concept of reentry has proved extraordinarily powerful in understanding cardiac arrhythmias. For example, in atrial flutter the wavefront rotates along an anatomically determined (macro)-reentrant circuit. In a perfused piece of normal rabbit atrial muscle, Allessie *et al.* demonstrated that an activation wavefront could also rotate in the absence of an anatomically determined circuit [4]. This "leading circle reentry" showed that reentry may be purely "functional," i.e., reentry can occur around a line of functional block (Figure 5.1d). An alternative description of a functional reentrant wave is based on the more general mathematical theory of "spiral waves" in excitable media [5]. This theory predicts the existence of "rotors" with a vortex-like pattern (Figure 5.1e), the maintenance of which depends critically on the curvature of the tip of the wavefront. The two theories differ with respect to what happens at the core of the circuit: in spiral wave reentry the core is excitable, but not excited whereas the central line of block in leading circle reentry is kept continuously refractory by centripetal waves. Secondly, in leading circle reentry, the circuit automatically assumes a size related to the WL. By contrast, the size of a rotor bears no simple relation to the ERP or CV, and can (in rare cases) have more than one wavefront rotating around one core, forming a rotor with more than one arm. When spreading away from a reentrant circuit, the wavefront may encounter refractory, slowly conducting or nonconducting tissue and break up, causing fibrillatory conduction in the rest of the atrium.

In 1924, Garrey already postulated that the likelihood of sustained AF is increased if several reentrant circuits are present at the same time [6]. Based on computer simulations, Moe and Abildskov presented an extension of this idea, proposing that reentrant waves do not necessarily have to travel along some fixed circuit, but can wander around refractory tissue in a seemingly chaotic pattern [7]. As depicted in Figure 5.1b, some wavelets may extinguish while others split up into separate daughter wavelets or fuse to become a single wavelet. As long as a certain number of wavelets remains present, AF will be sustained. The same factors which increased the likelihood of reentry in Mayer's jellyfish ring will stimulate multiple-wavelet reentry in the entire atrium: a shortened ERP, reduced CV, and a larger size of the substrate. All three factors will increase the number of wavelets that can be present simultaneously in the atrium and will therefore increase the stability of AF. Clinically, the hypothesis of multiple wavelet reentry is supported by the success of the maze procedure, in which the atria are divided surgically into compartments that by themselves are too small to sustain multiple wavelet reentry [8, 9].

In addition to these factors, there is the proarrhythmic effect of heterogeneity. Particularly at the rapid rates of AF, activation wavefronts will tend to move around areas with a relatively long ERP or low CV and will therefore take a more tortuous path. This "zig-zag" course of narrow individual wavelets will greatly increase the number of wavelets that can be present simultaneously within a certain area of tissue. Heterogeneity in conduction may be present at a very small scale, because electrical coupling between normal myocytes is stronger in the longitudinal than in the transverse direction. Computational [10] as well as experimental [11] studies have demonstrated that reduced cell-to-cell coupling can produce conduction which is at the same time very slow and very "safe" (i.e. unlikely to extinguish). The inhomogeneous distribution of gap junctions around myocytes, and the presence of fibrous tissue between (small strands of) myocytes will lead to "nonuniform anisotropy" in conduction, as Spach and coworkers have proposed [12]. This makes "micro"-reentry possible in very small areas of tissue. Possibly, this may explain that AF can, in some cases, occur in the tiny atria of the mouse heart, where the calculated WL is comparable to the circumference of the entire atrium [13]. In larger hearts, a small micro-reentrant area will appear very similar to an ectopic focus when viewed from a distance. The distinction between the two mechanisms can only be made based on high-resolution mapping of the area.

The two types of sources described above, focus and reentrant wave, may act either as a "driver" or as a "trigger" for AF (Figure 5.1a). In the case of a driver, its continuous presence is required for the maintenance of AF. If the driver stops or is stopped, this "hierarchical" form of AF terminates. In the case of a trigger, its initial activity sets off self-sustained multiple wavelet reentry in the rest of the atrium (the "substrate"). Even if the trigger is eliminated, the episode of "anarchical" AF it has initiated will continue. In this latter case, AF maintenance depends on the interplay between two factors: the incidence of activity of the trigger and the fertility of the substrate to independently sustain multiple wavelet reentry.

Experimental evidence of AF mechanisms in animal models

In many patients, AF is associated with some form of underlying heart disease. Congestive heart failure (CHF), hypertension, valvular pathologies, and aging are all strong clinical predictors of AF [14]. To unravel the mechanisms leading to AF, several of these predictors such as heart failure, atrial dilatation, and aging have been mimicked in animal models. However, in some patients, AF is observed in the absence of underlying structural heart disease or hypertension (so called "lone AF"). The analogous animal model is that of rapid atrial pacing (RAP), which has been used to address the effect on rapid activation rates on the atrium and which has helped to understand the progressive nature of AF. In some patients, AF may be caused by episodes of increased vagal activity, which has been mimicked in animal models by infusion of acetylcholine (ACh). Below, we give an overview of these animal models. Alterations in both atrial electrophysiology and tissue structure will be discussed to clarify the main differences between various models.

Cholinergic AF

It has long been recognized that cholinergic activity can promote AF [6]. This effect is instantaneous upon application of ACh or vagal stimulation and is mediated entirely by the effect of ACh on cellular electrophysiology. Mainly through a reduction in L-type calcium current ($I_{Ca,L}$) and an increase in the ACh sensitive inward rectifier (I_{KACh}), the action potential duration (APD) and atrial ERP (AERP) are shortened, thereby decreasing the WL [15]. The degree of AERP shortening depends on the ACh concentration applied or intensity of vagal stimulation. At very high concentrations of ACh, the AERP may become even shorter than 30 ms [15]. In addition, the effect of vagal stimulation on atrial refractoriness is heterogeneous because of heterogeneity in the distribution of parasympathetic nerve endings and/or ACh receptors [16, 17].

Although cholinergic AF has been investigated for decades, the exact mechanism is still controversial. In isolated atrial preparations from normal animals, AF can often not be induced. However, in the presence of ACh, prolonged periods of AF are frequently observed after a single premature beat. In isolated canine atrial preparations in the presence of 0.5–2 µM ACh, Allessie *et al.* mapped endocardial conduction during AF using two egg-shaped intracavitary electrode arrays. As illustrated in Figure 5.2, they described multiple wavelets wandering around chaotically in both atria, without any single tissue area dominating the activation pattern [18]. This observation provided experimental support for Moe's "multiple wavelet hypothe-

sis." In these preparations, AF was maintained as long as a critical minimal number of 4–6 wavelets was present simultaneously [18]. The number of wavelets could decrease due to fusion and collision of separate wavelets and block. It could increase due to division of an existing wavelet around an obstacle, either anatomical or functional (a refractory area). No sources of de novo formation of wavelets, such as a focus or microreentrant circuit were observed in this study.

Another scenario has been described by Jalife and coworkers for the isolated sheep heart, using Fourier analysis to determine activation frequencies. In the presence of 0.1–0.5 µM ACh, AF could be induced and there was a gradient in activation frequency across the atria, with the highest activation frequencies occurring in areas of the left atrium (LA) [19, 20]. These high frequencies (up to 30 Hz) were proposed to originate from stable microreentrant circuits or "rotors" [21], which may have a higher frequency in the LA because of a higher local expression of I_{KACh} [22]. In this view, multiple wavelets result from break-up of waves emanating from rotors. Multiple wavelets by themselves would not be sufficient to sustain AF, and AF would stop without rotors to form new wavelets [23].

Within a given experimental preparation, the mechanism of cholinergic AF may actually depend on the ACh concentration applied. Schuessler *et al.* have described conduction in a canine partial right atrial preparation [15]. Here, a premature stimulus caused multiple wavelet reentry at ACh concentration up to 1 µM. In this small preparation, multiple wavelet reentry did not sustain for longer than 2 seconds. Fibrillation was only sustained (>2 min) at very high ACh concentrations (>10 µM), due to the formation of small reentrant circuit with a fast cycle length of 30–50 ms that dominated activation in the entire preparation.

AF induced by RAP

An important finding in the understanding of AF was the observation that AF itself induces atrial electrophysiological changes that promote AF [24–26]. The AF goat model and dog model of RAP provided clear insight into this process of "electrical remodeling" that contributes to the progressive nature of AF. In both models, the duration of induced AF episodes increased after RAP. In the AF goat model, AF was

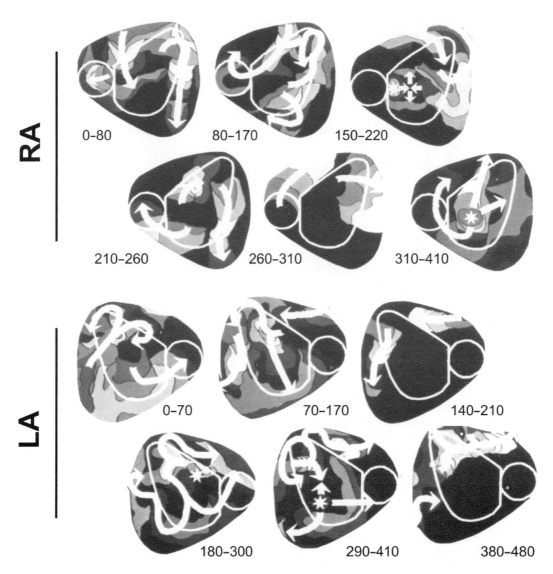

RA

0–80   80–170   150–220

210–260   260–310   310–410

LA

0–70   70–170   140–210

180–300   290–410   380–480

Figure 5.2 Multiple wavelets during infusion of 2 μM ACh. A series of consecutive activation maps covering the spread of excitation in the RA and LA during 0.5 seconds of AF. Consecutive time ranges in milliseconds are given below each panel. The propagation of wavelets is visualized by grayscale values, 10 ms apart. Black signifies areas not activated within that interval. The general direction of wavelets is indicated by white arrows. Asterisks indicate sites of breakthrough of wavelets from the epicardial surface or from the other atrium. Modified from [18].

maintained by an automatic fibrillation pacemaker that was activated as soon as sinus rhythm was detected. As shown in Figure 5.3, only seconds of AF could be induced by burst pacing in control goats, whereas AF episodes of hours were induced after 2 days of burst pacing. The episodes progressed into sustained AF (>24 h) after a week of artificially maintained AF. In the RAP canine model, it was demonstrated that continuous RAP (400 bpm) for 6 weeks increased the AF duration from seconds to minutes [25, 27, 28].

The progressive increase in AF stability upon sustained RAP was associated with changes in atrial refractoriness. After 1 week of RAP, the mean AERP was shortened to about 55% of baseline values in both goats and dogs [24, 26]. In the dog, the spatial

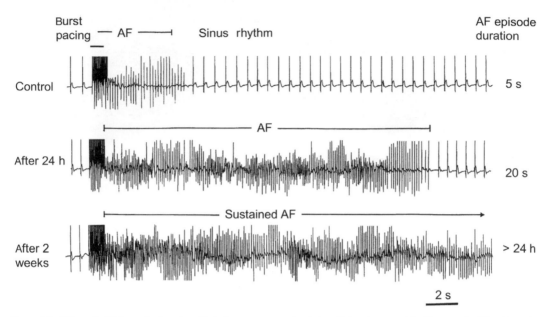

Figure 5.3 AF begets AF: in control goats, a high-frequency burst evokes only 5 seconds of AF. After 24 hours of artificially maintained AF with a "fibrillation pacemaker," episode length has increased to 20 seconds. After 2 weeks of AF, episodes last for more than 24 hours. Modified from [24].

heterogeneity of the AERP was increased by RAP, and this seemed to be an independent determinant of enhanced AF vulnerability [29]. Increased dispersion of refractoriness due to RAP was not observed in the goat [24].

As in atria infused with ACh, the decreased AERP can contribute to an increased stability of AF by a reduction of the WL. The AERP is largely determined by the APD. The action potential results from a complex interplay between depolarizing (sodium and calcium), repolarizing (potassium) currents, and various pump and exchanger currents (see Figure 5.4). In RAP models, alterations in current densities result in a shift of this balance toward the repolarizing currents, which causes shortening of the APD and a concomitant reduction of the AERP. Extensive studies have demonstrated that RAP is accompanied by a progressive decrease in the densities of the L-type calcium current (I_{CaL}) and transient outward current (I_{to}) (see Table 5.1). APD shortening is mainly caused by the reduction of I_{CaL} [28, 30].

Interestingly, the time course of the reduction of the AERP and the increase in AF stability diverge. In the goat, the AERP was already maximally reduced

after 24 hours of induced AF, whereas alterations in AF persistence developed more slowly and stabilized after 1–2 weeks [24]. Moreover, in goats subjected to sequential 4-week periods of AF separated by 1 week of sinus rhythm to allow full recovery of the AERP, a progressive increase in AF stability was measured independent of alterations in AERP [44]. These findings indicate that besides electrical remodeling at least one other factor contributes to the progression of AF.

Structural remodeling has been identified as a candidate for this "second factor" since it takes place in the same slower time domain (weeks, months). RAP induces structural alterations that develop progressively and include an increase in cell volume (hypertrophy), loss of sarcomers, accumulation of glycogen, and mitochondrial abnormalities [25, 45]. In contrast to the rapid recovery of the atrial AERP after restoration of sinus rhythm, recovery of morphological abnormalities was slow and incomplete [46]. Although these structural changes probably contribute to contractile dysfunction caused by AF, they are not likely to make the atria more vulnerable to AF, or at least their contribution is unknown at this moment.

Table 5.1 Overview of alterations in ionic currents in various animal models of AF and in myocytes from human AF patients.

	RAP	CHF	Aging	Human AF
I_{CaL}	↓ 61% [30]	↓ 30% [31]	↓ 47% [32]	↓ 63–73% [33-35]
I_{to}	↓ 49% [30]	↓ 50% [31]	↑ 31% [32]	↓ 70% [34, 36]
I_{K1}	↑ 72% [30]	↔ [31]		↑ 102–173% [34, 37, 38]
I_{Na}	↓ 52–68% [39, 40]			↔ [34]
I_{Ks}	↔ [30]	↓ 30% [31]		
I_{Kr}	↔ [41]	↔ [31]		
I_{Kur}		↔ [31]		↓ 55% [36]
I_{KACh}		↓ 45% [42]		↓ 47% [38] or ↑45% [34]
I_{NCX}	↑ 64% [30]	↑ 45% [31]		
I_{KATP}				↓ 53–59% [43]

Note that the reported decrease in I_{Na} in RAP is derived from a model of RAP without AV block, whereas the other entries in this column are based on studies of RAP with AV block and a controlled ventricular rate. I_{CaL}, L-type calcium current; I_{to}, transient outward potassium current; I_{K1}, inward rectifier potassium current; I_{Na}, sodium current; I_{Ks}, I_{Kr}, and I_{Kur}, slow, rapid, and ultra-rapid potassium currents; I_{KACh}, acetylcholine-sensitive potassium current; I_{NCX}, sodium–calcium exchanger; I_{KATP}, ATP-sensitive potassium current.

One of the characteristics of RAP models which may contribute to AF stability is the increase in substrate size due to atrial dilatation, although the extent of dilatation is modest compared to other models of AF (a 10 and 24% increase in LA systolic and diastolic area, respectively) [47]. It has also been demonstrated that fibrosis can contribute to AF stability by promoting heterogeneous

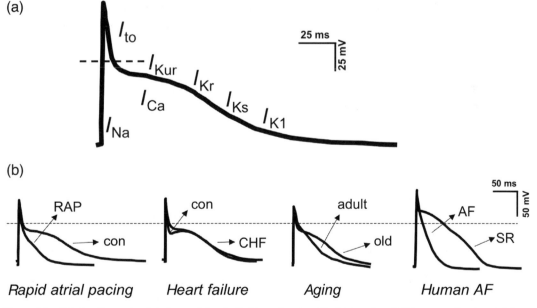

Figure 5.4 Atrial action potentials in models of AF. (a) Normal atrial action potential, illustrating the contribution of different ion currents. In reality, the contributions of these currents show a considerable overlap in time. (b) Superimposition of control action potentials with action potentials measured in atrial myocytes from canine models of rapid atrial pacing (RAP), congestive heart failure (CHF), aging, and in a myocyte from a patient with chronic AF. The dotted lines represent 0 mV. Action potentials are modified from References: RAP [28], CHF [31], aging [75], and human AF [34]. Stimulation frequency was 1 Hz in all cases.

(a)

(b)

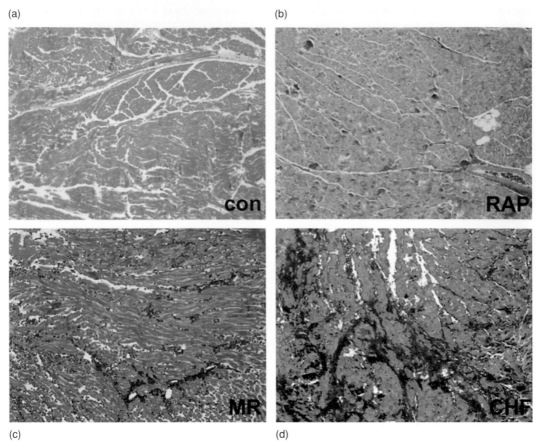

(c)

(d)

Figure 5.5 Histological changes in the left atrium of various canine models, Masson's trichrome staining with myocytes indicated in light gray and fibrous tissue in dark gray. (a) Control dog: adult mongrel dog, weighing 25–30 kg. (b) Rapid atrial pacing (RAP): atrial pacing at 600 bpm, with AV block and ventricular pacing at 100 bpm for 6 weeks. (c) Chronic left atrial dilatation following partial avulsion of the mitral valve, 4 weeks. (d) Congestive heart failure (CHF): ventricular pacing at 240 bpm for 4 weeks. At this scale, no abnormalities are apparent in the RAP left atrium compared to control dogs. In the MR model, inflammatory infiltrates and fibrosis are observed between strands of myocytes as small dark gray dots. In the CHF model, widespread fibrosis is present. Note the heterogeneous distribution of structural alterations in both the MR and CHF model.

conduction [12]. However, fibrosis is not increased in the atria of AF goats and dogs (Figure 5.5b) [26, 45]. Another factor that could directly impact myocardial conduction is electrical coupling between myocytes, which is mediated by gap junctions. Slowing of conduction by gap junctional remodeling has been considered as a factor contributing to the progression of AF [48]. However, data from several studies have shown diverging results. In the goat model, no quantitative changes in total gap junction proteins Cx40 and Cx43 levels were found, but the distribution of Cx40 became more heterogeneous during persistent AF [49]. In contrast, in the

dog model of RAP an increased expression of Cx43 has been reported [50]. Besides the variability in reported findings, the significance of altered gap junction patterns for AF is also unclear. Atrial impulse propagation depends on the expression and distribution of gap junction proteins in myocytes. However, a reduction of approximately 50% of Cx43 and Cx40 levels, respectively, in heterozygous Cx43 and Cx40 knock-out mice did not have an effect on CV [51, 52]. Complete elimination of Cx40 in mice resulted in a decrease of CV by about 30% [52]. In the goat RAP model, the increased heterogeneity in Cx40 also did not affect conduction patterns or overall CV [49]. These findings indicate that the number of gap junction proteins present between atrial myocytes is much higher than that required for normal conduction. However, it is not known how reduction in levels and increased heterogeneity of gap junction proteins impacts on conduction patterns during AF and how it contributes to AF stability.

For the interpretation of RAP animal models, the possible contribution of high and irregular ventricular rates to atrial structural remodeling should be considered. In the dog, most early studies were performed with only an atrial burst pacemaker and consequently a high ventricular rate. Most researchers now use an atrial burst pacemaker combined with complete AV block and a separate ventricular pacemaker set at a rate close to normal sinus rhythm (80–100 bpm). The differences between these models have never been investigated systematically, but in our experience, dogs with a single atrial pacemaker do develop heart failure (and atrial fibrosis) due to ventricular tachycardiomyopathy. This distinction among RAP models may explain some of the discrepancies in the literature. For example, dogs with a single atrial pacemaker show a progressive reduction in atrial CV [27] (and an underlying decrease in sodium current [39]), whereas the double pacemaker/AV block model does not [26, 53]. One study in goats has investigated the role of high ventricular rates in atrial structural remodeling and has shown that in goats with RAP and a controlled ventricular rate, the atrial structural abnormalities, observed with RAP alone, were virtually absent [54]. Both RAP models with and without AV block are relevant to human AF, corresponding to AF without and with an effective rate control, respectively.

Taken together, the increased stability of AF in models of RAP involves electrical remodeling by a reduction of the AERP and the contribution of a "second factor," which is likely to involve structural alterations. RAP alone is not associated with increased atrial fibrosis.

AF in animal models of heart failure

CHF is a clinical predictor of AF and the prevalence of AF increases with the severity of heart failure [55, 56]. To investigate the underlying mechanisms, an experimental model of CHF has been used by Nattel and coworkers to study atrial changes [26]. Overt heart failure was induced by pacing dogs with a ventricular pacemaker at a high rate (>200 bpm) for 5 weeks.

The duration of triggered AF episodes in these CHF-dogs was significantly increased to several minutes compared to a few seconds in control dogs. Electrophysiological studies demonstrated that CHF is accompanied by changes in a variety of ionic currents that contribute to the atrial action potential (see Table 5.1 and Figure 5.4). In particular, the depolarizing L-type calcium current and some repolarizing potassium currents were significantly reduced. However, the alterations in membrane currents observed in CHF did not result in a reduction of the APD. In clear contrast to RAP in dogs, CHF did not reduce the AERP or increase AERP heterogeneity. In addition, CHF did not alter the overall CV [26]. Therefore, the increased stability of AF in CHF models must be caused by a mechanism different from that in the RAP model.

Histological analysis of the atria of CHF dogs revealed dramatic interstitial fibrosis (Figure 5.5d) that was not observed in dogs subjected to RAP and control dogs [26]. Myofibers in CHF atria were less tightly packed and separated by thick layers of connective tissue composed of increased numbers of fibroblasts and large amounts of collagen. More connective tissue was also observed between individual myocytes from heart failure dogs. These structural abnormalities in CHF dogs were accompanied by regional conduction slowing. The resulting heterogeneous conduction would make the atrium more susceptible to AF. Studies that have addressed the reversibility of CHF confirm the key role of atrial fibrosis in the promotion of AF in this model [57, 58]. Ventricular pacing was followed by a recovery period of about 1 month to allow full recovery of ventricular function and atrial dimensions. This recovery was accompanied by a complete normalization of atrial cellular electrophysiology [57]. In contrast, atrial fibrosis as well as the conduction heterogeneities could not be reversed by this procedure [57, 58]. Moreover, the duration of induced AF episodes did not decrease after reversal from heart failure, indicating that atrial structural but not electrical remodeling determines the increased stability of AF in experimental CHF.

Remarkably, this dog model of CHF developed substantially (~25 times) more fibrosis in the atrium than in the ventricle [59]. Moreover, the time frame in which tissue damage emerged was different between atrium and ventricle. In the atria, a peak in inflammation, apoptosis, and necrosis was observed within 24 hours after activation of the ventricular pacemaker [59]. These indicators of tissue injury gradually disappeared in the following 5 weeks. In the ventricle these responses developed only slowly over the entire period of ventricular pacing. The reasons for these differences between atrium and ventricle are unknown.

It is widely accepted that the renin–angiotensin–aldosterone system (RAAS), and in particular angiotensin II (AT II) plays a major role in heart failure. In the atria of CHF dogs, tissue AT II levels were rapidly increased by rapid ventricular pacing and remained elevated thereafter [59]. Interestingly, inhibition of AT II production by the angiotensin-converting enzyme (ACE) blocker enalapril not only attenuated CHF-induced atrial fibrosis but also reduced the heterogeneity of conduction and AF promotion [60, 61]. This indicates that the renin–angiotensin system is an important mediator in the development of the substrate for AF in CHF.

In conclusion, it has been demonstrated in the CHF dog model that the mechanism by which heart failure promotes AF is completely different from RAP-induced AF. In contrast to RAP, the increased stability of AF is not caused by a shortening of the AERP but rather by more heterogeneous conduction patterns that result from widespread atrial fibrosis.

Animal models of atrial dilatation

Atrial size increases in animal models of CHF (80% LA area increase) and to a lesser extent in those of RAP (24% LA area increase) [47]. However, in these models the contribution of atrial dilatation in itself to the remodeling process cannot be determined.

The effects of atrial dilatation have been studied in several experimental settings that can be divided into models of acute and chronic atrial stretch. Data on effects of acute dilatation on atrial electrophysiology are diverging. In Langendorff-perfused rabbit hearts that were exposed to an increased atrial pressure, the AERP was reduced, which correlated with a decrease in the duration of monophasic action potentials (MAP) and enhanced AF inducibility [62]. These changes were reversible within 3 minutes upon release of atrial stretch. Also, in dogs in which acute LA dilatation was induced by inflation of a balloon catheter, a shortening of the AERP and concomitant increase in susceptibility to atrial arrhythmias was found [63]. However, a prolongation of atrial refractoriness was measured in dogs subjected to acute RA stretch by saline infusion [64], whereas acute atrial dilatation by rapid infusion of a blood-expanding fluid in goats did not change the AERP [65]. The mechanism by which acute dilatation increases the vulnerability to AF was studied in detail in rabbit atria using a mapping array of 240 electrodes on the right atrial wall [66]. In these experiments, it was demonstrated that conduction became more heterogeneous upon dilatation. Stretch-induced local conduction slowing and block seemed to create an atrial substrate susceptible to AF.

Different models of chronic atrial dilatation indicate that increased AF vulnerability by dilatation is not accompanied by a decrease in AERP [53, 67–69]. One of the first studies on chronic atrial dilatation was performed by Boyden and Hoffman [67]. Partial occlusion of the pulmonary artery and partial avulsion of the tricuspid valve resulted in enlarged and structurally remodeled right atria characterized by hypertrophied myocytes and increased interstitial fibrosis. These enlarged atria were more susceptible to arrhythmias but this was not due to electrical remodeling since action potentials were not significantly different from control.

In a canine model of mitral regurgitation (MR) the LA becomes significantly enlarged during the first minutes after MR, thereafter increasing more gradually to 129% of the baseline width during the first 3 weeks of MR (an area increase of 67%) [68]. Histological analysis demonstrated areas of inflammatory infiltrates and increased fibrosis in these MR dogs (Figure 5.5c). The increased duration of AF episodes in MR dogs could not be explained by a decrease in WL, because the AERP was homogeneously increased with no differences in the overall CV. High-resolution optical mapping revealed that conduction heterogeneity in LA was significantly increased during pacing at short cycle lengths and premature stimuli [13]. Together, these results indicate that the increased AF vulnerability in MR dogs is determined by structural changes which give rise to increased spatial heterogeneities in conduction.

In another model of chronic atrial dilatation, the relation between the time course of atrial dilatation and the stability of AF was studied [69]. Chronic complete AV block in goats resulted in a slow idioventricular rhythm and volume overload in the ventricle causing a progressive atrial enlargement and hypertrophy of atrial myocytes. In a time period of 4 weeks of AV block, the mean RA diameter gradually increased by 14%, corresponding to an area increase of 29%. Atrial dilatation was paralleled by a gradual increase in AF stability whereas the AERP and the dispersion of AERP remained constant. Atrial mapping during pacing at short cycle lengths showed that the incidence of areas with slow conduction was higher in dilated atria. Interestingly, in contrast to the MR dogs no signs of atrial fibrosis could be detected in atria from goats with AV block. This may be due to the slower time course of atrial dilatation in this model, which allows myocytes to undergo cellular hypertrophy. Thus, local conduction slowing in this model was not caused by increased fibrosis and also the expression of Cx40 and Cx43 was unchanged.

In summary, animal models of atrial dilatation demonstrate that atrial dilatation causes an increased stability of AF. This can occur in the absence of AERP shortening and involves increased heterogeneity of conduction.

The atria in animal models of aging

Although the clinical prevalence of AF strongly increases with age [70], the intrinsic contribution of aging to AF promotion is difficult to study in humans due to the long time span of senescence and the presence of numerous confounding factors. Several animal models have been used to investigate aging-related AF, but extrapolation of the results of these models to humans is hazardous. For example, spontaneous AF has never been observed in studies on old animals and the time frame of the animal studies is relatively short compared to a human lifetime.

Spach and coworkers studied conduction patterns in canine atria and found an age-dependent slowing of transverse propagation, which correlated with the development of extensive collagenous septa that separated small groups of fibers [71]. Similarly, a comparative study of young and old rats demonstrated large amounts of heterogeneous interstitial fibrosis in atria of old rats [72]. AF could only be induced in the old rat atria and this was not due to changes in AERP. Instead, the increased fibrosis caused age-dependent conduction slowing and enhanced AF vulnerability.

In a study on aging in dogs, Koura *et al.* demonstrated that with age, the amount of fibrosis and fatty infiltrates between adjacent strands of myocytes increased (Figure 5.6a) [73]. In addition, the gap junction protein Cx43 became increasingly concentrated at end-to-end connections between myocytes (Figure 5.6b), compared with a more homogeneous distribution in atria from infant and young dogs. Using high-resolution optical mapping of a tissue area with a highly organized, strongly anisotropic fiber orientation (Figure 5.6c), the authors demonstrated that aging of canine atria was accompanied by enhanced anisotropy of conduction patterns, while the APD was not altered [73]. Most notably, extremely slow transverse conduction, causing a "zig-zag" conduction pattern, was only observed in old atria (Figure 5.6d). It is conceivable that such "longitudinal dissociation" of conduction between adjacent fibers is a general characteristic of anisotropic atrial areas during aging.

At the cellular level, a study performed in adult (1–5 yr) and old (>8 yr) dogs showed an age-induced shift in membrane currents (see Table 5.1) that gave rise to a slight (~15%) increase in APD and AERP [74]. In addition, increased APD heterogeneity and slower conduction of premature beats was measured in aged atrial tissue [74, 75]. Despite these changes in atrial electrophysiology, the inducibility of AF was not significantly increased in this study [75].

Taken together, these studies show that even in the absence of any underlying pathology, the senescent heart possesses structural characteristics that predispose to AF. However, in these animal models, the extent of electrical and structural alterations is often not sufficient to lead to the increased AF vulnerability that is associated with aging in humans.

Mechanisms of AF in humans

Our knowledge of AF has increased enormously over the last decades as a result of both animal

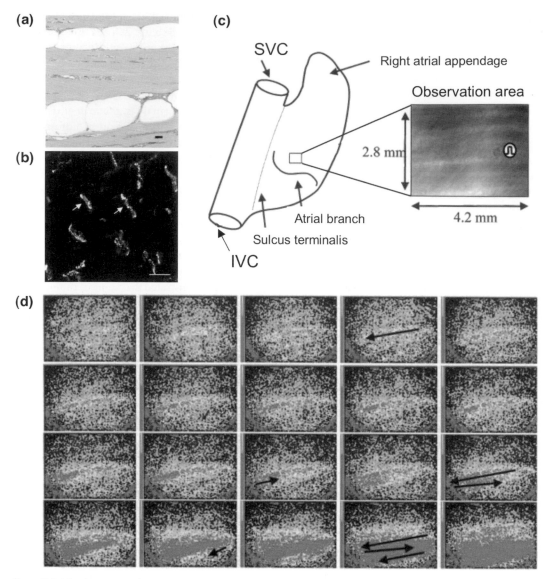

Figure 5.6 Histology, connexin expression, and conduction in old dogs. (a) Masson's trichrome staining, myocytes are indicated in light gray and fibrous tissue in dark gray. Large, vacant areas represent adipocytes. (b) Expression of the major gap junction protein Cx43. During aging, expression of Cx43 is increasingly confined to the intercalated discs at end-to-end connections between myocytes. (c) Tissue area stud-ied with high-resolution optical mapping, with the highly anisotropic fiber orientation visible in the inset. (d) Longi-tudinal dissociation between adjacent fibers leads to a "zig-zag" pattern of conduction. Resting tissue is colored light gray, activated tissue is colored dark gray. Each consecutive frame represents 2 ms. Modified from [73].

studies and clinical research. Although the ultimate goal is to understand human AF, clinical research is hampered by the fact that most studies provide no information on the baseline state of the patients or lack a true control group. Patient populations are mostly inhomogeneous and may include a variety of possible confounding factors.

The advantage of animal models is that hypotheses can be examined under controlled conditions with a limited number of confounders. This has provided opportunities to study separate factors contributing to AF, like rapid activation rates or dilatation, and to recognize the contribution of these factors in human AF. However, in humans these factors may be present in a mild form over prolonged periods of time and the final substrate of AF may have evolved very slowly over a period of decades. For practical purposes, stimuli in animals studies are applied in a more intense form, for example, creating acute severe MR to study chronic dilatation [68] and pronounced ventricular tachycardia causing a progression toward decompensating heart failure within only a couple of weeks [26]. Long-term animal studies in models of aging and long-standing hypertension, two of the most important clinical predictors of AF, are expensive and relatively rare.

In this final part of the chapter, we present an overview of important findings on mechanisms of human AF in light of the previously discussed animal models. Furthermore, we will discuss different types of substrates that may be responsible for initiation and perpetuation of human AF. One of the features of AF in patients is that it can become more and more "entrenched" with time. Initially, AF often occurs as paroxysms interrupted by long periods of sinus rhythm. In many patients, these paroxysms tend to become longer with time, until AF is "persistent" and the atria no longer convert spontaneously to sinus rhythm. Persistent AF can still be stopped by chemical or electrical cardioversion, but ultimately sinus rhythm can no longer be restored and AF is said to be "permanent."

The role of pulmonary veins in AF

In recent years, it has become apparent that paroxysmal AF is often focal in origin, with certain areas within the atria acting as drivers for AF. Such areas have sometimes been found in the crista terminalis or inferior and superior vena cava, but are located most often in the pulmonary veins (reviewed in Reference [76]). It has been demonstrated that the sleeves of atrial myocardium extending into the pulmonary veins may display focal activity that initiate and may perpetuate AF [77, 78].

The electrophysiological basis of rapid electrical activity originating from the pulmonary vein area is at this point unclear. Since the discovery of rapid "focal" activity in human PVs, the possible

contribution of the PVs in animal models of AF has received considerable attention. In the canine RAP model their contribution seems to be limited. Initially, it was suggested that chronic RAP in dogs can promote rapid PV activity [79] and various forms of abnormal and arrhythmogenic activity were measured in cardiomyocytes derived from control and RAP PVs [80]. However, more recent and extensive studies have demonstrated that PV myocytes do not display spontaneous automaticity [41, 81] and are not required for the maintenance of AF in atrial preparations of the dog RAP model [41]. Based on histological evidence, it has been argued that the myocardial sleeves in dogs may either contain pacemaker-like cells [82] or may be a fertile substrate for (micro)-reentry due to the peculiar fiber geometry of normal atrial myocytes [83]. Electrophysiologically, myocardial sleeves in dogs show slow, complex conduction with a propensity to reentry [84, 85], although some focus-like activation patterns have also been observed [85]. In general, the animal models of AF described in the previous part of this chapter do not display spontaneous AF episodes. Therefore, they allow study of the substrate of perpetuation of AF, rather than the mechanism of AF initiation and paroxysmal AF.

Since the initial description of focal PV activity in AF patients, targeted or circumferential pulmonary vein ablation has become a widely used, but still experimental, treatment of AF. Several studies in patients with permanent AF have suggested that drivers in the LA may be responsible for the perpetuation of AF [86–88]. However, in a recent study it was demonstrated that in patients with paroxysmal AF the sites with a dominant AF frequency were clustered in the PVs, whereas in patients with permanent AF, these dominant sites were distributed throughout both atria [88]. Nevertheless, isolation of the PVs in patients with persistent and permanent AF has been reported to be successful in stopping AF in 60–80% of patients [89, 90].

Todd *et al.* showed that AF could be maintained in a PV region disconnected by ablation, whereas the remaining atrial tissue was unable to sustain AF. They suggested that the likely mechanisms responsible for the perpetuation of AF in the PV area may be triggered activity or self-sustaining rotors [91]. However, as discussed in the first part of this chapter, a structurally heterogeneous substrate may also sustain "microreentry" in a very small tissue area. Other studies showed that complete isolation of the PV area after circumferential PV ablation is relatively rare. Less than 20% of the circumferentially ablated pulmonary veins were truly electrically isolated [89, 92]. Kottkamp *et al.* showed that restoration of sinus rhythm was not related to complete PV isolation [89]. This raises the question whether complete isolation of the PVs is required for the treatment of AF. Several alternative explanations for the success of pulmonary vein isolation in permanent and persistent AF treatment are possible. First of all, encircling lesions around the pulmonary veins may impair multiple wavelet reentry in a substantial part of the LA and may resemble a maze procedure because the encircled posterior wall of the LA accounts for approximately 40–50% of the left atrial tissue mass [93]. Secondly, the PV may embody an anatomical substrate for AF that facilitates micro-reentry and may act as a perpetuator of AF.

We are currently performing intraoperative high-density mapping in patients with persistent AF and mitral valve disease. Preliminary data of this study indicate that in this diseased population, the substrate of AF shows a high variability in spatial distribution. Considerable spatial dispersion in AF cycle length was present in most patients. However, with careful mapping of conduction pathways, we did not find preferential sites with a shortest and most regular AF cycle length. Also, a high degree of fractionation and dissociation of fibrillation waves was observed in the pulmonary vein area, and at Bachmann's bundle, particularly in patients with chronic AF. Figure 5.7 depicts an example of the degree of dissociated fibrillation and fractionation in a patient with permanent AF and mitral valve disease. It is conceivable that the PV area, which has a highly organized fiber orientation [94], is a substrate for longitudinal dissociation in AF patients. Such a substrate may support zig-zag conduction, similar to that shown in Figure 5.6, and thereby act as a perpetuator of AF.

Electrical remodeling in humans

In patients, paroxysms of AF often tend to become longer with time, ultimately leading to persistent or permanent AF. Animal models of RAP, which may be comparable to "lone AF" in humans in many respects, have helped to understand this progressive nature: AF itself leads to changes which increase the stability of AF [24]. It is now widely accepted that "electrical remodeling" plays an important role in this process: the rapid rates of AF cause a decrease in AERP and a loss of rate adaptation of the AERP [24, 27]. In patients, the existence of electrical remodeling is well established. Several clinical studies have shown that patients with AF have shorter atrial action potentials than patients in sinus rhythm [95–99]. In addition to AERP shortening, Boutjdir *et al.* have shown a loss of rate adaptation of the AERP in tissue from AF patients [96]. Franz *et al.* confirmed this observation by showing reduced rate adaptation of the MAP duration in patients with AF or atrial flutter [98]. This loss of rate adaptation may constitute an independent predictor of vulnerability to AF, as was shown by Attuel *et al.* [95]. Other studies have found not only AERP shortening, but also dispersion of the AERP, which may also contribute to the persistent nature of AF [100–103]. Interestingly, some studies did not find a shortening of the MAP/AERP in patients with AF [104, 105]. In addition, Simpson *et al.* did not find an association between the AERP and the inducibility of AF by premature beats [105]. The underlying molecular mechanisms that cause APD shortening are believed to occur at the level of expression and/or phosphorylation of ion channels responsible for the inward (depolarizing) and outward (repolarizing) currents. The L-type Ca^{2+} ion channel density, responsible for the major inward current during the plateau phase, is reduced in chronic AF and will contribute to the shortening of the APD (see Table 5.1 and Figure 5.4) [106]. Changes in outward currents consist of a reduction of the rapidly activated potassium currents I_{to} and I_{kur} and an increase in the inward rectifier I_{K1} (see Table 5.1 and the references therein).

Does the process of electrical remodeling explain the progressive nature of AF in patients? Often, AF can be cardioverted by agents that prolong the atrial APD. This indicates that a prolongation of the AERP is antiarrhythmic, but does not show to which extent the AERP shortening contributes to AF stability. Importantly, the success rate of chemical cardioversion is relatively high in recent onset AF but its efficacy decreases with longer AF durations [107–110]. The

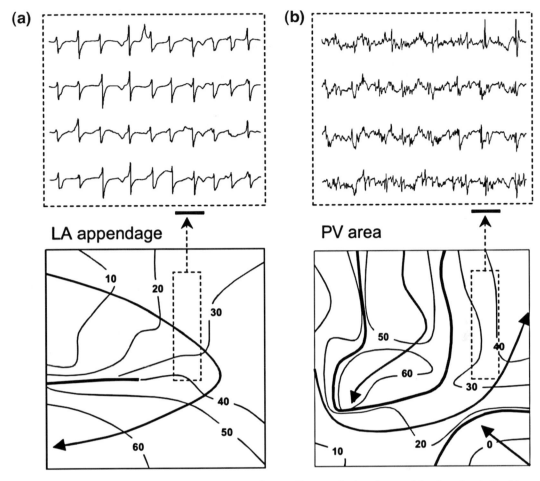

(a) LA appendage

(b) PV area

Figure 5.7 Intraoperative mapping of human AF: recordings were made using a 1 by 1 cm electrode containing an array of 64 electrodes in a patient with persistent AF and mitral valve disease. (a) Recording from the LA appendage. (b) Recording from the area in between the PVs. In the upper panels, a selection of 5 electrograms is shown to illustrate the low degree of fractionation in the LA appendage whereas the PV area shows highly fractionated electrograms. Correspondingly, the LA appendage has a relatively simple activation pattern, and the PV area a more complex activation pattern (lower panels).

exact time course of electrical remodeling during AF in humans is unknown, but in animal models it is complete within at most a few days. The limited efficacy of ion channel blockers in the treatment of chronic AF indicates that other processes occurring more slowly than electrical remodeling contribute to the stability of AF in many patients.

Several studies reported that a short right atrial MAP duration directly after cardioversion correlated to a higher recurrence of AF [111, 112]. The question is how long this effect persists. In most patients with recent onset of paroxysmal AF, the time spent in sinus rhythm between two AF episodes may be long enough to completely reverse electrical remodeling. In animal models, complete reversal of electrical remodeling takes place within 2–3 days of sinus rhythm with a gradual prolongation of the AERP and progressive return of the rate adaptation response [44, 65, 113]. A number of clinical studies have demonstrated that after cardioversion of persistent AF in patients, the AERP also gradually increases and is reversible within several days [99, 114, 115]. Interestingly, several other studies showed that increased vulnerability to AF after cardioversion still exists 2–4 weeks after reversal of electrical remodeling [116, 117]. This discrepancy in time course indicates that the effect of other processes than just electrical remodeling remain present after cardioversion of AF.

Structural abnormalities and human AF

Taken together, the observations above indicate that, in analogy to animal models of RAP [24], there is also a "second factor" in human AF. This "second factor" may similarly entail alterations in atrial tissue structure. However, comparison of these animal models to "lone AF" in humans is not straightforward. No data are available on biopsies from the baseline state of "lone AF" patients, before AF occurred. This makes it impossible at this point to determine whether structural abnormalities in these patients are a cause or a consequence of AF.

In one group of patients with chronic "lone AF," Frustaci et al. have described evidence of occult atrial pathology, such as myocyte necrosis, myocarditis, and fibrosis [118, 119], indicating that some AF patients without clinically detectable underlying heart disease may suffer from occult, underlying pathology. However, the majority of chronic AF patients is of advanced age or suffers from cardiovascular diseases such as hypertension, ischemic heart disease, valvular diseases, or CHF. Animal models of heart failure, chronic atrial dilatation, and aging all show structural changes of the atrial myocardium. It is likely that in the corresponding human patient populations, these pathologies also lead to alterations in atrial tissue structure. Figure 5.8 depicts examples of atrial pathology in patients with persistent or permanent AF. The observed atrial structural changes such as fibrosis and fatty infiltration may predispose the atria to AF by causing heterogeneity in conduction [12]. From the dog CHF model, it has become apparent that the renin–angiotensin system may be an important mediator for atrial myocardial fibrosis [60]. Interestingly, several recent studies have shown that angiotensin converting enzyme inhibitors interfere with atrial remodeling and can prevent AF in patients with structural heart disease [117, 120–124].

Degenerative changes of the atrial myocardium with aging have been associated with an increased prevalence of AF. Spach and Dolber found an age-related electrical uncoupling of side-to-side fiber connections in human cardiac muscle [125]. More recently, Lie et al. reported atrial pathology associated with AF, such as degenerative necrosis, fibrosis, and fibrofatty myocardial infiltration [126]. Kostin et al. also reported augmentation of fibrosis in patients with AF [127]. Fibrofatty replacement with a patchy distribution within the atrial myocardium was the most common finding in postmortem histological study of 10 patients without and 10 patients with AF, but this phenomenon was much more pronounced in the hearts of the AF patients [128]. Becker has also suggested that structural changes in fast conducting pathways such as Bachmann's bundle may play a crucial role in the pathogenesis of AF. In some patients with a history of AF, Becker observed total replacement of Bachmann's bundle by fibrofatty tissue [128]. In addition to these large-scale changes, several studies showed degeneration and apoptosis of atrial myocytes from patients with AF [119, 129, 130]. Overall, the frequency and degree of histological abnormalities encountered in AF patients suggest that structural remodeling may be an important contributor to AF persistence in humans.

An additional relevant factor for altered conduction in AF may be changes in atrial connexin expression. Several studies have reported alterations in Cx40 and/or Cx43 in patients with AF, but the observations are not consistent. In patients with chronic AF, both higher [131] and lower [132] levels of Cx40 were reported. Another study found increased heterogeneity in the distribution of Cx40, along with a reduction of Cx43 [127]. Kanagaratnam et al. reported that the total level of connexin expression did not correlate with CV but that lower levels were associated with a more complex activation pattern during AF [133]. In patients undergoing open chest surgery, higher Cx40 levels were found to be correlated with an increased incidence of postoperative AF [134]. Although altered connexin distribution patterns may play a role in forming a substrate for (micro)-reentry in AF, their exact contribution requires further investigation.

The electroanatomic substrate of human AF

High-density mapping of human AF has been an important tool to provide insight into the substrates responsible for the sustained nature of the arrhythmia. Konings et al. studied conduction in the right atrium during electrically induced AF in patients undergoing surgery for WPW syndrome [135, 136].

(a)   (b)

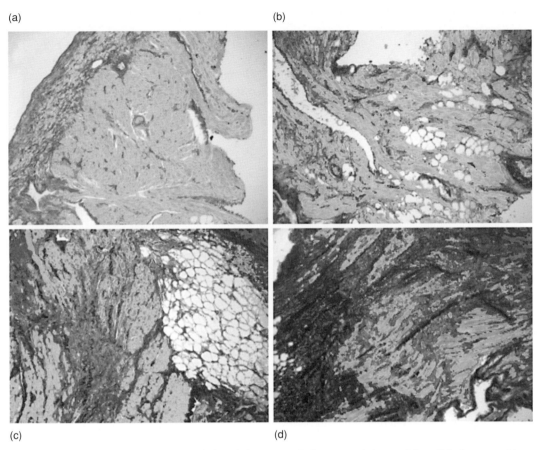

(c)   (d)

Figure 5.8 Variability of atrial structural pathology in human patients with a history of AF. Masson's trichrome staining with myocytes indicated in light gray and fibrous tissue in dark gray. (a) Area of comparatively normal atrial myocardium. (b) Interstitial fibrosis and fatty infiltrates in an adjacent area in the same patient, illustrating the heterogeneity in structural abnormalities within the same atrium. (c) Extensive fibrosis and large fatty area in another patient. (d) Widespread fibrosis and fiber disarray in a third patient. All samples were taken from right atrial appendages of patients undergoing open chest surgery for bypass surgery or valvular repair.

As illustrated in Figure 5.9, three types of AF in the right atrium were classified, based on the complexity of atrial activation. From type I to type III, the frequency and irregularity of AF increased, and the incidence reentry became higher. The more complex form of AF was characterized by a higher number and smaller dimension of the reentrant circuits [135]. The morphology of single unipolar electrograms in the right atrium during AF reflected the occurrence of various specific patterns of conduction. Mapping of electrogram fragmentation may therefore allow identification of regions with structural conduction disturbances involved in perpetuation of chronic AF [136]. Nademanee *et al.* have mapped patients with paroxysmal and chronic AF

and demonstrated that complex fractionated electrograms occur more frequently in the interatrial septum, pulmonary veins, and the roof of the LA [137]. Ablation of all areas with complex fractionated electrograms resulted in restoration of sinus rhythm in 91% of the patients after a follow-up of 1 year. The concept of targeting the local substrate by ablation of fractionated areas represents a novel strategy in the treatment of AF.

Some aspects of the atrial architecture itself, apart from pathological structural changes, may play a role in creating a substrate for AF. Schuessler *et al.* showed by endo- and epicardial mapping in canine hearts that the epicardial and endocardial activation can be markedly different and that the epicardial

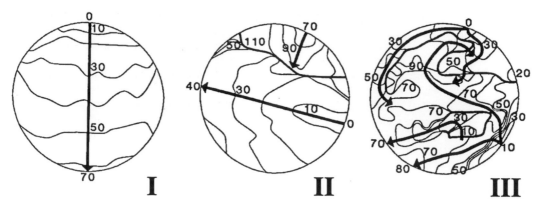

Figure 5.9 Illustration of three types of activation during atrial fibrillation. The mapping electrode had a diameter of 3.6 cm and was positioned on the free wall of the right atrium. During type I fibrillation the free wall of the right atrium was activated by single broad, uniformly propagat-ing waves. In contrast, during type III fibrillation a high degree of dissociation was present and the right atrium was activated by multiple wandering wavelets. Adapted from [135].

layer plays a leading role in atrial wave propagation during sinus rhythm [138]. In a study on isolated sheep right atria, Berenfeld *et al.* have shown how the endocardial network of trabeculae increases the complexity of activation patterns during AF [139]. Recently, Houben *et al.* have suggested that with a loss of continuity in the thin epicardial layer of the atrial wall, the trabeculated endocardial structure may become dominant, resulting in a more disorganized and stable type III AF [140] (Figure 5.9). One of the challenges ahead is to link the various conduction patterns during AF to the underlying tissue architecture and pathological changes in order to elucidate the electropathological substrate for perpetuation of AF.

References

1 Scherf D, Romano FJ, Terranova R. Experimental studies on auricular flutter and auricular fibrillation. *Am Heart J* 1948; **36**(36): 241–251.

2 Mayer AG. *Rhythmical Pulsation in Scyphomedusae.* Carnegie Institute of Washington, Washington, DC, 1906: 1–62.

3 Wiener N, Rosenblueth A. The mathematical formulation of the problem of conduction of impulses in a network of connected excitable elements, specifically in cardiac muscle. *Arch Inst Cardiol Mex* 1946; **16**(16): 205–265.

4 Allessie MA, Bonke FI, Schopman FJ. Circus movement in rabbit atrial muscle as a mechanism of tachycardia. III. The "leading circle" concept: a new model of circus movement in cardiac tissue without the involvement of an anatomical obstacle. *Circ Res* 1977; **41**(1): 9–18.

5 Pertsov AM, Davidenko JM, Salomonsz R, Baxter WT, Jalife J. Spiral waves of excitation underlie reentrant activity in isolated cardiac muscle. *Circ Res* 1993; **72**(3): 631–650.

6 Garrey WE. Auricular fibrillation. *Physiol Rev* 1924; **4**(4): 215–250.

7 Moe GK, Abildskov JA. Atrial fibrillation as a self-sustaining arrhythmia independent of focal discharge. *Am Heart J* 1959; **58**(1): 59–70.

8 Cox JL, Schuessler RB, D'Agostino HJ, Jr *et al.* The surgical treatment of atrial fibrillation. III. Development of a definitive surgical procedure. *J Thorac Cardiovasc Surg* 1991; **101**(4): 569–583.

9 Cox JL, Boineau JP, Schuessler RB *et al.* Successful surgical treatment of atrial fibrillation. Review and clinical update. *JAMA* 1991; **266**(14): 1976–1980.

10 Shaw RM, Rudy Y. Ionic mechanisms of propagation in cardiac tissue. Roles of the sodium and L-type calcium currents during reduced excitability and decreased gap junction coupling. *Circ Res* 1997; **81**(5): 727–741.

11 Rohr S, Kucera JP, Kleber AG. Slow conduction in cardiac tissue. I. Effects of a reduction of excitability versus a reduction of electrical coupling on microconduction. *Circ Res* 1998; **83**(8): 781–794.

12 Spach MS, Boineau JP. Microfibrosis produces electrical load variations due to loss of side-to-side cell connections: a major mechanism of structural heart disease arrhythmias. *Pacing Clin Electrophysiol* 1997; **20**(2, pt 2): 397–413.

13 Verheule S, Sato T, Everett Tt *et al.* Increased vulnerability to atrial fibrillation in transgenic mice with selective atrial fibrosis caused by overexpression of TGF-beta1. *Circ Res* 2004; **94**(11): 1458–1465.

14 Kannel WB, Wolf PA, Benjamin EJ, Levy D. Prevalence, incidence, prognosis, and predisposing conditions for

atrial fibrillation: population-based estimates. *Am J Cardiol* 1998; **82**(8A): 2N–9N.

15 Schuessler RB, Grayson TM, Bromberg BI, Cox JL, Boineau JP. Cholinergically mediated tachyarrhythmias induced by a single extrastimulus in the isolated canine right atrium. *Circ Res* 1992; **71**(5): 1254–1267.

16 Alessi R, Nusynowitz M, Abildskov JA, Moe GK. Nonuniform distribution of vagal effects on the atrial refractory period. *Am J Physiol* 1958; **194**(2): 406–410.

17 Ninomiya I. Direct evidence of nonuniform distribution of vagal effects on dog atria. *Circ Res* 1966; **19**(3): 576–583.

18 Allessie MA, Lammers WJEP, Bonke FIM, Hollen J. Experimental evaluation of Moe's multiple wavelet hypothesis of atrial fibrillation. In: Zipes DP & Jalife J, eds. *Cardiac Arrhythmias.* Grune & Stratton, New York, 1985:265–276.

19 Skanes AC, Mandapati R, Berenfeld O, Davidenko JM, Jalife J. Spatiotemporal periodicity during atrial fibrillation in the isolated sheep heart. *Circulation* 1998; **98**(12): 1236–1248.

20 Mansour M, Mandapati R, Berenfeld O, Chen J, Samie FH, Jalife J. Left-to-right gradient of atrial frequencies during acute atrial fibrillation in the isolated sheep heart. *Circulation* 2001; **103**(21): 2631–2636.

21 Mandapati R, Skanes A, Chen J, Berenfeld O, Jalife J. Stable microreentrant sources as a mechanism of atrial fibrillation in the isolated sheep heart. *Circulation* 2000; **101**(2): 194–199.

22 Sarmast F, Kolli A, Zaitsev A *et al.* Cholinergic atrial fibrillation: I(K,ACh) gradients determine unequal left/right atrial frequencies and rotor dynamics. *Cardiovasc Res* 2003; **59**(4): 863–873.

23 Chen J, Mandapati R, Berenfeld O, Skanes AC, Gray RA, Jalife J. Dynamics of wavelets and their role in atrial fibrillation in the isolated sheep heart. *Cardiovasc Res* 2000; **48**(2): 220–232.

24 Wijffels MC, Kirchhof CJ, Dorland R, Allessie MA. Atrial fibrillation begets atrial fibrillation. A study in awake chronically instrumented goats. *Circulation* 1995; **92**(7): 1954–1968.

25 Morillo CA, Klein GJ, Jones DL, Guiraudon CM. Chronic rapid atrial pacing. Structural, functional, and electrophysiological characteristics of a new model of sustained atrial fibrillation. *Circulation* 1995; **91**(5): 1588–1595.

26 Li D, Fareh S, Leung TK, Nattel S. Promotion of atrial fibrillation by heart failure in dogs: atrial remodeling of a different sort. *Circulation* 1999; **100**(1): 87–95.

27 Gaspo R, Bosch RF, Talajic M, Nattel S. Functional mechanisms underlying tachycardia-induced sustained atrial fibrillation in a chronic dog model. *Circulation* 1997; **96**(11): 4027–4035.

28 Yue L, Feng J, Gaspo R, Li GR, Wang Z, Nattel S. Ionic remodeling underlying action potential changes in a canine model of atrial fibrillation. *Circ Res* 1997; **81**(4): 512–525.

29 Fareh S, Villemaire C, Nattel S. Importance of refractoriness heterogeneity in the enhanced vulnerability to atrial fibrillation induction caused by tachycardia-induced atrial electrical remodeling. *Circulation* 1998; **98**(20): 2202–2209.

30 Cha TJ, Ehrlich JR, Zhang L, Nattel S. Atrial ionic remodeling induced by atrial tachycardia in the presence of congestive heart failure. *Circulation* 2004; **110**(12): 1520–1526.

31 Li D, Melnyk P, Feng J *et al.* Effects of experimental heart failure on atrial cellular and ionic electrophysiology. *Circulation* 2000; **101**(22): 2631–2638.

32 Dun W, Yagi T, Rosen MR, Boyden PA. Calcium and potassium currents in cells from adult and aged canine right atria. *Cardiovasc Res* 2003; **58**(3): 526–534.

33 Van Wagoner DR, Pond AL, Lamorgese M, Rossie SS, McCarthy PM, Nerbonne JM. Atrial L-type Ca^{2+} currents and human atrial fibrillation. *Circ Res* 1999; **85**(5): 428–436.

34 Bosch RF, Zeng X, Grammer JB, Popovic K, Mewis C, Kuhlkamp V. Ionic mechanisms of electrical remodeling in human atrial fibrillation. *Cardiovasc Res* 1999; **44**(1): 121–131.

35 Skasa M, Jungling E, Picht E, Schondube F, Luckhoff A. L-type calcium currents in atrial myocytes from patients with persistent and non-persistent atrial fibrillation. *Basic Res Cardiol* 2001; **96**(2): 151–159.

36 Brandt MC, Priebe L, Bohle T, Sudkamp M, Beuckelmann DJ. The ultrarapid and the transient outward K(+) current in human atrial fibrillation. Their possible role in postoperative atrial fibrillation. *J Mol Cell Cardiol* 2000; **32**(10): 1885–1896.

37 Dobrev D, Graf E, Wettwer E *et al.* Molecular basis of downregulation of G-protein-coupled inward rectifying K(+) current (I(K,ACh) in chronic human atrial fibrillation: decrease in GIRK4 mRNA correlates with reduced I(K,ACh) and muscarinic receptor-mediated shortening of action potentials. *Circulation* 2001; **104**: 2551–2557.

38 Dobrev D, Wettwer E, Kortner A, Knaut M, Schuler S, Ravens U. Human inward rectifier potassium channels in chronic and postoperative atrial fibrillation. *Cardiovasc Res* 2002; **54**(2): 397–404.

39 Gaspo R, Bosch RF, Bou-Abboud E, Nattel S. Tachycardia-induced changes in Na+ current in a chronic dog model of atrial fibrillation. *Circ Res* 1997; **81**(6): 1045–1052.

40 Yagi T, Pu J, Chandra P *et al.* Density and function of inward currents in right atrial cells from chronically fibrillating canine atria. *Cardiovasc Res* 2002; **54**(2): 405–415.

41 Cha TJ, Ehrlich JR, Zhang L, Chartier D, Leung TK, Nattel S. Atrial tachycardia remodeling of pulmonary vein cardiomyocytes: comparison with left atrium and potential relation to arrhythmogenesis. *Circulation* 2005; **111**(6): 728–735.

42 Shi H, Wang H, Li D, Nattel S, Wang Z. Differential alterations of receptor densities of three muscarinic acetylcholine receptor subtypes and current densities of the corresponding K+ channels in canine atria with atrial fibrillation induced by experimental congestive heart failure. *Cell Physiol Biochem* 2004; **14**(1–2):31–40.

43 Balana B, Dobrev D, Wettwer E, Christ T, Knaut M, Ravens U. Decreased ATP-sensitive K(+) current density during chronic human atrial fibrillation. *J Mol Cell Cardiol* 2003; **35**: 1399–1405.

44 Todd DM, Fynn SP, Walden AP, Hobbs WJ, Arya S, Garratt CJ. Repetitive 4-week periods of atrial electrical remodeling promote stability of atrial fibrillation: time course of a second factor involved in the self-perpetuation of atrial fibrillation. *Circulation* 2004; **109**(11): 1434–1439.

45 Ausma J, Wijffels M, Thone F, Wouters L, Allessie M, Borgers M. Structural changes of atrial myocardium due to sustained atrial fibrillation in the goat. *Circulation* 1997; **96**(9): 3157–3163.

46 Ausma J, van der Velden HM, Lenders MH *et al.* Reverse structural and gap-junctional remodeling after prolonged atrial fibrillation in the goat. *Circulation* 2003; **107**(15): 2051–2058.

47 Shi Y, Ducharme A, Li D, Gaspo R, Nattel S, Tardif JC. Remodeling of atrial dimensions and emptying function in canine models of atrial fibrillation. *Cardiovasc Res* 2001; **52**(2): 217–225.

48 Kanagaratnam P, Peters NS. Conduction, gap junctions, and atrial fibrillation: an eternal triangle? *Heart Rhythms* 2004; **1**(6): 746–749.

49 van der Velden HM, van Kempen MJ, Wijffels MC *et al.* Altered pattern of connexin40 distribution in persistent atrial fibrillation in the goat. *J Cardiovasc Electrophysiol* 1998; **9**(6): 596–607.

50 Elvan A, Huang XD, Pressler ML, Zipes DP. Radiofrequency catheter ablation of the atria eliminates pacing-induced sustained atrial fibrillation and reduces connexin 43 in dogs. *Circulation* 1997; **96**(5): 1675–1685.

51 Thomas SA, Schuessler RB, Berul CI *et al.* Disparate effects of deficient expression of connexin43 on atrial and ventricular conduction: evidence for chamber-specific molecular determinants of conduction. *Circulation* 1998; **97**(7): 686–691.

52 Verheule S, van Batenburg CA, Coenjaerts FE, Kirchhoff S, Willecke K, Jongsma HJ. Cardiac conduction abnormalities in mice lacking the gap junction protein connexin40. *J Cardiovasc Electrophysiol* 1999; **10**(10): 1380–1389.

53 Verheule S, Wilson E, Banthia S *et al.* Direction-dependent conduction abnormalities in a canine model of atrial fibrillation due to chronic atrial dilatation. *Am J Physiol Heart Circ Physiol* 2004; **287**(2): H634–H644.

54 Schoonderwoerd BA, Ausma J, Crijns HJ, Van Veldhuisen DJ, Blaauw EH, Van Gelder IC. Atrial ultrastructural changes during experimental atrial tachycardia depend on high ventricular rate. *J Cardiovasc Electrophysiol* 2004; **15**(10): 1167–1174.

55 Dries DL, Exner DV, Gersh BJ, Domanski MJ, Waclawiw MA, Stevenson LW. Atrial fibrillation is associated with an increased risk for mortality and heart failure progression in patients with asymptomatic and symptomatic left ventricular systolic dysfunction: a retrospective analysis of the SOLVD trials. Studies of left ventricular dysfunction. *J Am Coll Cardiol* 1998; **32**(3): 695–703.

56 Stevenson WG, Stevenson LW, Middlekauff HR *et al.* Improving survival for patients with atrial fibrillation and advanced heart failure. *J Am Coll Cardiol* 1996; **28**(6): 1458–1463.

57 Cha TJ, Ehrlich JR, Zhang L *et al.* Dissociation between ionic remodeling and ability to sustain atrial fibrillation during recovery from experimental congestive heart failure. *Circulation* 2004; **109**(3): 412–418.

58 Shinagawa K, Shi YF, Tardif JC, Leung TK, Nattel S. Dynamic nature of atrial fibrillation substrate during development and reversal of heart failure in dogs. *Circulation* 2002; **105**(22): 2672–2678.

59 Hanna N, Cardin S, Leung TK, Nattel S. Differences in atrial versus ventricular remodeling in dogs with ventricular tachypacing-induced congestive heart failure. *Cardiovasc Res* 2004; **63**(2): 236–244.

60 Li D, Shinagawa K, Pang L *et al.* Effects of angiotensin-converting enzyme inhibition on the development of the atrial fibrillation substrate in dogs with ventricular tachypacing-induced congestive heart failure. *Circulation* 2001; **104**(21): 2608–2614.

61 Shi Y, Li D, Tardif JC, Nattel S. Enalapril effects on atrial remodeling and atrial fibrillation in experimental congestive heart failure. *Cardiovasc Res* 2002; **54**(2): 456–461.

62 Ravelli F, Allessie M. Effects of atrial dilatation on refractory period and vulnerability to atrial fibrillation in the isolated Langendorff-perfused rabbit heart. *Circulation* 1997; **96**(5): 1686–1695.

63 Solti F, Vecsey T, Kekesi V, Juhasz-Nagy A. The effect of atrial dilatation on the genesis of atrial arrhythmias. *Cardiovasc Res* 1989; **23**(10): 882–886.

64 Satoh T, Zipes DP. Unequal atrial stretch in dogs increases dispersion of refractoriness conducive to developing atrial fibrillation. *J Cardiovasc Electrophysiol* 1996; **7**(9): 833–842.

65 Wijffels MC, Kirchhof CJ, Dorland R, Power J, Allessie MA. Electrical remodeling due to atrial fibrillation in

chronically instrumented conscious goats: roles of neu-rohumoral changes, ischemia, atrial stretch, and high rate of electrical activation. *Circulation* 1997; **96**(10): 3710–3720.

66 Eijsbouts SC, Majidi M, van Zandvoort M, Allessie MA. Effects of acute atrial dilation on heterogeneity in conduction in the isolated rabbit heart. *J Cardiovasc Electrophysiol* 2003; **14**(3): 269–278.

67 Boyden PA, Hoffman BF. The effects on atrial elec-trophysiology and structure of surgically induced right atrial enlargement in dogs. *Circ Res* 1981; **49**(6): 1319–1331.

68 Verheule S, Wilson E, Everett Tt, Shanbhag S, Golden C, Olgin J. Alterations in atrial electrophysiology and tissue structure in a canine model of chronic atrial dilatation due to mitral regurgitation. *Circulation* 2003; **107**(20): 2615–2622.

69 Neuberger HR, Schotten U, Verheule S *et al.* Develop-ment of a substrate of atrial fibrillation during chronic atrioventricular block in the goat. *Circulation* 2005; **111**(1): 30–37.

70 Feinberg WM, Blackshear JL, Laupacis A, Kronmal R, Hart RG. Prevalence, age distribution, and gender of pa-tients with atrial fibrillation. Analysis and implications. *Arch Intern Med* 1995; **155**(5): 469–473.

71 Spach MS, Miller WT, III, Dolber PC, Kootsey JM, Som-mer JR, Mosher CE, Jr. The functional role of structural complexities in the propagation of depolarization in the atrium of the dog. Cardiac conduction disturbances due to discontinuities of effective axial resistivity. *Circ Res* 1982; **50**(2): 175–191.

72 Hayashi H, Wang C, Miyauchi Y *et al.* Aging-related in-crease to inducible atrial fibrillation in the rat model. *J Cardiovasc Electrophysiol* 2002; **13**(8): 801–808.

73 Koura T, Hara M, Takeuchi S *et al.* Anisotropic con-duction properties in canine atria analyzed by high-resolution optical mapping: preferential direction of conduction block changes from longitudinal to trans-verse with increasing age. *Circulation* 2002; **105**(17): 2092–2098.

74 Anyukhovsky EP, Sosunov EA, Plotnikov A *et al.* Cellular electrophysiologic properties of old canine atria provide a substrate for arrhythmogenesis. *Cardiovasc Res* 2002; **54**(2): 462–469.

75 Anyukhovsky EP, Sosunov EA, Chandra P *et al.* Age-associated changes in electrophysiologic remodeling: a potential contributor to initiation of atrial fibrillation. *Cardiovasc Res* 2005; **66**(2): 353–363.

76 Jais P, Shah DC, Haissaguerre M, Hocini M, Peng JT, Clementy J. Catheter ablation for atrial fibrillation. *Annu Rev Med* 2000; **51**: 431–441.

77 Jais P, Haissaguerre M, Shah DC *et al.* A focal source of atrial fibrillation treated by discrete radiofrequency ablation. *Circulation* 1997; **95**(3): 572–576.

78 Haissaguerre M, Jais P, Shah DC *et al.* Spontaneous ini-tiation of atrial fibrillation by ectopic beats originating in the pulmonary veins. *N Engl J Med* 1998; **339**(10): 659–666.

79 Wu TJ, Ong JJ, Chang CM *et al.* Pulmonary veins and ligament of Marshall as sources of rapid activations in a canine model of sustained atrial fibrillation. *Circulation* 2001; **103**(8): 1157–1163.

80 Chen YJ, Chen SA, Chen YC *et al.* Effects of rapid atrial pacing on the arrhythmogenic activity of single car-diomyocytes from pulmonary veins: implication in ini-tiation of atrial fibrillation. *Circulation* 2001; **104**(23): 2849–2854.

81 Wang TM, Chiang CE, Sheu JR, Tsou CH, Chang HM, Luk HN. Homogenous distribution of fast response ac-tion potentials in canine pulmonary vein sleeves: a con-tradictory report. *Int J Cardiol* 2003; **89**(2–3): 187–195.

82 Perez-Lugones A, McMahon JT, Ratliff NB *et al.* Evidence of specialized conduction cells in human pulmonary veins of patients with atrial fibrillation. *J Cardiovasc Elec-trophysiol* 2003; **14**(8): 803–809.

83 Verheule S, Wilson EE, Arora R, Engle SK, Scott LR, Olgin JE. Tissue structure and connexin expression of canine pulmonary veins. *Cardiovasc Res* 2002; **55**(4): 727–738.

84 Hocini M, Ho SY, Kawara T *et al.* Electrical conduc-tion in canine pulmonary veins: electrophysiological and anatomic correlation. *Circulation* 2002; **105**(20): 2442–2448.

85 Arora R, Verheule S, Scott L *et al.* Arrhythmogenic sub-strate of the pulmonary veins assessed by high-resolution optical mapping. *Circulation* 2003; **107**(13): 1816–1821.

86 Sueda T, Imai K, Ishii O, Orihashi K, Watari M, Okada K. Efficacy of pulmonary vein isolation for the elimination of chronic atrial fibrillation in cardiac valvular surgery. *Ann Thorac Surg* 2001; **71**(4): 1189–1193.

87 Sahadevan J, Ryu K, Peltz L *et al.* Epicardial mapping of chronic atrial fibrillation in patients: preliminary obser-vations. *Circulation* 2004; **110**(21): 3293–3299.

88 Sanders P, Berenfeld O, Hocini M *et al.* Spectral analysis identifies sites of high-frequency activity maintaining atrial fibrillation in humans. *Circulation* 2005; **112**(6): 789–797.

89 Kottkamp H, Tanner H, Kobza R *et al.* Time courses and quantitative analysis of atrial fibrillation episode number and duration after circular plus linear left atrial lesions: trigger elimination or substrate modification: early or delayed cure? *J Am Coll Cardiol* 2004; **44**(4): 869–877.

90 Benussi S, Pappone C, Nascimbene S *et al.* A simple way to treat chronic atrial fibrillation during mitral valve surgery: the epicardial radiofrequency approach. *Eur J Cardiothorac Surg* 2000; **17**(5): 524–529.

91 Todd DM, Skanes AC, Guiraudon G *et al.* Role of the pos-terior left atrium and pulmonary veins in human lone

atrial fibrillation: electrophysiological and pathological data from patients undergoing atrial fibrillation surgery. *Circulation* 2003; **108**(25): 3108–3114.

92 Cappato R, Negroni S, Pecora D *et al.* Prospective assessment of late conduction recurrence across radiofrequency lesions producing electrical disconnection at the pulmonary vein ostium in patients with atrial fibrillation. *Circulation* 2003; **108**(13): 1599–1604.

93 Pappone C, Oreto G, Rosanio S *et al.* Atrial electroanatomic remodeling after circumferential radiofrequency pulmonary vein ablation: efficacy of an anatomic approach in a large cohort of patients with atrial fibrillation. *Circulation* 2001; **104**(21): 2539–2544.

94 Ho SY, Sanchez-Quintana D, Cabrera JA, Anderson RH. Anatomy of the left atrium: implications for radiofrequency ablation of atrial fibrillation. *J Cardiovasc Electrophysiol* 1999; **10**(11): 1525–1533.

95 Attuel P, Childers R, Cauchemez B, Poveda J, Mugica J, Coumel P. Failure in the rate adaptation of the atrial refractory period: its relationship to vulnerability. *Int J Cardiol* 1982; **2**(2): 179–197.

96 Boutjdir M, Le Heuzey JY, Lavergne T *et al.* Inhomogeneity of cellular refractoriness in human atrium: factor of arrhythmia? *Pacing Clin Electrophysiol* 1986; **9**(6, pt 2): 1095–1100.

97 Daoud EG, Bogun F, Goyal R *et al.* Effect of atrial fibrillation on atrial refractoriness in humans. *Circulation* 1996; **94**(7): 1600–1606.

98 Franz MR, Karasik PL, Li C, Moubarak J, Chavez M. Electrical remodeling of the human atrium: similar effects in patients with chronic atrial fibrillation and atrial flutter. *J Am Coll Cardiol* 1997; **30**(7): 1785–1792.

99 Yu WC, Lee SH, Tai CT *et al.* Reversal of atrial electrical remodeling following cardioversion of long-standing atrial fibrillation in man. *Cardiovasc Res* 1999; **42**(2): 470–476.

100 Michelucci A, Padeletti L, Fradella GA. Atrial refractoriness and spontaneous or induced atrial fibrillation. *Acta Cardiol* 1982; **37**(5): 333–344.

101 Misier AR, Opthof T, van Hemel NM *et al.* Increased dispersion of "refractoriness" in patients with idiopathic paroxysmal atrial fibrillation. *J Am Coll Cardiol* 1992; **19**(7): 1531–1535.

102 Gaita F, Calo L, Riccardi R *et al.* Different patterns of atrial activation in idiopathic atrial fibrillation: simultaneous multisite atrial mapping in patients with paroxysmal and chronic atrial fibrillation. *J Am Coll Cardiol* 2001; **37**(2): 534–541.

103 Firouzi M, Ramanna H, Kok B *et al.* Association of human connexin40 gene polymorphisms with atrial vulnerability as a risk factor for idiopathic atrial fibrillation. *Circ Res* 2004; **95**(4): e29–e33.

104 Luck JC, Engel TR. Dispersion of atrial refractoriness in patients with sinus node dysfunction. *Circulation* 1979; **60**(2): 404–412.

105 Simpson RJ, Jr, Amara I, Foster JR, Woelfel A, Gettes LS. Thresholds, refractory periods, and conduction times of the normal and diseased human atrium. *Am Heart J* 1988; **116**(4): 1080–1090.

106 Brundel BJ, Van Gelder IC, Henning RH *et al.* Ion channel remodeling is related to intraoperative atrial effective refractory periods in patients with paroxysmal and persistent atrial fibrillation. *Circulation* 2001; **103**(5): 684–690.

107 Antman EM, Beamer AD, Cantillon C, McGowan N, Goldman L, Friedman PL. Long-term oral propafenone therapy for suppression of refractory symptomatic atrial fibrillation and atrial flutter. *J Am Coll Cardiol* 1988; **12**(4): 1005–1011.

108 Crijns HJ, van Wijk LM, van Gilst WH, Kingma JH, van Gelder IC, Lie KI. Acute conversion of atrial fibrillation to sinus rhythm: clinical efficacy of flecainide acetate. Comparison of two regimens. *Eur Heart J* 1988; **9**(6): 634–638.

109 Van Gelder IC, Crijns HJ, Van Gilst WH, Verwer R, Lie KI. Prediction of uneventful cardioversion and maintenance of sinus rhythm from direct-current electrical cardioversion of chronic atrial fibrillation and flutter. *Am J Cardiol* 1991; **68**(1): 41–46.

110 Reimold SC, Cantillon CO, Friedman PL, Antman EM. Propafenone versus sotalol for suppression of recurrent symptomatic atrial fibrillation. *Am J Cardiol* 1993; **71**(7): 558–563.

111 Olsson SB, Cotoi S, Varnauskas E. Monophasic action potential and sinus rhythm stability after conversion of atrial fibrillation. *Acta Med Scand* 1971; **190**(5): 381–387.

112 Cotoi S, Gavrilescu S, Pop T, Vicas E. The prognostic value of right astrium monophasic action potential after conversion of atrial fibrillation. *Eur J Clin Invest* 1972; **2**(6): 472–474.

113 Schotten U, Duytschaever M, Ausma J, Eijsbouts S, Neuberger HR, Allessie M. Electrical and contractile remodeling during the first days of atrial fibrillation go hand in hand. *Circulation* 2003; **107**(10): 1433–1439.

114 Raitt MH, Kusumoto W, Giraud G, McAnulty JH. Reversal of electrical remodeling after cardioversion of persistent atrial fibrillation. *J Cardiovasc Electrophysiol* 2004; **15**(5): 507–512.

115 Manios EG, Kanoupakis EM, Chlouverakis GI, Kaleboubas MD, Mavrakis HE, Vardas PE. Changes in atrial electrical properties following cardioversion of chronic atrial fibrillation: relation with recurrence. *Cardiovasc Res* 2000; **47**(2): 244–253.

116 Tieleman RG, Van Gelder IC, Crijns HJ *et al.* Early recurrences of atrial fibrillation after electrical cardioversion:

a result of fibrillation-induced electrical remodeling of the atria? *J Am Coll Cardiol* 1998; **31**(1): 167–173.

117 Ueng KC, Tsai TP, Yu WC *et al.* Use of enalapril to facilitate sinus rhythm maintenance after external cardioversion of long-standing persistent atrial fibrillation. Results of a prospective and controlled study. *Eur Heart J* 2003; **24**(23): 2090–2098.

118 Frustaci A, Caldarulo M, Buffon A, Bellocci F, Fenici R, Melina D. Cardiac biopsy in patients with "primary" atrial fibrillation. Histologic evidence of occult myocardial diseases. *Chest* 1991; **100**(2): 303–306.

119 Frustaci A, Chimenti C, Bellocci F, Morgante E, Russo MA, Maseri A. Histological substrate of atrial biopsies in patients with lone atrial fibrillation. *Circulation* 1997; **96**(4): 1180–1184.

120 Kumagai K, Nakashima H, Urata H, Gondo N, Arakawa K, Saku K. Effects of angiotensin II type 1 receptor antagonist on electrical and structural remodeling in atrial fibrillation. *J Am Coll Cardiol* 2003; **41**(12): 2197–2204.

121 L'Allier PL, Ducharme A, Keller PF, Yu H, Guertin MC, Tardif JC. Angiotensin-converting enzyme inhibition in hypertensive patients is associated with a reduction in the occurrence of atrial fibrillation. *J Am Coll Cardiol* 2004; **44**(1): 159–164.

122 Bourassa MG. Angiotensin II inhibition and prevention of atrial fibrillation and stroke. *J Am Coll Cardiol* 2005; **45**(5): 720–721.

123 Healey JS, Baranchuk A, Crystal E *et al.* Prevention of atrial fibrillation with angiotensin-converting enzyme inhibitors and angiotensin receptor blockers: a meta-analysis. *J Am Coll Cardiol* 2005; **45**(11): 1832–1839.

124 Wachtell K, Lehto M, Gerdts E *et al.* Angiotensin II receptor blockade reduces new-onset atrial fibrillation and subsequent stroke compared to atenolol: the Losartan Intervention for End Point reduction in hypertension (LIFE) study. *J Am Coll Cardiol* 2005; **45**(5): 712–719.

125 Spach MS, Dolber PC. Relating extracellular potentials and their derivatives to anisotropic propagation at a microscopic level in human cardiac muscle. Evidence for electrical uncoupling of side-to-side fiber connections with increasing age. *Circ Res* 1986; **58**(3): 356–371.

126 Lie JT, Falk RH. Pathology of atrial fibrillation: insights from autopsy studies. In: Falk RH ed. *Atrial Fibrillation: Mechanisms and Management.* Raven Press, New York, 1992: 1–39.

127 Kostin S, Klein G, Szalay Z, Hein S, Bauer EP, Schaper J. Structural correlate of atrial fibrillation in human patients. *Cardiovasc Res* 2002; **54**(2): 361–379.

128 Becker AE. How structurally normal are human atria in patients with atrial fibrillation? *Heart Rhythms* 2004; **1**(5): 627–631.

129 Aime-Sempe C, Folliguet T, Rucker-Martin C *et al.* Myocardial cell death in fibrillating and dilated human right atria. *J Am Coll Cardiol* 1999; **34**(5): 1577–1586.

130 Thijssen VL, Ausma J, Borgers M. Structural remodelling during chronic atrial fibrillation: act of programmed cell survival. *Cardiovasc Res* 2001; **52**(1): 14–24.

131 Polontchouk L, Haefliger JA, Ebelt B *et al.* Effects of chronic atrial fibrillation on gap junction distribution in human and rat atria. *J Am Coll Cardiol* 2001; **38**(3): 883–891.

132 Nao T, Ohkusa T, Hisamatsu Y *et al.* Comparison of expression of connexin in right atrial myocardium in patients with chronic atrial fibrillation versus those in sinus rhythm. *Am J Cardiol* 2003; **91**(6): 678–683.

133 Kanagaratnam P, Cherian A, Stanbridge RD, Glenville B, Severs NJ, Peters NS. Relationship between connexins and atrial activation during human atrial fibrillation. *J Cardiovasc Electrophysiol* 2004; **15**(2): 206–216.

134 Dupont E, Ko Y, Rothery S *et al.* The gap-junctional protein connexin40 is elevated in patients susceptible to postoperative atrial fibrillation. *Circulation* 2001; **103**(6): 842–849.

135 Konings KT, Kirchhof CJ, Smeets JR, Wellens HJ, Penn OC, Allessie MA. High-density mapping of electrically induced atrial fibrillation in humans. *Circulation* 1994; **89**(4): 1665–1680.

136 Konings KT, Smeets JL, Penn OC, Wellens HJ, Allessie MA. Configuration of unipolar atrial electrograms during electrically induced atrial fibrillation in humans. *Circulation* 1997; **95**(5): 1231–1241.

137 Nademanee K, McKenzie J, Kosar E *et al.* A new approach for catheter ablation of atrial fibrillation: mapping of the electrophysiologic substrate. *J Am Coll Cardiol* 2004; **43**(11): 2044–2053.

138 Schuessler RB, Kawamoto T, Hand DE *et al.* Simultaneous epicardial and endocardial activation sequence mapping in the isolated canine right atrium. *Circulation* 1993; **88**(1): 250–263.

139 Berenfeld O, Zaitsev AV, Mironov SF, Pertsov AM, Jalife J. Frequency-dependent breakdown of wave propagation into fibrillatory conduction across the pectinate muscle network in the isolated sheep right atrium. *Circ Res* 2002; **90**(11): 1173–1180.

140 Houben RP, de Groot NM, Smeets JL, Becker AE, Lindemans FW, Allessie MA. S-wave predominance of epicardial electrograms during atrial fibrillation in humans: indirect evidence for a role of the thin subepicardial layer. *Heart Rhythms* 2004; **1**(6): 639–647.

6 CHAPTER 6

Pulmonary and thoracic vein sources: the focal theory of atrial fibrillation

Prashanthan Sanders, Mélèze Hocini, Pierre Jaïs, Yoshihide Takahashi, Thomas Rostock, Fréderic Sacher, Anders Jonsson, Martin Rotter, Li-Fern Hsu, & Michel Haïssaguerre

Introduction

The most prevalent theory of atrial fibrillation (AF) has been the "multiple wavelet" hypothesis. Hypothesized by Gordon Moe on the basis of computer simulations, this postulate suggested that a grossly irregular wavefront becomes fractionated as it divides around islets or strands of refractory tissue, each of the daughter wavelets could then be considered independent offspring [1]. In this model, fully developed AF would be a state in which many such randomly wandering wavelets coexist. Allessie *et al.* subsequently demonstrated this hypothesis by mapping the activation wavefronts during pacing induced AF in isolated blood perfused canine atria in which acetylcholine was added to the perfusate [2]. Multiple wavelets were seen to extinguish, divide, and combine with neighboring wavelets. These investigators observed considerable variation in the size of the wave and the direction of activation. Based on their observations they estimated that the maintenance of AF in the canine atrium required a critical number of four to six coexisting wavelets. Subsequent intraoperative mapping studies have also demonstrated this phenomenon

in humans [3]. The existence and importance of multiple wavelets during AF was further confirmed by the clinical observation that AF could be cured in patients by the placement of multiple surgical lesions (maze) to compartmentalize the atria into regions, which were presumably unable to sustain the multiple wavelets [4].

However, as early as the beginning of the twentieth century, Sir Thomas Lewis [5] advanced the concept that a localized source of rapid activity could maintain the atria in fibrillation. More recently, the important interaction between the triggers, perpetuators, and substrate in the initiation and maintenance of AF has been recognized [6]. This chapter will review the evidence for focal sources from the pulmonary and thoracic veins in the initiation and maintenance of AF.

Atrial ectopy in the initiation of AF

It has long been recognized that AF could arise from degeneration of other supraventricular tachycardias such as accessory pathways or atrial flutter [7]. However, the importance of atrial ectopy or triggers for the conversion to AF has only been recently recognized [8, 9]. Furthermore, it is now appreciated that spontaneous episodes of AF are initiated by atrial ectopy [10, 11]. Atrial ectopy from a number of sites have now been found to be capable of

Manual of Surgical Treatment of Atrial Fibrillation.
Edited by Hauw T. Sie *et al.* © 2008 Blackwell Publishing, ISBN: 978-1-4051-4032-4.

initiating AF in a variety of clinical scenarios. These have included the pulmonary veins [11–13], the vein/ligament of Marshall [14], the coronary sinus [10, 11, 15], the crista terminalis [11, 15], the superior vena cava [10, 16, 17], and the inferior vena cava [18]. However, the vast majority of atrial ectopy that initiate AF originates in the pulmonary veins [12].

Pulmonary vein as a source of triggers initiating AF

In a consecutive series of patients with highly symptomatic paroxysmal AF, selected on the basis of frequent atrial ectopy, we observed that 94% of ectopy at the time of electrophysiological study were of pulmonary vein origin [12]. Spontaneous activity arising from these structures were observed to manifest in a spectrum of atrial arrhythmias; single discharges may manifest as isolated atrial ectopy, repetitive discharge with a long cycle length may manifest as slow atrial rhythms, and shorter cycle length discharges may manifest as an atrial tachycardia [12]. Rapid sustained focal discharges (sometimes for hours, days, or even longer) may drive sustained AF (focal AF—implicating the focus in both the trigger and substrate for AF) [11] or, more commonly, ectopy or bursts initiate AF (focally initiated AF) in patients with the appropriate substrate [12]. Mapping of these ectopic beats identified the earliest local activity to a point 2–4 cm within the main pulmonary vein or one of its branches, with depolarization marked by a spike (pulmonary vein potential) preceding the onset of atrial activation by 35–45 ms. Our initial experience in a select group, experiencing ≥1 episode of AF per 48 hours and with 4377 ± 3629 atrial ectopics per 24 hours found that, focal ablation at the site of earliest activity eliminated AF in 62% of patients at a follow-up of 8 ± 6 months. However, as this technique was applied to a greater number of patients, two major limitations became identified: the infrequent or even the lack of spontaneous ectopy during the procedure in many patients, and/or the occurrence of new foci at the ostial side after apparently successful ablation of venous foci.

Several techniques evolved in an attempt to overcome this, including pattern recognition of the right atrial endocardial activation sequence during ectopy, algorithms to predict the arrhythmogenic pulmonary vein based on P wave ectopic morphology with or without QRST subtraction to reveal the morphology of the "P on T" ectopics, utilization of multielectrode mapping catheters to enhance the density of mapping during ectopy, and the mapping of postcardioversion immediate recurrences of AF [19]. However, it was soon realized that patients prone to AF may also have multiple veins and multiple foci within any given vein that were capable of producing spontaneous triggers [20], necessitating further procedures [21, 22]. These ectopics have been observed to interact with the atrial substrate by conduction utilizing discrete or wide fascicles connecting the pulmonary veins and the left atrium. As such, the focal approach has been progressively expanded with the evolution of ostial ablation aimed at electrical isolation of all pulmonary veins. Interestingly, even after electrical isolation, these structures have been observed to have spontaneous dissociated slow rhythms (in up to 33%; Figure 6.1) and can sustain spontaneous or induced tachycardia within the pulmonary vein, further highlighting their arrhythmogenic potential (Figure 6.2) [23–25].

Localized sources of activity maintaining AF

The notion that a localized source of activity could maintain AF was put forth by early investigators such as Lewis [5] and Scherf [26]. More recently, others have provided corroborative evidence to suggest a greater role of such sources in the maintenance of AF. Schuessler *et al.* demonstrated in isolated canine right atrial preparations with increasing concentrations of acetylcholine, activation patterns characterized by multiple reentrant circuits converted to a single, relatively stable, high-frequency reentrant circuit that resulted in fibrillatory conduction [27]. In a sterile pericarditis model Kumagai *et al.* identified unstable reentrant circuits of very short cycle length at the septum maintaining AF and performed focal ablation to terminate AF [28, 29]. Recent studies have not only demonstrated that the dominant frequencies were found in the left atrium [30–32] but also that there was a significant left to right atrial gradient in fibrillatory

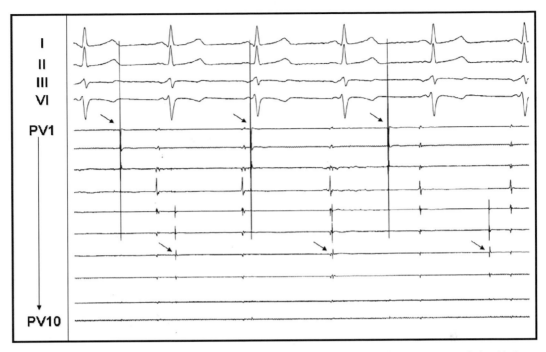

Figure 6.1 Spontaneous, dissociated pulmonary vein activity after electrical isolation of the pulmonary vein by ablation. The arrows indicate the two dissociated fascicles.

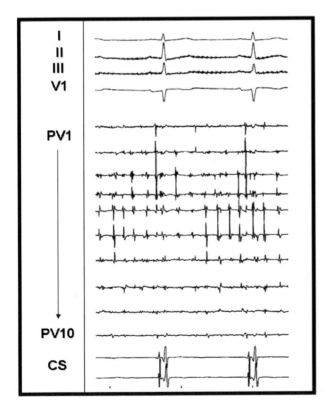

Figure 6.2 Persistent pulmonary vein tachycardia after electrical isolation of the pulmonary vein by ablation. In this patient, AF terminated during ablation of the pulmonary vein and in this example the vein persists in tachycardia with the atria in sinus rhythm; implicating this pulmonary vein activity in the maintenance of AF in this patient.

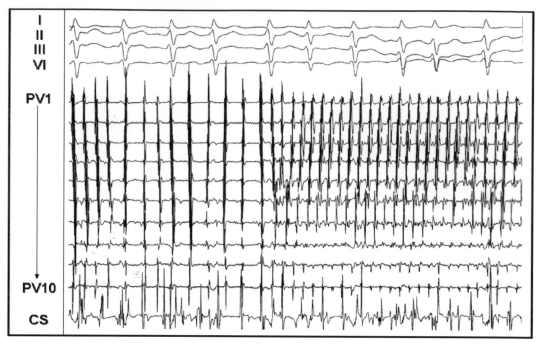

Figure 6.3 Paroxysmal short cycle length activity within the pulmonary vein during ongoing AF has been suggested to be evidence of a continual refueling of the fibrillatory process by the pulmonary veins.

intervals [32–35]. Based on these findings, Mansour *et al.* postulated that these sources of high-frequency waves within the left atrium might act as drivers or a dominant rotor that maintains AF [33]. Support for this theory is provided in a canine rapid atrial pacing model of AF in which cryoablation, targeting areas of the shortest cycle length in the posterior left atrium, resulted in termination of arrhythmia [36].

Pulmonary veins in the maintenance of AF

In addition to acting as a source of triggers, the pulmonary veins have also been implicated in the maintenance of AF in some patients. Jais *et al.* reported a small series of patients with irregular rapid focal discharges, persisting sometimes for hours, days, or even longer, driving sustained AF; this represents the true "focally driven AF" [11]. These patients were cured of their arrhythmia by focal application of radiofrequency energy. Thus, in these cases, foci in the pulmonary veins, left atrium, or the coro-

nary sinus formed not only the trigger but also the substrate maintaining AF.

More recently, investigators have observed paroxysmal short cycle length activity within the pulmonary veins during AF and suggested that this may represent a continual fuelling of the fibrillatory process from the pulmonary veins (Figure 6.3) [37–39]. Such paroxysmal bursts of activity demonstrate a distal-to-proximal activation sequence, implicating the distal pulmonary vein in their origin [40]. Others have demonstrated a gradient of high-frequency activity emanating from the pulmonary veins during paroxysmal AF and suggested that activity from these structures may maintain AF [34, 35]. We have provided further evidence to demonstrate the direct participation of pulmonary vein activity in the maintenance of paroxysmal AF [41]. Pulmonary vein isolation performed during AF in patients with paroxysmal AF produced progressive slowing of the AF process (prolongation of the AF cycle length; Figure 6.4), varying in extent from vein-to-vein and between individuals, culminating in the termination of AF in 75% of patients [41]. A subsequent study demonstrated that ablation

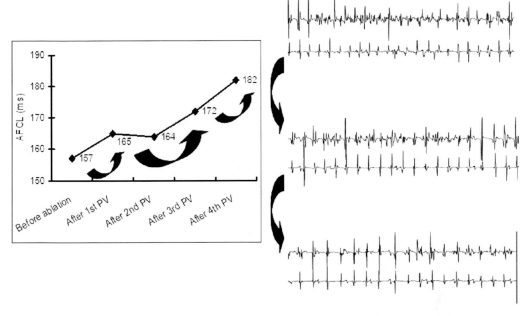

Figure 6.4 Effect of pulmonary vein electrical isolation on the global fibrillatory process. In this case the AF cycle length has been determined in the coronary sinus and demonstrates that with each vein isolated there is a gradual slow-ing of fibrillation (or prolongation of the AF cycle length). The right panels show representative examples of the coronary sinus electrograms at each stage of ablation.

performed of a pulmonary vein harboring a site of dominant frequency activity resulted in slowing or termination of paroxysmal AF whereas ablation at sites without dominant frequency activity had no impact on the fibrillatory process (Figure 6.5) [35]. Remarkably, pulmonary vein isolation in these patients rendered AF noninducible in 57%, providing evidence that the pulmonary veins or the pulmonary vein—left atrial junction form the perpetuators and substrate of AF in this significant proportion of patients with paroxysmal AF [41]. Indeed, activity within the pulmonary veins has been observed to persist even after isolation of these structures from the atria [23–25]. In concert, these observations have led us to posit a much greater role of the pulmonary veins in the maintenance of AF, which we have termed "the venous wave hypothesis" (Figure 6.6) [42].

Mechanisms of pulmonary vein arrhythmogenicity

Why the pulmonary veins are a source of arrhythmogenic triggers in patients with AF is a subject of intense investigation. The atrial myocardium extends a variable distance into each pulmonary vein [43]. Anatomical studies have identified that the atrial muscle fibers at the atriovenous junction are variably arranged (sphincter-like) and that the peripheral zones of these myocardial sleeves are variably associated with connective tissue, providing regions of anisotropy and therefore the substrate for micro-reentry [43–45]. Hocini et al. using canine pulmonary veins found significant conduction delay within the pulmonary veins, which was correlated with myocardial fiber orientation producing nonuniform anisotropy and fractionated electrograms [46]. Hamabe et al. correlated intra-pulmonary vein conduction delay and block with the complex muscle fiber orientation and at the pulmonary vein—left atrial junction, with areas of discrete connective tissue and altered muscle fiber orientation [47]. Indeed, patients with AF demonstrated significantly greater deposition of fibrous tissue and altered myocardial fiber orientation, implicating these changes in the arrhythmogenicity of the pulmonary veins [48]. These latter conditions may be further exacerbated by conditions

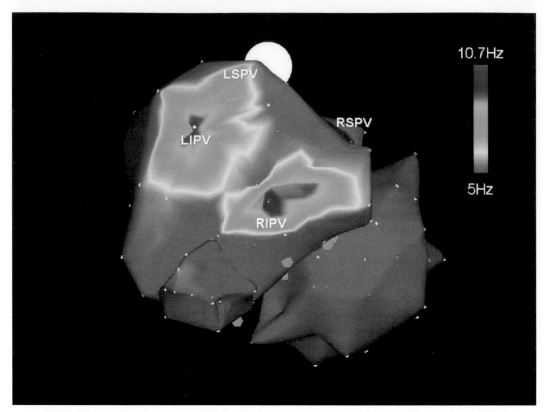

Figure 6.5 Dominant frequency three-dimensional map of the atria and coronary sinus in a patient with paroxysmal AF. This map was created using the electroanatomic mapping system and by performing spectral analysis of the local electrograms. The posterior-anterior view is presented. Areas of high frequency (rapid rates) are dark and low-frequency activity (slow rates) are lighter . In this patient the three dominant frequency sites were found to be within the pulmonary veins. Ablation of the veins resulted in not only termination of AF but also the atria could no longer sustain AF.

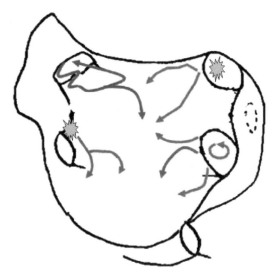

Figure 6.6 Venous wave hypothesis for paroxysmal AF. This postulate recognizes the importance of the pulmonary veins and the venoatrial junction in the maintenance of AF.

predisposed to the development of AF [49]. Arora et al. demonstrated that these changes were capable of sustaining reentry within the pulmonary vein [50].

Clinical studies have suggested that larger or dilated pulmonary veins may be a marker of arrhythmogenicity at the time of ablation [51]. This is further corroborated by evidence suggesting that patients with AF have significantly larger pulmonary vein diameters compared to those without AF [52, 53]. These findings have been extended by the demonstration of structural changes within the pulmonary veins of patients with AF, with greater degrees of discontinuous myocardium, hypertrophic myocytes, and fibrosis [48], suggesting that dilatation may in fact be a marker of structural changes that are capable of promoting pulmonary vein arrhythmogenesis.

The pulmonary veins and the venoatrial region have been identified to have distinctive electrophysiological properties. Chen et al. demonstrated that the distal pulmonary vein had significantly shorter effective refractory periods (ERP) than the adjacent left atrium [13]. Jais et al. demonstrated significantly shorter ERP of the pulmonary vein in patients with paroxysmal AF (in some as short as 80 ms) compared with patients without a history of AF [54]. Interestingly, while the pulmonary vein ERP was shorter, the ERP of the pulmonary vein—atrial junction and the left atrium were without significant differences. A comparison of patients with paroxysmal AF treated with amiodarone to those without an antiarrhythmic treatment emphasized these distinctive electrophysiological properties of the pulmonary veins, with amiodarone producing a heterogeneous alteration of pulmonary vein electrophysiology with decreased ERPs of the superior but not inferior veins [55]. In addition, these patients had more frequent and greater degree of decremental conduction to the left atrium with a tendency for pulmonary vein extrastimuli to initiate AF [54]. In a clinical study in patients with known AF, Kumagai et al. have extended these observations by demonstrating preferential conduction, unidirectional conduction block, and reentry within the pulmonary veins [56]. These clinical studies have implicated reentry as the predominant mechanism of pulmonary vein arrhythmogenesis. Takahashi et al. have also demonstrated features to suggest

reentry within the pulmonary vein after electrical isolation of these structures [24].

Evidence also exists that suggests that the pulmonary veins may have tissue that is able to sustain automaticity. Blom et al. studying the human embryo using monoclonal antibodies to stain conducting tissue, demonstrated the presence of cardiac conduction tissue within the pulmonary veins during embryonic development [57]. However, although node-like cells have been found in the pulmonary veins of rats [58], detailed histology of the atrial myocardial sleeves of the pulmonary veins in human hearts has thus far failed to reveal any node-like structures [45]. Cheung found spontaneous activity from the pulmonary vein in the guinea pig [59], and Chen et al. demonstrated spontaneous electrical activity in canine pulmonary vein musculature and observed a higher incidence of early and delayed after-depolarization and automatic high-frequency irregular rhythms after several weeks of rapid atrial pacing [60, 61]. However, while similar observations have been made in experimental models following rapid atrial pacing [62–64] and congestive heart failure [49], they have not been consistently observed in normal pulmonary vein musculature [46, 63].

Identifying patients in whom the pulmonary veins maintain AF

An accumulating body of evidence has demonstrated the value of ablation targeting the pulmonary veins for the cure of AF. Thus, ablation of these structures forms the central theme in all strategies currently utilized for AF ablation. While many patients with paroxysmal AF can be cured by pulmonary vein ablation alone, some patients with paroxysmal AF and most patients with persistent or permanent AF require additional substrate modification indicating that, in these latter patients, the pulmonary veins are not the only structures with a role in the maintenance of AF [65–68]. However, substrate modification in the form of left atrial lines is technically challenging, associated with increased risk, and can be proarrhythmic in the setting of incomplete lesions [69–71]. Thus, it is important to identify patients who have a significant benefit from pulmonary vein ablation alone in order that a rationalized approach targeting the individual rather than a "one size fits all" approach being applied to substrate modification in paroxysmal AF.

The ideal modality to identify these patients and individualize our approach is still evolving. Potentially, this could be based on the cycle length of activation, change of cycle length with ablation, inducibility of AF, or on clinical outcome [41]. To identify patients who will benefit from pulmonary vein isolation alone, we have been evaluating the role of the inducibility of AF. We utilize a standardized protocol of AF induction consisting of burst atrial pacing at maximum output (20 mA) for 5–10 seconds commencing at a cycle length of approximately 250 ms and decreasing to refractoriness. This is performed three times from ≥ 2 sites. Sustained AF, thought to indicate the presence of potential atrial substrate capable of maintaining AF, is defined as AF lasting ≥ 10 minutes. Using this approach several baseline characteristics may be identified to predict the likelihood that a given patient's AF is maintained by the pulmonary veins (that is, of the patient being cured by pulmonary vein ablation alone). In 181 consecutive patients with paroxysmal AF undergoing ablation at our institution the following factors were identified by multivariate analysis as being associated with noninducibility of sustained AF after pulmonary vein isolation: short episodes (<24 h) of paroxysmal AF, absence of left ventricular hypertrophy (or structural heart disease), and normal left atrial size [72]. In these patients with paroxysmal AF, pulmonary vein activity is responsible for triggering and maintaining AF [25].

Coronary sinus in the initiation and the maintenance of AF

In a recent series of patients, we have observed evidence to support a role for localized sources of activity in the maintenance of persistent or permanent AF [67, 68]. Of these 60 patients ablation was performed utilizing all described strategies focusing on pulmonary vein ablation, linear ablation, and electrogram-guided atrial substrate modification. Using this strategy AF was terminated in 87% of patients either directly in sinus rhythm in 7 or following ablation of 1–6 intermediate atrial tachycardia in 45 patients. Conversion of AF was preceded by prolongation of AFCL by

39 ± 9 ms. Interestingly, the sites identified as resulting in the greatest effect on the fibrillatory process were the anterior left atrium (at the base of the appendage), coronary sinus, and the pulmonary veins. Indeed each of these regions was sites that are annexed to the atria, having complex atrial muscular architecture.

The region of the coronary sinus itself has been well characterized. Anatomical studies have demonstrated that the right atrial myocardium surrounds and extends into the coronary sinus for a variable distance from its ostium and is connected distally to the left atrial myocardium [73]. This musculature is electrically connected to the right and left atria in canine hearts and forms the inferior interatrial connection [74]. Clinical studies have also demonstrated that the inferior interatrial connections are in the region of the coronary sinus ostium [75], and these have been implicated in the mechanism of atrial arrhythmia [76, 77]. We have observed both focal ectopy from this structure initiating AF and also persistent activity driving AF [78, 79]. Oral *et al.* have observed intermittent bursts of activity within the coronary sinus during AF [80]. However, disconnection of the coronary sinus, by ablation of the numerous muscular connections between this structure and the left atrium, requires ablation along the inferior left atrium and also from within the coronary sinus. In our laboratory, disconnection of the coronary sinus is commenced along the endocardial aspect and completed from within the vessel as required. The catheter was dragged along the endocardial inferior left atrium by looping the catheter to be positioned parallel to the coronary sinus catheter. After achieving this loop, it allowed gradual withdrawal of the catheter starting from the septal area anterior to the right veins to the inferior left atrium along the posterior mitral annulus to the lateral left atrium. Ablation within the coronary sinus is started at the most distal position (4 o'clock in left anterior oblique position) and pursued to the ostium by targeting local sharp potentials [67, 68]. Both the ablation endocardially and from within the coronary sinus has been observed to have an effect on the fibrillatory process. In addition, often permanent AF converts to an atrial tachycardia which was also localized to this region or the coronary sinus ostium (Figure 6.7). Interestingly, these tachycardias are frequently observed

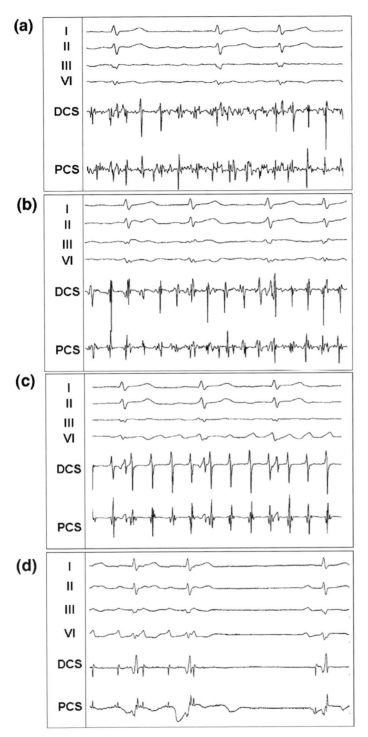

Figure 6.7 Effect on the AF process of inferior left atrial and coronary sinus ablation. Panels (a) to (c) demonstrate the effect of endocardial ablation along the endocardial aspect of the posterior mitral annulus. Note the progressive slowing, organization, and then conversion of AF to an atrial tachycardia. The final panel (d) demonstrates ablation from within the coronary sinus itself, which terminates the atrial tachycardia to sinus rhythm.

to have an unexpected positive P-wave morphology in the inferior leads due to the altered conduction created by ablation.

Other thoracic veins have also been implicated in the initiation and maintenance of AF. These have involved the vein of Marshall [14], and the superior vena cava [17, 81] and also the inferior vena cava [18].

Conclusion

The pulmonary veins are a dominant source of triggers initiating AF in a number of clinical situations. In addition, these structures have a role in perpetuation of arrhythmia. Preliminary evidence suggests that such localized activity from structures including the pulmonary veins, coronary sinus, and the left atrial appendage also have a documented role in persistent and permanent AF. The clustering of these sites to structures appended to the atria suggests that the mechanisms by which these regions promote the maintenance of AF is partly related to the complex muscular architecture.

Acknowledgments

Dr Sanders is the recipient of the Neil Hamilton Fairley Fellowship funded by the National Health and Medical Research Council of Australia and the Ralph Reader Fellowship funded by the National Heart Foundation of Australia. Dr Rostock is supported by the German Cardiac Society. Dr Rotter is supported by the Swiss National Foundation for Scientific Research, Bern, Switzerland. Dr Jonsson is supported by the Swedish Cardiac Society.

References

1 Moe GK. On the multiple wavelet hypothesis of atrial fibrillation. *Arch Int Pharmacodyn Ther* 1962; **140**: 183–188.

2 Allessie MA, Lammers WJEP, Bonke FIM, Hollen J. Experimental evaluation of Moe's multiple wavelet hypothesis of atrial fibrillation. In: Zipes DP & Jalife J, eds. *Cardiac Arrhythmias.* Grune & Stratton, Inc, New York, 1985: 265–275.

3 Konings KT, Kirchhof CJ, Smeets JR *et al.* High-density mapping of electrically induced atrial fibrillation in humans. *Circulation* 1994; **89**: 1665–1680.

4 Cox JL, Schuessler RB, Boineau JP. The development of the maze procedure for the treatment of atrial fibrillation. *Semin Thorac Cardiovasc Surg* 2000; **12**: 2–14.

5 Lewis T. The nature of clinical fibrillation of the auricles. In: *The Mechanism and Graphic Registration of the Heart Beat.* Shaw & Sons, London, UK, 1925: 319–374.

6 Allessie MA, Boyden PA, Camm AJ *et al.* Pathophysiology and prevention of atrial fibrillation. *Circulation* 2001; **103**: 769–777.

7 Haissaguerre M, Fischer B, Labbe T *et al.* Frequency of recurrent atrial fibrillation after catheter ablation of overt accessory pathways. *Am J Cardiol* 1992; **69**: 493–497.

8 Roithinger FX, Karch MR, Steiner PR, Sippens Groenewegen A, Lesh MD. Relationship between atrial fibrillation and typical atrial flutter in humans: activation sequence changes during spontaneous conversion. *Circulation* 1997; **96**: 3484–3491.

9 Morton JB, Byrne MJ, Power JM, Raman J, Kalman JM. Electrical remodeling of the atrium in an anatomic model of atrial flutter: relationship between substrate and triggers for conversion to atrial fibrillation. *Circulation* 2002; **105**: 258–264.

10 Haissaguerre M, Marcus FI, Fischer B, Clementy J. Radiofrequency catheter ablation in unusual mechanisms of atrial fibrillation: report of three cases. *J Cardiovasc Electrophysiol* 1994; **5**: 743–751.

11 Jais P, Haissaguerre M, Shah DC *et al.* A focal source of atrial fibrillation treated by discrete radiofrequency ablation. *Circulation* 1997; **95**: 572–576.

12 Haissaguerre M, Jais P, Shah DC *et al.* Spontaneous initiation of atrial fibrillation by ectopic beats originating in the pulmonary veins. *N Engl J Med* 1998; **339**: 659–666.

13 Chen SA, Hsieh MH, Tai CT *et al.* Initiation of atrial fibrillation by ectopic beats originating from the pulmonary veins: electrophysiological characteristics, pharmacological responses, and effects of radiofrequency ablation. *Circulation* 1999; **100**: 1879–1886.

14 Hwang C, Wu TJ, Doshi RN, Peter CT, Chen PS. Vein of Marshall cannulation for the analysis of electrical activity in patients with focal atrial fibrillation. *Circulation* 2000; **101**: 1503–1505.

15 Chen SA, Tai CT, Yu WC *et al.* Right atrial focal atrial fibrillation: electrophysiologic characteristics and radiofrequency catheter ablation. *J Cardiovasc Electrophysiol* 1999; **10**: 328–335.

16 Tsai CF, Tai CT, Hsieh MH *et al.* Initiation of atrial fibrillation by ectopic beats originating from the superior vena cava: electrophysiological characteristics and results of radiofrequency ablation. *Circulation* 2000; **102**: 67–74.

17 Hsu LF, Jais P, Keane D *et al.* Atrial fibrillation originating from persistent left superior vena cava. *Circulation* 2004; **109**: 828–832.

18 Scavee C, Jais P, Weerasooriya R, Haissaguerre M. The inferior vena cava: an exceptional source of atrial fibrillation. *J Cardiovasc Electrophysiol* 2003; **14**: 659–662.

19 Lau CP, Tse HF, Ayers GM. Defibrillation-guided radiofrequency ablation of atrial fibrillation secondary to an atrial focus. *J Am Coll Cardiol* 1999; **33**: 1217–1226.

20 Hocini M, Haissaguerre M, Shah D *et al*. Multiple sources initiating atrial fibrillation from a single pulmonary vein identified by a circumferential catheter. *Pacing Clin Electrophysiol* 2000; **23**: 1828–1831.

21 Gerstenfeld EP, Guerra P, Sparks PB, Hattori K, Lesh MD. Clinical outcome after radiofrequency catheter ablation of focal atrial fibrillation triggers. *J Cardiovasc Electrophysiol* 2001; **12**: 900–908.

22 Sanders P, Morton JB, Deen VR *et al*. Immediate and long-term results of radiofrequency ablation of pulmonary vein ectopy for cure of paroxysmal atrial fibrillation using a focal approach. *Intern Med J* 2002; **32**: 202–207.

23 Weerasooriya R, Jais P, Scavee C *et al*. Dissociated pulmonary vein arrhythmia: incidence and characteristics. *J Cardiovasc Electrophysiol* 2003; **14**: 1173–1179.

24 Takahashi Y, Iesaka Y, Takahashi A *et al*. Reentrant tachycardia in pulmonary veins of patients with paroxysmal atrial fibrillation. *J Cardiovasc Electrophysiol* 2003; **14**: 927–932.

25 Ouyang F, Bansch D, Ernst S *et al*. Complete isolation of left atrium surrounding the pulmonary veins. New insights from the double-lasso technique in paroxysmal atrial fibrillation. *Circulation* 2004; **110**: 2090–2096.

26 Scherf D. Studies on auricular tachycardia caused by aconitine administration. *Proc Soc Exp Biol Med* 1947; **64**: 233–239.

27 Schuessler RB, Grayson TM, Bromberg BI, Cox JL, Boineau JP. Cholinergically mediated tachyarrhythmias induced by a single extrastimulus in the isolated canine right atrium. *Circ Res* 1992; **71**: 1254–1267.

28 Kumagai K, Khrestian C, Waldo AL. Simultaneous multisite mapping studies during induced atrial fibrillation in the sterile pericarditis model. Insights into the mechanism of its maintenance. *Circulation* 1997; **95**: 511–521.

29 Kumagai K, Uno K, Khrestian C, Waldo AL. Single site radiofrequency catheter ablation of atrial fibrillation: studies guided by simultaneous multisite mapping in the canine sterile pericarditis model. *J Am Coll Cardiol* 2000; **36**: 917–923.

30 Skanes AC, Mandapati R, Berenfeld O, Davidenko JM, Jalife J. Spatiotemporal periodicity during atrial fibrillation in the isolated sheep heart. *Circulation* 1998; **98**: 1236–1248.

31 Mandapati R, Skanes A, Chen J, Berenfeld O, Jalife J. Stable microreentrant sources as a mechanism of atrial fibrillation in the isolated sheep heart. *Circulation* 2000; **101**: 194–199.

32 Wu TJ, Doshi RN, Huang HL *et al*. Simultaneous biatrial computerized mapping during permanent atrial fibrillation in patients with organic heart disease. *J Cardiovasc Electrophysiol* 2002; **13**: 571–577.

33 Mansour M, Mandapati R, Berenfeld O *et al*. Left-to-right gradient of atrial frequencies during acute atrial fibrillation in the isolated sheep heart. *Circulation* 2001; **103**: 2631–2636.

34 Lazar S, Dixit S, Marchlinski FE, Callans DJ, Gerstenfeld EP. Presence of left-to-right atrial frequency gradient in paroxysmal but not persistent atrial fibrillation in humans. *Circulation* 2004; **110**: 3181–3186.

35 Sanders P, Berenfeld O, Hocini M *et al*. Spectral analysis identifies sites of high frequency activity maintaining atrial fibrillation in humans. *Circulation* 2005; **112**: 789–797.

36 Morillo CA, Klein GJ, Jones DL, Guiraudon CM. Chronic rapid atrial pacing. Structural, functional, and electrophysiological characteristics of a new model of sustained atrial fibrillation. *Circulation* 1995; **91**: 1588–1595.

37 Kumagai K, Yasuda T, Tojo H *et al*. Role of rapid focal activation in the maintenance of atrial fibrillation originating from the pulmonary veins. *Pacing Clin Electrophysiol* 2000; **11**: 1823–1827.

38 O'Donnell D, Furniss SS, Bourke JP. Paroxysmal cycle length shortening in the pulmonary veins during atrial fibrillation correlates with arrhythmogenic triggering foci in sinus rhythm. *J Cardiovasc Electrophysiol* 2002; **13**: 124–128.

39 Oral H, Ozaydin M, Tada H *et al*. Mechanistic significance of intermittent pulmonary vein tachycardia in patients with atrial fibrillation. *J Cardiovasc Electrophysiol* 2002; **13**: 645–650.

40 Haissaguerre M, Shah DC, Jais P *et al*. Mapping-guided ablation of pulmonary veins to cure atrial fibrillation. *Am J Cardiol* 2000; **86**: K9–K19.

41 Haissaguerre M, Sanders P, Hocini M *et al*. Changes in atrial fibrillation cycle length and inducibility during catheter ablation and their relation to outcome. *Circulation* 2004; **109**: 3007–3013.

42 Haissaguerre M, Sanders P, Hocini M, Jais P, Clementy J. Pulmonary veins in the substrate for atrial fibrillation: the "venous wave" hypothesis. *J Am Coll Cardiol* 2004; **43**: 2290–2292.

43 Nathan H, Eliakim M. The junction between the left atrium and the pulmonary veins. An anatomic study of human hearts. *Circulation* 1966; **34**: 412–422.

44 Nathan H, Gloobe H. Myocardial atrio-venous junctions and extensions (sleeves) over the pulmonary and caval veins. Anatomical observations in various mammals. *Thorax* 1970; **25**: 317–324.

45 Saito T, Waki K, Becker AE. Left atrial myocardial extension onto pulmonary veins in humans: anatomic

observations relevant for atrial arrhythmias. *J Cardiovasc Electrophysiol* 2000; **11**: 888–894.

46 Hocini M, Ho SY, Kawara T *et al.* Electrical conduction in canine pulmonary veins: electrophysiological and anatomic correlation. *Circulation* 2002; **105**: 2442–2448.

47 Hamabe A, Okuyama Y, Miyauchi Y *et al.* Correlation between anatomy and electrical activation in canine pulmonary veins. *Circulation* 2003; **107**: 1550–1555.

48 Hassink RJ, Aretz HT, Ruskin J, Keane D. Morphology of atrial myocardium in human pulmonary veins. A postmortem analysis in patients with and without atrial fibrillation. *J Am Coll Cardiol* 2003; **42**: 1108–1114.

49 Okuyama Y, Miyauchi Y, Park AM *et al.* High resolution mapping of the pulmonary vein and the vein of Marshall during induced atrial fibrillation and atrial tachycardia in a canine model of pacing-induced congestive heart failure. *J Am Coll Cardiol* 2003; **42**: 348–360.

50 Arora R, Verheule S, Scott L *et al.* Arrhythmogenic substrate of the pulmonary veins assessed by high-resolution optical mapping. *Circulation* 2003; **107**: 1816–1821.

51 Yamane T, Shah DC, Jais P *et al.* Dilatation as a marker of pulmonary veins initiating atrial fibrillation. *J Interv Card Electrophysiol* 2002; **6**: 245–249.

52 Lin WS, Prakash VS, Tai CT *et al.* Pulmonary vein morphology in patients with paroxysmal atrial fibrillation initiated by ectopic beats originating from the pulmonary veins: implications for catheter ablation. *Circulation* 2000; **101**: 1274–1281.

53 Tsao HM, Yu WC, Cheng HC *et al.* Pulmonary vein dilation in patients with atrial fibrillation: detection by magnetic resonance imaging. *J Cardiovasc Electrophysiol* 2001; **12**: 809–813.

54 Jais P, Hocini M, Macle L *et al.* Distinctive electrophysiological properties of pulmonary veins in patients with atrial fibrillation. *Circulation* 2002; **106**: 2479–2485.

55 Rostock T, Servatius H, Risius T *et al.* Impact of amiodarone on electrophysiological properties of pulmonary veins in patients with paroxysmal atrial fibrillation. *J Cardiovasc Electrophysiol* 2005; **16**: 39–44.

56 Kumagai K, Ogawa M, Noguchi H *et al.* Electrophysiologic properties of pulmonary veins assessed using a multielectrode basket catheter. *J Am Coll Cardiol* 2004; **43**: 2281–2289.

57 Blom NA, Gittenberger-de Groot AC, DeRuiter MC *et al.* Development of the cardiac conduction tissue in human embryos using HNK-1 antigen expression: possible relevance for understanding of abnormal atrial automaticity. *Circulation* 1999; **99**: 800–806.

58 Masani F. Node-like cells in the myocardial layer of the pulmonary vein of rats: an ultrastructural study. *J Anat* 1986; **145**: 133–142.

59 Cheung DW. Electrical activity of the pulmonary vein and its interaction with the right atrium in the guinea-pig. *J Physiol* 1980; **314**: 445–456.

60 Chen YJ, Chen SA, Chen YC *et al.* Effects of rapid atrial pacing on the arrhythmogenic activity of single cardiomyocytes from pulmonary veins: implication in initiation of atrial fibrillation. *Circulation* 2001; **104**: 2849–2854.

61 Chen YJ, Chen SA, Chang MS, Lin CI. Arrhythmogenic activity of cardiac muscle in pulmonary veins of the dog: implication for the genesis of atrial fibrillation. *Cardiovasc Res* 2000; **48**: 265–273.

62 Wu TJ, Ong JJ, Chang CM *et al.* Pulmonary veins and ligament of Marshall as sources of rapid activations in a canine model of sustained atrial fibrillation. *Circulation* 2001; **103**: 1157–1163.

63 Honjo H, Boyett MR, Niwa R *et al.* Pacing-induced spontaneous activity in myocardial sleeves of pulmonary veins after treatment with ryanodine. *Circulation* 2003; **107**: 1937–1943.

64 Schauerte P, Scherlag BJ, Patterson E *et al.* Focal atrial fibrillation: experimental evidence for a pathophysiologic role of the autonomic nervous system. *J Cardiovasc Electrophysiol* 2001; **12**: 592–599.

65 Kanagaratnam L, Tomassoni G, Schweikert R *et al.* Empirical pulmonary vein isolation in patients with chronic atrial fibrillation using a three-dimensional nonfluoroscopic mapping system: long-term follow-up. *Pacing Clin Electrophysiol* 2001; **24**: 1774–1779.

66 Oral H, Knight BP, Tada H *et al.* Pulmonary vein isolation for paroxysmal and persistent atrial fibrillation. *Circulation* 2002; **105**: 1077–1081.

67 Haissaguerre M, Sanders P, Hocini M *et al.* Catheter ablation of long lasting persistent atrial fibrillation: critical structures for termination. *J Cardiovasc Electrophysiol* 2005; **16**: 1125–1137.

68 Haissaguerre M, Hocini M, Sanders P *et al.* Catheter ablation of long lasting persistent atrial fibrillation: clinical outcome and mechanisms of subsequent arrhythmias. *J Cardiovasc Electrophysiol* 2005; **16**: 1138–1147.

69 Jais P, Hocini M, Hsu LF *et al.* Technique and results of linear ablation at the mitral isthmus. *Circulation* 2004; **110**: 2996–3002.

70 Sanders P, Jais P, Hocini M *et al.* Electrophysiologic and clinical consequence of linear catheter ablation to transect the anterior left atrium in patients with atrial fibrillation. *Heart Rhythms* 2004; **1**: 176–184.

71 Ernst S, Ouyang F, Lober F, Antz M, Kuck KH. Catheter-induced linear lesions in the left atrium in patients with atrial fibrillation: an electroanatomic study. *J Am Coll Cardiol* 2003; **42**: 1271–1282.

72 Rotter M, Jais P, Garrigue S *et al.* Clinical predictors of noninducibility of sustained atrial fibrillation after

pulmonary vein isolation. *J Cardiovasc Electrophysiol* 2005; **16**: 1298–1303.

73 Chauvin M, Shah DC, Haissaguerre M, Marcellin L, Brechenmacher C. The anatomic basis of connections between the coronary sinus musculature and the left atrium in humans. *Circulation* 2000; **101**: 647–652.

74 Antz M, Otomo K, Arruda M *et al.* Electrical conduction between the right atrium and the left atrium via the musculature of the coronary sinus. *Circulation* 1998; **98**: 1790–1795.

75 Roithinger FX, Cheng J, SippensGroenewegen A *et al.* Use of electroanatomic mapping to delineate transseptal atrial conduction in humans. *Circulation* 1999; **100**: 1791–1797.

76 Olgin JE, Jayachandran JV, Engesstein E, Groh W, Zipes DP. Atrial macroreentry involving the myocardium of the coronary sinus: a unique mechanism for atypical flutter. *J Cardiovasc Electrophysiol* 1998; **9**: 1094–1099.

77 Sun Y, Arruda M, Otomo K *et al.* Coronary sinus-ventricular accessory connections producing posteroseptal and left posterior accessory pathways: incidence and electrophysiological identification. *Circulation* 2002; **106**: 1362–1367.

78 Sanders P, Jais P, Hocini M, Haissaguerre M. Electrical disconnection of the coronary sinus by radiofrequency catheter ablation to isolate a trigger of atrial fibrillation. *J Cardiovasc Electrophysiol* 2004; **15**: 364–368.

79 Rotter M, Sanders P, Takahashi Y *et al.* Images in cardiovascular medicine. Coronary sinus tachycardia driving atrial fibrillation. *Circulation* 2004; **110**: e59–e60.

80 Oral H, Ozaydin M, Chugh A *et al.* Role of the coronary sinus in maintenance of atrial fibrillation. *J Cardiovasc Electrophysiol* 2003; **14**: 1329–1336.

81 Lin WS, Tai CT, Hsieh MH *et al.* Catheter ablation of paroxysmal atrial fibrillation initiated by non-pulmonary vein ectopy. *Circulation* 2003; **107**: 3176–3183.

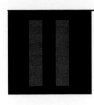

PART II

Surgical approach to atrial fibrillation

CHAPTER 7

Surgical treatment of atrial fibrillation: a retrospection

Gerard M. Guiraudon

"The insolubility of a problem has never deterred men and women from confidently propounding solutions. The method adopted is always the same: that of over-simplification. Thus, all but the immediate antecedents of the event under consideration are ignored. At the same time, all embarrassing complexities are mentally abolished. The event is thus made to seem simple enough to admit explanation in terms of a very few "causes", perhaps."

Aldous Huxley [1]

Introduction

Claude Bernard in his book *Introduction to the Study of Experimental Medicine* [2] made it clear that scientific publications become obsolete as rapidly as the publications become outdated by new discoveries and concepts, while literature or philosophy can still be current and of great interest years after their publications. Plato, Shakespeare, and Flaubert are still a great source of personal pleasure and growth. The historical view of science does not share this privilege for the scientist. Bernard, in 1857, thought that scientific publications were outdated after few years. Nowadays the pace of science is faster than the pace of editing and publishing, making today papers obsolete before publication.

Science is a team effort. The whole group is more important than the individuals who, at best, are the final pathway of a complex neuro-scientific stochastic process and never the sole creator of their

Manual of Surgical Treatment of Atrial Fibrillation.
Edited by Hauw T. Sie *et al.* © 2008 Blackwell Publishing, ISBN: 978-1-4051-4032-4.

eponymic contribution(s) even if they feel otherwise.

These premises explain my reluctance to address the title of my chapter in a conventional retrospection. On the one hand, I am disqualified as an historian because I was involved in the conspiracy and on the other hand, my many friends, colleagues, and I who participated in the group-process do not want to become "history."

Karl Popper considers self-criticism, which is better and less painful than critique by others, as the core of the scientific attitude [3]. Therefore, instead of telling a story of the people and their achievements, this chapter will address a series of theses on atrial fibrillation (AF) surgery.

Thesis one: why was AF, the most common cardiac arrhythmia, the first to be identified and studied [4], the last to be surgically approached?

Hypothesis 1

There was not one mechanism but a complex set of mechanisms for AF. These hypothetical mechanisms have been continuously discussed since 1870 [4]: the primacy of the cardiac intrinsic autonomic system or neurogenic AF [5–10]; the myocardial substrate hypothesis or myogenic AF [11, 12]; the critical mass hypothesis [13]; the single ectopic focal activity hypothesis; and the reentrant wave hypothesis [14–16] with a single rotor or self-sustained multiple wavelet mechanism [17–24]. Each hypothesis was not exclusive of the other. It could be anticipated that a single "grand manipulator" would be recognized: the cardiac autonomic system being the favored candidate [25]) as the sole initiating and perpetuating mechanism(s). In addition, it was impossible to dissociate fibrillatory activation from its mechanism: AF was preventing the study of AF. It was concluded that the complexity of the mechanisms with so many vicarious factors could not be neutralized by a gross surgical approach in the absence of a clear target site determined by an electrophysiological study. All those speculative mechanisms were waiting to be validated by clinical data. This would be the feat of Michel Haïssaguerre [26–28]; but in the mean time, the world had to wait.

Hypothesis 2

The other cardiac arrhythmias that were surgically treated were fraught with significant difficulties in that exciting but stressful pioneering period. A single well-defined target, such as the AV accessory connection associated with the Wolf–Parkinson–White (WPW) syndrome was associated with failure to interrupt the pathway, and significant morbidity [29–37]. Surgery for ventricular tachycardia produced great results in terms of confirming the mechanism and the interventional concepts of ablation or exclusion, but with the prohibitive risk and morbidity [38–45]. Improving the current approaches seemed a reasonable task before addressing other challenges.

Hypothesis 3

"The no solution no problem principle." If one revisits the short story of interventional electrophysiology, one discovers a trend to adjust the problem to the solution. A condition is deemed and documented to be life-threatening when the intervention is itself life-threatening [46]. When the intervention is deemed trivial and very effective, asymptomatic WPW patients are offered "curative" catheter-based intervention. AF might have fallen into the nonsolution trap; even if during the early eighties its morbidity and mortality were well documented. This "no problem no solution" attitude was well illustrated in the eighties when the first surgical technique for AF, the corridor operation, was presented at the AHA meeting and heckled by the audience upset by an unconscionable surgeon having the au-

dacity to propose open heart surgery for a benign electrocardiographic curiosity [47].

Thesis two: the irresistible attraction of linear thinking

In the early years of surgery for cardiac arrhythmia surgeons and cardiologists, working for the first time, together in the operating room were learning the new discipline with the WPW syndrome which was a simple model of linear reentry with an anatomically defined atrioventricular accessory pathway. Intraoperative cardiac mapping did not localize the actual site of the accessory pathway connection but a wide region of the atrioventricular sulcus. Surgeons and cardiologists were learning the functional anatomy and inventing the best surgical rationale in daunting circumstances. At the same time surgery for ventricular arrhythmia was developing amid even more grueling challenges. AF, without a well-defined target, seems beyond any organized strategy: "No discrete target! No surgery!" In the meantime, there were other well-defined targets to be surgically addressed before: atrioventricular nodal reentrant tachycardia and atrial flutter. Surprisingly, we failed to convince our colleagues that surgery was a safe and effective option for problematic atrial flutter, despite good evidence of safety and effectiveness produced in the seventies and in the eighties [48–51]. Only when cardiologists became interventionists did atrial flutter become an arrhythmia worth ablating.

Thesis three: posing the wrong question without an answer

In the seventies, Philippe Coumel [6] described the atrial arrhythmia syndrome of vagal origin with no demonstrable underlying cardiac disease. The condition developed slowly over the course of years toward daily attacks of AF or flutter. Stormy vagal activity was deemed the initiating factor. The beginning of each attack, with a long sinus pause and sinus bradycardia was very suggestive of vagal participation. This arrhythmia responded poorly to antiarrhythmic drugs and atrial pacing. Philippe thought that intervention on extracardiac thoracic innervation should be effective in preventing the initiation of AF. We therefore embarked in exploring cardiac denervation in the dog. The surgical technique of extensive dissection of arterial and venous pedicles of the heart was successful in suppressing markers of cardiac vagal response: sinus bradycardia and/or PR prolongation. This experiment was supported by other published animal experiments [52–55]. The same dissection in patients was not effective, even aggravating. After six disappointing interventions, the experience was abandoned with the simple conclusion that "it did not work" and considered unpublishable. This first novel surgical approach to AF, which is deemed nowadays the next best approach, was abandoned because the wrong question was asked. We were satisfied by the unscientific yes–no answer: "Does it work or not?" while we should have investigated the cause of failure, identified a new physiology and target, and designed a new rationale. The neurological nature of the mechanism was correct; but the target was misguided because, at that time, the current concept of anatomy and physiology of the cardiac intrinsic autonomic system (the small cardiac brain) [56–61] was ignored by clinical electrophysiologists and rediscovered only recently [25, 62, 63]. Thirty years has been lost before the cardiac intrinsic autonomic system was recognized a prime mechanism and prime target for interventions for AF. Success–failure is not a valid criterion; it does not belong to the scientific method because it neglects the basic tenet: testing and self-criticism and does not provide evidence for change and progress. It either freezes a "successful" technique or eliminates a failed one without due scientific process that might have identified the flaws and transformed a failure into a success. The right question is: Why it did work or why it did not?

Thesis four: the scientific attitude

Surgery for cardiac arrhythmia had a unique privilege in the history of cardiac surgery. Arrhythmia surgery was challenged by defined mechanisms and targets, with the additional benefit of testing before, during, and after ablation of target. Most cardiac surgical targets did not provide that intellectual luxury. Albeit arrhythmia surgery started with a solution, implementation of the solution was not easy. Failures of neutralizing the target and the magnitude of side effects put a dire burden on the pioneers

[32–35, 37, 64–69]. That experience provided the opportunity to apply the tenets of scientific surgery [2, 3]. Surgery must be designed as an experiment [2]. Every therapy, specially instrumental intervention, is composed of three parts. The target, the bullet, and the gun [70, 71]. The *target* is determined by the degree of knowledge of the pathophysiology. It is the necessary condition for the mechanism of the disease or symptom under consideration to be effective, such as the accessory atrioventricular connection in the WPW syndrome. The *bullet* is the action on target in order to neutralize, repair, remove, or ablate. This action must be as target-specific as possible. The *gun* is the complete system for delivery of the bullet on target. The delivery in cardiac surgery can be highly complex with sophisticated technology: heart–lung machine, cardiac arrest, myocardial preservation, etc. Unfortunately, if every effect that does not affect the target is a side effect, it becomes obvious that much of the delivery system is essentially a side effect of high magnitude when considering surgery for the WPW syndrome. This consideration leads us, in London, to change our surgical practice for less invasiveness or side effects when we described the epicardial approach on the close beating heart [72–78]. Delivery (the gun) has two additional components that have been confused for a very long time: access and visualization. In conventional surgical approach, opening is performed to expose, as well as to operate, on the target: this has paved the way to our new approach to AF [79–81].

But the most important feature of a scientific surgical intervention is the design of a testable rationale. Testability documents the completeness of the intervention: a basic requirement before any further assessment. Testability allows refutability of the rationale, better understanding of pathophysiology, and improvement of rationale. Testability allows evaluation of the side effects on the target organ or structure. In all, testability can elucidate the cause of success or failure. Better results than anticipated must be thoroughly studied to identify the lurking compounding factor. Canguillem, a philosopher of medicine, claimed that the main difference between a physician scientist and a medicine man is that the former takes the scientific method as the sole guidance, and the latter takes success as sole criteria; an old trick as old as humanity!

As far as AF is concerned, the absence of a well-defined pathophysiology encourages a return to empiricism with the inherent difficulties of testing hypotheses and learning [82–87]. Thanks to remarkable recent progress in pathophysiology, learning again while cutting, or ablating [88] may return.

Thesis five: how well did we use the scientific method in clinical practice?

Surgical rationales for the treatment of AF have long been empirical in the absence of documented discrete mechanism(s). The corridor operation and the maze operation were based on the multiple wavelet theory proposed by Moe [17–21, 89].

Postoperative electrophysiological testing of the corridor operation documented two important features: the left atrium was the site of the fibrillatory mechanism, while the coronary sinus was a conducting interatrial bundle and therefore a cause of incomplete isolation of the left atrium [50, 82, 84, 85, 90]. Consequently, all or parts of the left atrium were the therapeutic target to eliminate AF. This observation was good evidence that treatment of the right atrium was unwarranted for AF. The fact that an isolated normal left atrium could sustain AF was evidence that the multiple wavelet mechanism was not the operative mechanism (J. Jarife, personal communication). The maze operation, based on the multi-wavelet theory was subsequently developed. It was a complex intervention with multiple left atrial and right atrial incisions. It has undergone multiple changes based on empirical clinical results but without supportive postoperative electrophysiological evidence. The maze operation was progressively accepted as the gold standard (it will be extensively discussed in the next chapter by its inventor: J. L. Cox). There are few reports of electrophysiological testing of the maze intervention [86]. A meta-analysis performed by Khargi *et al.* failed to provide evidence on completeness of the surgical technique and causes of failure [91]. The maze operation remains largely unchanged, although empirical variants or simplifications have been reported [92–94].

In the late 1990s, we designed the corridor III operation based on the new documented pathophysiology that located the sites of origin of AF in the pulmonary vein region. In the early 1990s, our laboratories reported a canine chronic pacing model study of AF with evidence of a focal origin of AF in the left superior pulmonary vein region [95]. But Michel Haïssaguerre was the first to document that foci situated in the pulmonary veins were the primary triggering factors of lone AF and their ablation interrupted the arrhythmia [28]. The corridor III comprised *en bloc* cryo-exclusion of the pulmonary vein region combined with a line of block across the left atrial isthmus not aimed at ablating fibrillatory sites but preventing iatrogenic left atrial flutter around the mitral valve annulus [83]. Postoperative electrophysiological studies in 14 patients, performed using temporary pacing electrodes, documented that only the excluded atrial segment could exhibit fibrillatory activity while the non-excluded segment of the atria did not exhibit any arrhythmia either spontaneously or by programmed electrical stimulations. Two types of recurrences of atrial arrhythmia were observed. One was associated with incomplete exclusion and the other was a left atria flutter associated with incomplete block of the left atrial isthmus. Both were interrupted by application of RF energy. Results of postoperative testing exemplifies its value in providing unique information on the mechanism of success (critical value of isolation of fibrillatory process) and the mechanisms of failure (incomplete intervention), while validating the interventional rationale. The most striking feature was the inability to induce AF in the non-excluded segments of the atria. This result suggested that the pulmonary vein region may be the only segment that could initiate and perpetuate AF [96].

Thesis six: never be first

In any retrospective view, there should be room for humor and provocation. A recent paper about innovation and its various breeds from disruptive to benign, argues that the pioneer, in the business world, is never the final winner: never be first [97]. Although this is a strong statement without much room for nuance, the author gives convincing examples that the second may be the winner. The disruptive innovator (creator) runs the risk of feeling lonely in the wild with no hope of rescue. Because innovations improve existing technologies or techniques without breaking any paradigm they are safe and accepted. But the innovator runs a different risk of becoming an expert at doing the wrong operation for to long. J. Diamond, looking at the larger picture spanning the last 15,000 years after humanity got out of the ice age, support the same conclusion [98]. "Necessity is mother of invention" but invention does not invent necessarily its own necessity. The most important is not to be first but to be in synchrony with the cultural milieu. These remarks put in perspective the vanity of being first or successful. The early decades of cardiac surgery were productive, because there were no obstructive established paradigms. Nowadays, cardiac surgeons feel that the future is somber and that the end nearing. But the future is unpredictable and only fools, according to Erasmus, dare believing their predictions. The reasonable attitude is to rely on creativity and imagination for discovering new solutions for old problems, or more importantly anticipating new problems and their solutions, while expecting that a fool will do the pioneering.

Thesis six: the heart is arrhythmogenic

This thesis raises the issue of function and physiology. This conundrum is made clear by answering the following statements: (1) the purpose of the heart is to pump blood; (2) the function of the heart is to pump blood; (3) an effect of the heart is to pump blood [99]. The first two statements are dismissed because of their teleological bias; the first implies a conscious purpose and the second a preexisting design. Those considerations are beyond the scientific domain. The third statement implies that pumping blood is one of many cardiac features: heart sounds, excretion of ANF, arrhythmias, etc. The model for physiology is a stochastic or highly complex system, which gives the impression of working within the cause-and-effect pattern and self-regulation but is not, albeit its actions can be counterproductive from the individual point of view. The cardiac intrinsic autonomic system (the small cardiac brain) is a prime example of arrhythmogenic feature capable of initiating and perpetuating AF in the so-called normal heart.

The "intrinsic" cardiac neuronal elements are organized and collected in fat pads of sulcuses to form ganglionated plexuses (GPs) connected by nerves. These GPs contain afferent and efferent somata of parasympathetic or sympathetic neurons with connective neurons that comprise about 80% of the cellular population and constitute the *little brain on the heart*, transducing centripetal and centrifugal inputs and representing the final common pathway for modulation of electrical and mechanical cardiac events. There is good experimental evidence of the role of the cardiac ganglionated plexuses on cardiac electrophysiology [100–102] and its role in producing AF. Excessive release of cholinergic and adrenergic neurotransmitters can shorten refractoriness and induce triggered fast firing sufficient to cause AF. The combination of the two produces a self-sustained mechanism for the perpetuation of AF via atrial remodeling that involves the autonomic system and the atrial myocardium. Remodeling produces a new pathophysiology via emergent properties.

The small cardiac brain has very special features: (a) the intrinsic cardiac nervous system is the *final common pathway* for the neurological control of regional cardiac function; (b) neurons belonging to a given GP module participate in modulating diverse cardiac segments, while having a preferential and predominant control over one cardiac region or structure; (c) the macroscopic anatomy-based nomenclature of GPs does not imply any specific function and has only practical topographical value; (d) naming GPs after their target is misleading, as exemplified by the study of AV node function [102–104]. These studies documented that multiple pathways travel to and from a single target; and (e) *remodeling of the intrinsic cardiac autonomic system* is inherent to its physiology, specially in response to cardiac diseases and their progression such as AF, cardiac failure, or any other condition or stress [105–109]. Remodeling of the intrinsic cardiac autonomic system involves *reorganization and remodeling* of the systems itself, remodeling of the neurons which exhibit a new physiology, reorganization of the myocytes and their connections [110] as well as the collagenous-elastic framework [111]. Remodeling transforms the anatomy and function of heart and its GPs, but this remodeled pathophysiology with new emergent properties is *more a self-aggravating rather than a regulatory process* [107].

Recent publications have shown in patients with altered vagal response after intervention for AF where the GPs were targeted or were inadvertently modified that a significant increase in AF control was observed [112–116]. But controlling such a complex system is going to be a daunting challenge for the surgeon since the cardiac autonomic system can change its anatomy (hardware) and physiology (software) at the same time: a very elusive arrhythmogenic anatomical substrate.

Thesis seven: the future is already present

If cardiac surgery is to flourish, cardiac surgeons have to reinvent surgery by reinventing themselves. This involves dismissing the pervasive disenchantment of cardiac surgeons based on three assumptions: (1) cardiac surgery is the last resort for the hopeless cases abandoned by cardiologist, therefore surgery will die with the dying; (2) the quality of reasonable effective treatment for most cardiac conditions is not giving the credit it deserves: a way to say that we are the best and therefore cannot get better; (3) innovation comes now from industry rather than academia. Therefore, we have lost our brainpower for adaptable innovation and creativity (V. Gaudiani, 2005, Internet communication.). There are few paths to renewal:

1 *Strict usage of the scientific method.* The critique and testing should apply to every component of practice: pathophysiology, mechanisms, pathology, surgical rationale that must be testable, since surgery must be designed as an experiment as discussed above. Randomized controlled clinical trials (RCTs) are not a substitute for science: comparing is not understanding: the quality of the mathematics is not transferable to the processed clinical material. The impediments of the surgical practice explain why no surgical RCT meets the criteria of CONSORT [117, 118]. Valid conclusions cannot be drawn from invalid trials. Claude Bernard, in his book [2] (page 137), made comments on clinical trials that are still valid today. "Well, I say that this ratio means literally nothing scientifically and gives us no certainty in performing the next operation; for we do not know whether the next case will be among the recoveries or the deaths. What really should be done, instead of gathering facts empirically, is to study them more accurately, each in its special determinism. We must study cases of death with great care and try to discover in them the cause of mortal accidents, so as to master the cause and avoid the accidents. Thus if we accurately know the cause of recovery and the cause of death, we shall always have a recovery in a definite case. We cannot, indeed, admit that cases with different endings were identical at every point." These comments apply well to RCT of surgery for AF, that quantify the number of failures without shedding any light on their cause. "...statistics...never can...teach anything about the nature [mechanism] of phenomena [disease]."

2 *Suppression of barriers between disciplines.* It is time to suppress the mosaic of closed boxes where each subspecialty confines itself. We should all jump out of the boxes to think in the open field with free connection and collaboration with all. The brain is only connections not partitions. This renaissance man attitude must be shared by every participant, since productive collaboration requires an intelligent understanding of other disciplines.

3 *The surgeon is no longer the sole operator.* Indeed the surgeon is going to be only one actor in the team of electrophysiologists, anesthesiologists, imagist, engineers, interventionists, etc. At the end of the day, it may be difficult to determine who or what was the final effector, as new surgeons may like to describe themselves.

4 *Searching for new targets and surgical rationale.* The intrinsic cardiac autonomic nervous system seems to be the designated surrogate target but the multiplicity of mechanisms suggest that we are not running out of targets in the foreseeable future.

Conclusion

We feel that surgeons must break the old surgical paradigm and develop minimally invasive approaches that can be performed on the closed off pump, beating heart and allow access to all epicardial and endocardial targets via minimal access with the gentleness of the catheter but without compromising effectiveness. New access implies revisiting surgical rationales as well. What we do, should not be determined how we get on target, but what is the best action on target in term of effectiveness and side effects on target! This is our current project, the description of which is beyond the framework of this chapter. The actual goal of our research is not to develop a substitute to catheter-based techniques, but provide a safe and effective, but minimally invasive, back-up to failures or limitations of catheter-based interventions while at the same time developing technologies that will be transferable to catheter-based interventions. In other words, our project follows the tradition of surgery for cardiac arrhythmia that paved the way to effective development of catheter-based interventions for the WPW syndrome, AV nodal reentrant tachycardia, atrial flutter, ventricular tachycardia, and AF.

References

1 Aldous Huxley. *Grey Eminence: A Study in Religion and Politics*. The MacMillan Co., Canada, Toronto, 1941.

2 Bernard C. *Introduction to the Study of Experimental Medicine* (Trans. Green HC). Dover edition, New York, 1957.

3 Popper K. *Conjectures and Refutations. The Growth of Scientific Knowledge*. Routledge Classics, London and New York, 2002.

4 Efimov IR, Fedorov VV. Chessboard of atrial fibrillation: reentry or focus? Single or multiple source(s)? Neurogenic or myogenic? *Am J Physiol Heart Circ Physiol* September 2005; **289**(3): H977–H979.

5 Hoffa M, Ludwig C. Einige neueversuche uber herzbewegung. *Zeitschrift Rationellen Medizin* 1850; **9**: 107–144.

6 Coumel P, Attuel P, Lavallee J *et al.* The atrial arrhythmia syndrome of vagal origin. *Arch Mal Coeur Vaiss* 1978; **71**: 645–656.

7 Nattel S. Age, gender, and supraventricular arrhythmias: roles of ion channels, connexins, and tissue architecture? *Heart Rhythm* October 2004; **1**(4): 397–398.

8 Zipes DP, Mihalick MJ, Robbins GT. Effects of selective vagal and stellate ganglion stimulation of atrial refractoriness. *Cardiovasc Res* September 1974; **8**(5): 647–655.

9 Chang CM, Wu TJ, Zhou S *et al.* Nerve sprouting and sympathetic hyperinnervation in a canine model of atrial fibrillation produced by prolonged right atrial pacing. *Circulation* 2001; **103**(1): 22–25.

10 Liu L, Nattel S. Differing sympathetic and vagal effects on atrial fibrillation in dogs: role of refractoriness heterogeneity. *Am J Physiol* 1997; **273**(2, pt 2): H805–H816.

11 MacWilliam JA. Fibrillar contraction of the heart. *J Physiol* 1887; **8**: 296.

12 Vulpian A. Note sur les effets de la faradisation directe des ventricules du coeur le chien. *Arch Physiol* 1874; **i**: 975.

13 Garrey WE. The nature of fibrillary contraction of the heart. Its relations to tissue mass and form. *Am J Physiol* 1914; **33**: 397–414.

14 Garrey WE. Auricular fibrillation. *Physiol Rev* 1924; **4**: 215–250.

15 Lewis T, Drury AN, Iliescu CC. Further observations upon the state of rapid re-excitation of the auricles. *Heart* 1921; **8**: 311–340.

16 Lewis T. *The Mechanism and Graphic Registration of the Heart Beat*. Shaw and Sons, London, 1925.

17 Moe GK, Abildskov JA. Atrial fibrillation as a self-sustaining arrhythmia independent of focal discharge. *Am Heart J* July 1959; **58**(1): 59–70.

18 Moe GK, Rheinboldt WC, Abildskov JA. A computer model of atrial fibrillation. *Am Heart J* February 1964; **67**: 200–220.

19 Allessie MA, Lammers W, Bonke F. Experimental evaluation of Moe's multiple wavelet hypothesis of atrial fibrillation. In: Zipes DP & Jarife J, eds. *Cardiac Electrophysiology and Arrhythmias*. Grune & Stratton Inc., New York, 1985: 265–275.

20 Moe GK. On the multiple wavelet hypothesis of atrial fibrillation. *Arch Int Pharmacol* 1962; **140**: 183–188.

21 Zipes DP. The seventh annual Gordon K. Moe Lecture. Atrial fibrillation: from cell to bedside. *J Cardiovasc Electrophysiol* August 1997; **8**(8): 927–938.

22 Jalife J, Berenfeld O, Skanes A, Mandapati R. Mechanisms of atrial fibrillation: mother rotors or multiple daughter wavelets, or both? *J Cardiovasc Electrophysiol* August 1998; **9**(suppl 8): S2–S12.

23 Skanes AC, Mandapati R, Berenfeld O, Davidenko JM, Jalife J. Spatiotemporal periodicity during atrial fibrillation in the isolated sheep heart. *Circulation* September 22, 1998; **98**(12): 1236–1248.

24 Mandapati R, Skanes A, Chen J, Berenfeld O, Jalife J. Stable microreentrant sources as a mechanism of atrial fibrillation in the isolated sheep heart. *Circulation* January 18, 2000; **101**(2): 194–199.

25 Armour JA, Ardell JL eds. *Basic and Clinical Neurocardiology*. Oxford University Press, New York, 2004.

26 Weerasooriya R, Jais P, Scavee C *et al.* Dissociated pulmonary vein arrhythmia: incidence and characteristics. *J Cardiovasc Electrophysiol* November 2003; **14**(11): 1173–1179.

27 Haissaguerre M, Sanders P, Hocini M, Jais P, Clementy J. Pulmonary veins in the substrate for atrial fibrillation: the "venous wave" hypothesis. *J Am Coll Cardiol* June 16, 2004; **43**(12): 2290–2292.

28 Haissaguerre M, Jais P, Shah DC *et al.* Spontaneous initiation of atrial fibrillation by ectopic beats originating in the pulmonary veins. *N Engl J Med* September 3, 1998; **339**(10): 659–666.

29 Selle JG, Sealy WC, Gallagher JJ *et al.* The complex posterior septal space in the Wolff–Parkinson–White syndrome. Surgical experience with 47 patients. *Thorac Cardiovasc Surg* October 1989; **37**(5): 299–304.

30 Svenson RH, Gallagher JJ, Sealy WC, Wallace AG. An electrophysiologic approach to the surgical treatment of the Wolff–Parkinson–White syndrome. Report of two cases utilizing catheter recording and epicardial mapping techniques. *Circulation* May 1974; **49**(5): 799–804.

31 Boineau JP, Moore EN, Sealy WC, Kasell JH. Epicardial mapping in Wolff–Parkinson–White syndrome. *Arch Intern Med* March 1975; **135**(3): 422–431.

32 Sealy WC. The evolution of the surgical methods for interruption of right free wall Kent bundles. *Ann Thorac Surg* July 1983; **36**(1): 29–36.

33 Sealy WC, Wallace AJ, Ramming KP, Gallagher JJ, Svenson RH. An improved operation for the definitive treatment of the Wolff–Parkinson–White syndrome. *Ann Thorac Surg* February 1974; **17**(2): 107–113.

34 Sealy WC. Kent bundles in the anterior septal space. *Ann Thorac Surg* August 1983; **36**(2): 180–186.

35 Cobb FR, Blumenschein SD, Sealy WC, Boineau JP, Wagner GS, Wallace AG. Successful surgical interruption of the bundle of Kent in a patient with Wolff–Parkinson–White syndrome. *Circulation* December 1968; **38**(6): 1018–1029.

36 Selle JG, Gallagher JJ, Colavita PG, Smith RT, Jr, Sealy WC. Surgical division of posterior septal accessory pathways in the Wolff–Parkinson–White syndrome: a new modified approach. *J Card Surg* June 1991; **6**(2): 311–316, discussion.

37 Gallagher JJ, Gilbert M, Svenson RH, Sealy WC, Kasell J, Wallace AG. Wolff–Parkinson–White syndrome. The problem, evaluation, and surgical correction. *Circulation* May 1975; **51**(5): 767–785.

38 Guiraudon GM, Fontaine G, Frank R *et al.* Circular exclusion ventriculotomy. Surgical treatment of ventricular tachycardia following myocardial infarction [French]. *Arch Mal Coeur Vaiss* November 1978; **71**(11): 1255–1262.

39 Guiraudon GM, Fontaine G, Frank R, Escande G, Etievent P, Cabrol C. Encircling endocardial ventriculotomy: a new surgical treatment for life-threatening ventricular tachycardias resistant to medical treatment following myocardial infarction 166. *Ann Thorac Surg* November 1978; **26**(5): 438–444.

40 Guiraudon GM, Fontaine G, Frank R, Cabrol C, Grosgogeat Y. Encircling endocardial ventriculotomy in the treatment of recurrent ventricular tachycardia after myocardial infarction [French]. *Arch Mal Coeur Vaiss* September 1982; **75**(9): 1013–1021.

41 Fontaine G, Guiraudon G, Frank R *et al.* Epicardial cartography and surgical treatment by simple ventriculotomy of certain resistant re-entry ventricular tachycardias [French]. *Arch Mal Coeur Vaiss* February 1975; **68**(2): 113–124.

42 Guiraudon GM, Franck R, Fontaine G. Letter: value of cartographies in the surgical treatment of recurrent intractable ventricular tachycardia [French]. *Nouv Presse Med* February 9, 1974; **3**(6): 321.

43 Vedel J, Frank R, Fontaine G *et al.* Recurrent ventricular tachycardia and parchment right ventricle in the adult. Anatomical and clinical report of 2 cases [French]. *Arch Mal Coeur Vaiss* September 1978; **71**(9): 973–981.

44 Jones DL, Guiraudon GM, Klein GJ. Total disconnection of the right ventricular free wall: physiological consequences in the dog 124. *Am Heart J* June 1984; **107**(6): 1169–1177.

45 Guiraudon GM, Klein GJ, Gulamhusein SS *et al.* Total disconnection of the right ventricular free wall: surgical treatment of right ventricular tachycardia associated with right ventricular dysplasia. *Circulation* February 1983; **67**(2): 463–470.

46 Gallagher JJ, Wallace AG, Sealy WC. Surgery in the Wolff–Parkinson–White syndrome. *J Electrocardiol* 1976; **9**(4): 293–294.

47 Guiraudon GM, Campbell CS, Jones DL. Combined sino-atrial node atrioventricular node isolation: a surgical alternative to His bundle ablation in patients with atrial fibrillation [Abstract]. *Circulation* 1985; **72**(suppl 12): III220.

48 Guiraudon GM, Klein GJ, van HN, Guiraudon CM, de Bakker JM. Atrial flutter: lessons from surgical interventions (musing on atrial flutter mechanism). *Pacing Clin Electrophysiol* November 1996; **19**(11, pt 2): 1933–1938.

49 Klein GJ, Guiraudon GM, Sharma AD, Milstein S. Demonstration of macroreentry and feasibility of operative therapy in the common type of atrial flutter. *Am J Cardiol* March 1, 1986; **57**(8): 587–591.

50 Guiraudon GM, Klein GJ, Yee R. Supraventricular tachycardias: the role of surgery. *Pacing Clin Electrophysiol* March 1993; **16**(3, pt 2): 658–670.

51 Guiraudon GM, Klein GJ, Sharma AD, Yee R, McLellan DG. Surgical treatment of supraventricular tachycardia: a five-year experience 109. *Pacing Clin Electrophysiol* November 1986; **9**(6, pt 2): 1376–1380.

52 Geis WP, Tatooles CJ, Kaye MP, Randall WC. Complete cardiac denervation without transplantation: a simple and reliable technique. *J Appl Physiol* 1971; **30**(2): 289–293.

53 Priola DV, Spurgeon HA, Geis WP. The intrinsic innervation of the canine heart: a functional study. *Circ Res* 1977; **40**(1): 50–56.

54 Kaye MP, Hageman GR, Randall WC, Isobe J. One stage cardiac denervation without transplantation. *J Surg Res* 1973; **15**(5): 357–362.

55 Schaal SF, Wallace AG, Sealy WC. Protective influence of cardiac denervation against arrhythmias of myocardial infarction. *Cardiovasc Res* 1969; **3**(3): 241–244.

56 Scarpa A. *Abulae neurologicae; Ad illustrandum anatomiam cardiacorum nervosum, novi nervorum cerebri glosso-pharingali et octavocerebri.* T Ticini, Italy, 1794.(As cited in Mitchell GAG, Brown R, Cookson FB. 1952. Ventricular nerve cells in mammals. *Nature* **172**: 812.)

57 Mitchell G, Brown R, Cookson F. Ventricular nerve cells in mammals. *Nature* 1952; **172**: 812.

58 Kuntz A. *The Autonomic Nervous System.* Lea and Febiger, Philadelphia, 1934.

59 Robb JS. *Comparative Basic Cardiology.* Grune and Stratton, New York, 1965.

60 Dogiel AS. Zur Frage über den feineren Bau der Herzganglien des Menschen und der Säugetiere. *Arch MIkrosc Anat* 1899; **53**: 237–281.

61 Davies F, Francis E, King T. Neurological studies of the cardiac ventricles of mammals. *J Anat* 1952; **86**: 130–143.

62 Nakagawa H, Sherlag BJ, Lockwood D *et al.* Localization of left atrial ganglionated plexuses using endocardial and epicardial high frequency stimulation in patients with atrial fibrillation. *Heart Rhythm* 2005; **2**(suppl 1): S10–S11.

63 Sherlag BJ, Tamanasi E, Edwards J, Geng NPS, Lazzra R, Jackmann WM. Mapping the onset of atrial fibrillation arising from pulmonary vein and non-pulmonary vein sites in the dog heart. *Heart Rhythms* 2005; **2**(suppl 1): S218.

64 Sealy WC. Reminiscences of the beginning of clinical electrophysiology at Duke. *Pacing Clin Electrophysiol* February 1997; **20**(2, pt 2): 382–387.

65 Sealy WC, Mikat EM. Anatomical problems with identification and interruption of posterior septal Kent bundles. *Ann Thorac Surg* November 1983; **36**(5): 584–595.

66 Sealy WC. Effectiveness of surgical management of the Wolff–Parkinson–White syndrome. *Am J Surg* June 1983; **145**(6): 756–762.

67 Sealy WC, Gallagher JJ. Surgical treatment of left free wall accessory pathways of atrioventricular conduction of the Kent type. *J Thorac Cardiovasc Surg* May 1981; **81**(5): 698–706.

68 Sealy WC, Gallagher JJ. The surgical approach to the septal area of the heart based on experiences with 45 patients with Kent bundles. *J Thorac Cardiovasc Surg* April 1980; **79**(4): 542–551.

69 Sealy WC, Gallagher JJ, Pritchett EL. The surgical anatomy of Kent bundles based on electrophysiological mapping and surgical exploration. *J Thorac Cardiovasc Surg* December 1978; **76**(6): 804–815.

70 Guiraudon GM. Musing while cutting 13. *J Card Surg* March 1998; **13**(2): 156–162.

71 Guiraudon GM. Surgery without interventions?. *Pacing Clin Electrophysiol* November 1998; **21**(11, pt 2): 2160–2165.

72 Guiraudon GM, Klein GJ. Closed heart surgery for Wolff–Parkinson–White syndrome. *Int J Cardiol* March 1984; **5**(3): 387–391.

73 Guiraudon GM, Klein GJ, Sharma AD, Milstein S, McLellan DG. Closed-heart technique for Wolff–Parkinson–White syndrome: further experience and potential limitations. *Ann Thorac Surg* December 1986; **42**(6): 651–657.

74 Guiraudon GM, Guiraudon CM, Klein GJ, Sharma AD, Yee R. The coronary sinus diverticulum: a pathologic entity associated with the Wolff–Parkinson–White syndrome. *Am J Cardiol* October 1, 1988; **62**(10, pt 1): 733–735.

75 Jones DL, Klein GJ, Guiraudon GM, Yee R, Brown JE, Sharma AD. Effects of lidocaine and verapamil on defibrillation in humans 59. *J Electrocardiol* October 1991; **24**(4): 299–305.

76 Guiraudon GM, Klein GJ, Sharma AD, Yee R, McLellan DG. Surgery for the Wolff–Parkinson–White syndrome: the epicardial approach. *Semin Thorac Cardiovasc Surg* July 1989; **1**(1): 21–33.

77 Guiraudon GM, Klein GJ, Sharma AD, Jones DL, McLellan DG. Surgical ablation of posterior septal accessory pathways in the Wolff–Parkinson–White syndrome by a closed heart technique. *J Thorac Cardiovasc Surg* September 1986; **92**(3, pt 1): 406–413.

78 Guiraudon GM, Klein GJ, Sharma AD, Yee R, Pineda EA, McLellan DG. Surgical approach to anterior septal accessory pathways in 20 patients with the Wolff–Parkinson–White syndrome. *Eur J Cardiothorac Surg* 1988; **2**(4): 201–206.

79 Guiraudon GM, Jones DL, Skanes AC *et al.* Effects of pulmonary vein region isolation on inducibility of atrial fibrillation in an acute pig model. *Heart Rhythm* 2005; **2**(suppl 1): S90.

80 Guiraudon GM, Jones DL, Skanes AC *et al.* Intracardiac cryo-ablation on the off pump beating heart, combined with or replacing the epicardial approach for minimally invasive surgery for atrial fibrillation. *Heart Rhythm* 2005; **2**(suppl 1): S91.

81 Guiraudon GM, Jones DL, Bainbridge D *et al.* En bloc exclusion of pulmonary vein region using off pump closed beating intracardiac approach. A pilot study for mini-invasive surgical ablation of atrial fibrillation. *Can J Cardiol* 2004; **20**(suppl D): 115D.

82 Leitch JW, Klein G, Yee R, Guiraudon G. Sinus node-atrioventricular node isolation: long-term results with the "corridor" operation for atrial

fibrillation. *J Am Coll Cardiol* March 15, 1991; **17**(4): 970–975.

83 Todd DM, Skanes AC, Guiraudon G *et al*. Role of the posterior left atrium and pulmonary veins in human lone atrial fibrillation: electrophysiological and pathological data from patients undergoing atrial fibrillation surgery. *Circulation* December 23, 2003; **108**(25): 3108–3114.

84 van Hemel NM, Defauw JJ, Guiraudon GM, Kelder JC, Jessurun ER, Ernst JM. Long-term follow-up of corridor operation for lone atrial fibrillation: evidence for progression of disease? *J Cardiovasc Electrophysiol* September 1997; **8**(9): 967–973.

85 van Hemel NM, Defauw JJ, Kingma JH *et al*. Long-term results of the corridor operation for atrial fibrillation. *Br Heart J* February 1994; **71**(2): 170–176.

86 Defauw JA, Ballaux P, Geuzebrock G *et al*. Surgery for atrial fibrillation—Questions after 20 years of experience. In: van Hemel NM, Vermeulen F & de Bakker J, eds. *Exclusion or Targeting-Proceedings of the Conference on Cardiac Arrhythmias and Treatment to Honor Gerard Guiraudon, MD*. Grafishe Producties Budde-Elinkwijk, Utrecht, The Netherlands; Nieuwegen, The Netherlands; February 24, 2005: 199–210.

87 Guiraudon CM, Campbell CS, Jones DL, McLellan DG, MacDonald JL. Combined sino-atrial node atrioventricular isolation: a surgical alternative to His bundle ablation in patients with atrial fibrillation. *Circulation* 1985; **72**(suppl III): III-220.

88 Guiraudon GM. Musing while cutting. *J Card Surg* March 1998; **13**(2): 156–162.

89 Moe GK. A conceptual model of atrial fibrillation. *J Electrocardiol* 1968; **1**(2): 145–146.

90 Defauw JJ, Guiraudon GM, van Hemel NM, Vermeulen FE, Kingma JH, de Bakker JM. Surgical therapy of paroxysmal atrial fibrillation with the "corridor" operation. *Ann Thorac Surg* April 1992; **53**(4): 564–570.

91 Khargi K, Hutten BA, Lemke B, Deneke T. Surgical treatment of atrial fibrillation; a systematic review. *Eur J Cardiothorac Surg* February 2005; **27**(2): 258–265.

92 Imai K, Sueda T, Orihashi K, Watari M, Matsuura Y. Clinical analysis of results of a simple left atrial procedure for chronic atrial fibrillation. *Ann Thorac Surg* February 2001; **71**(2): 577–581.

93 Sueda T, Imai K, Orihashi K, Okada K, Ban K, Hamamoto M. Midterm results of pulmonary vein isolation for the elimination of chronic atrial fibrillation. *Ann Thorac Surg* February 2005; **79**(2): 521–525.

94 Sueda T, Shikata H, Orihashi K, Mitsui N, Nagata H, Matsuura Y. A modified maze procedure performed only on the left atrium for chronic atrial fibrillation associated with mitral valve disease: report of a case. *Surg Today* 1996; **26**(2): 135–137.

95 Morillo CA, Klein GJ, Jones DL, Guiraudon CM. Chronic rapid atrial pacing. Structural, functional, and electrophysiological characteristics of a new model of sustained atrial fibrillation. *Circulation* March 1, 1995; **91**(5): 1588–1595.

96 Popper K. Science: conjectures and refutations. In: *Conjectures and Refutations*. Routledge, London and New York, 2004: 42–86.

97 Ganascia J-G. Le futur conjugè au mode interactif (The future is intricated with multiple factors). *Le banquet Revue du CERAP* September, 2005 ; **22**: 183–195.

98 Diamond J. *Guns Germs and Steel: The Fate of Human Societies*. W.W. Norton & company Inc., New York, 1999.

99 Grinnell F. *The Scientific Attitude*, 2nd edn. The Guilford Press, New York, 1992.

100 Lazzara R, Herlag BJ, Obinson MJ, Amet P. Selective in situ parasympathetic control of the canine sinoatrial and atrioventricular nodes. *Circ Res* 1973; **32**: 393–401.

101 Page PL, Dandan N, Savard P, Nadeau R, Armour JA, Cardinal R. Regional distribution of atrial electrical changes induced by stimulation of extracardiac and intracardiac neural elements. *J Thorac Cardiovasc Surg* February 1995; **109**(2): 377–388.

102 Cardinal R, Pagè P. Neuronal regulation of atrial and ventricular electrical properties. In: Armour JA & Ardell JL, eds. *Basic and Clinical Neurocardiology*. Oxford University Press, New York, 2004: 315–339.

103 Pagè P, Dandan N, Savard P, Nadeau R, Armour JA, Cardinal R. Regional distribution of atrial electrical changes induced by stimulation of extracardiac and intracardiac neural elements. *J Thorac Cardiovasc Surg* 1995; **109**: 377–388.

104 Yuan B, Ardell JL, Hopkins DA, Armour JA. Differential cardiac responses induced by nicotine sensitive canine atrial and ventricular neurons. *Cardiovasc Res* 1993; **27**: 760–769.

105 Jones DL, Kadishevitz L. Insights into the organization of the stellate ganglia of myopathic Syrian hamsters (Bio 14.6) from *in vitro* intracellular studies. *Can J Physiol Pharmacol* 1996; **74**(Axv).

106 Armour JA. Myocardial ischaemia and the cardiac nervous system. *Cardiovasc Res* January 1999; **41**(1): 41–54.

107 Ardell JL, Dell'Italia LJ, Armour JA. Epilogue: relevance of the cardiac neuronal hierarchy in heart disease. In: Armour JA & Ardell JL, eds. *Basic and Clinical Neurocardiology*. Oxford University Press, New York, 2004: 419–424.

108 Cardin S, Li D, Thorin-Trescases N, Leung TK, Thorin E, Nattel S. Evolution of the atrial fibrillation substrate in experimental congestive heart failure: angiotensin-dependent and -independent pathways. *Cardiovasc Res* November 1, 2003; **60**(2): 315–325.

109 Arora RC, Cardinal R, Smith FM, Ardell JL, Dell'Italia LJ, Armour JA. Intrinsic cardiac nervous system in tachycardia induced heart failure. *Am J Physiol Regul Integr Comp Physiol* November 2003; **285**(5): R1212–R1223.

110 Severs NJ, Copper SR, Dupont E, Yeh HI, Ko YS, Matsushita T. Gap junction alterations in human cardiac disease. *Cardiovasc Res* 2004; **62**: 368–377.

111 Weber KT, Pick R, Silver MA *et al.* Fibrillar collagen and remodeling of dilated canine left ventricle. *Circulation* 1990; **82**: 1387–1401.

112 Pappone C, Santinelli V, Manguso F *et al.* Pulmonary vein denervation enhances long-term benefit after circumferential ablation for paroxysmal atrial fibrillation. *Circulation* January 27, 2004; **109**(3): 327–334.

113 Pappone C, Rosanio S, Oreto G *et al.* Circumferential radiofrequency ablation of pulmonary vein ostia: a new anatomic approach for curing atrial fibrillation. *Circulation* November 21, 2000; **102**(21): 2619–2628.

114 Nakagawa H, Sherlag BJ, Wu AW *et al.* Addition of selective ablation of autonomic ganglia to pulmonary vein antrum ablation for treatment of paroxysmal and persistent atrial fibrillation. *Circulation* 2005; **110**(17): III-543.

115 Platt M, Mandapati R, Sherlag BJ *et al.* Limiting the number and extend of radiofrequency applications to terminate atrial fibrillation and subsequently prevent its inducibility [Abstract]. *Heart Rhythm* 2004; **1**(suppl 1): S11.

116 Nakagawa H, Sherlag BJ, Aoyama H *et al.* Catheter ablation of cardiac autonomic system for preventing atrial fibrillation in a canine model [Abstract]. *Heart Rhythm* 2004; **1**(suppl 1): S10.

117 Rennie D. How to report randomized controlled trials. The CONSORT statement. *JAMA* 1996; **276**: 6492.

118 Anyanwu A, Treasure T. Surgical research: clinical trials in the cardiothoracic surgical literature. *Eur J Cardiol-Thorac Surg* 2004; **25**(299): 303.

CHAPTER 8

The maze procedure: past, present, and future

Niv Ad

Introduction

Atrial fibrillation is considered by many to be a mild arrhythmia; however, its associated morbidity and mortality directly relate with its detrimental sequelae: loss of atrial transport, irregular cardiac rhythm, and increased incidence of systemic thromboembolism. Each of these can serve as an indication for intervention, with the most important one being the elevated risk for thromboembolism.

Pharmacological treatment for atrial fibrillation is targeted to gain either rate or rhythm control. Recent reports comparing the two strategies showed no clear advantage of rhythm control over rate control in such patients. However, a significant number of patients in both groups was in atrial fibrillation when the reports were made and the follow-up is relatively short. Although the ventricular response rate can usually be controlled medically and relieve some of the symptoms, it is important to recognize the fact that the atrium is still fibrillating and the patient is still at a high risk for a stroke and heart failure. Therefore, in large number of patients with atrial fibrillation, pharmacological therapy is not optimal.

Surgery for atrial fibrillation: past

In 1980, Cox *et al.* described the left atrial isolation procedure. The procedure was capable in significant number of patients to confine atrial fibrillation to

the left atrium leaving the right atrium and the ventricles synchronized in sinus rhythm.

This procedure was relatively effective in restoring regular ventricular rhythm without the need for a permanent pacemaker. Interestingly, it also restored normal cardiac hemodynamics in patients with normal left ventricular function. This is due to the fact that the right atrium and the right ventricle beat in synchrony following the procedure. This results in normal right-sided cardiac output that is then delivered to the left side of the heart. Although the left atrium is isolated it can still serve as a conduit and delivers the normal right-sided output to the left ventricle that, if normally functioning, can adapt and deliver a normal forward cardiac output. Unfortunately, because the left atrium may continue to fibrillate the risk for systemic thromboembolism is not reduced by the procedure.

The other valid option available in the early 80s was surgical ablation of the His bundle and implantation of a VVI pacemaker [1]. This approach now utilizes a transvenous catheter ablation using radiofrequency energy in a very effective way [2]. It is designed mainly to control symptoms directly related to high ventricular response, palpitation, and tachycardia induced cardiomyopathy, but do not address the increased risk for thromboembolism and the loss of the atrial kick.

Therefore, it was a necessity to design a more complete surgical treatment for atrial fibrillation that should address the following goals: (1) abolishing atrial fibrillation and reestablishing sinus rhythm, (2) maintenance of A-V synchrony, (3) restitution of atrial transport function, and (4) elimination of the risk for thromboembolic event.

Manual of Surgical Treatment of Atrial Fibrillation.
Edited by Hauw T. Sie *et al.* © 2008 Blackwell Publishing,
ISBN: 978-1-4051-4032-4.

The maze procedure: from theory to clinical experience

The concept of the maze procedure is based on findings using a variety of canine models that were developed in the laboratory at Washington University, St Louis. They all had in common a series of atrial surgical incisions that were placed on the atria in an effort to prevent the ability of the atria to fibrillate [3–7]. Initially, the electrophysiology findings suggested that atrial flutter resulted from the presence of a large reentrant circuit in the right atrium revolving around the orifices of the inferior and the superior vena cava. The suggested mechanism for atrial fibrillation was similar and it was a large macro-reentrant circuit around the orifices of the left atrial appendage and the ostia of the four pulmonary veins [3, 5]. Based on these findings the first surgical procedure tried was the atrial transection procedure that involves an incision at the dorsal aspect of the atria from the annulus of the tricuspid valve to the annulus of the mitral valve. The procedure was performed on a patient in 1986 and the patient remained in sinus rhythm for 5 months with marked improvement of his symptom [8]. Despite the failure of this procedure to cure atrial fibrillation, the initial success suggested that it was, in fact, feasible to surgically modify the atria and prevent the development of atrial fibrillation. It was clear that human electrophysiological mapping inpatients with atrial fibrillation would enhance the understanding of the mechanisms underlying atrial fibrillation.

In addition, as with other arrhythmias, it was very unlikely that an effective surgical procedure to cure atrial fibrillation could be developed without a better understanding of the relationship between atrial anatomy and atrial electrophysiology in both normal and pathological circumstances. By combining computerized mapping data in humans and data recorded in animal model, a better picture of the mechanisms of atrial flutter and fibrillation evolved [7, 9, 10]. It was documented that all types of atrial flutter and fibrillation have three components: (1) macro-reentrant circuit(s), (2) passive atrial conduction, in atrial portion not involved in the macro-reentrant circuit(s), and (3) atrioventricular conduction. The electrophysiological characteristics of these three components define a spectrum of atrial arrhythmias, from simple atrial flutter to complex atrial fibrillation. Because of the fact that the macro-reentrant circuits responsible for atrial flutter and atrial fibrillation are fleeting in nature, the application of activation maps to guide surgery with on-line maps is extremely difficult to apply. A surgical procedure capable of interrupting any and all macro-reentrant circuits that might potentially develop in the atria was designed. The procedure was designed to allow the sinoatrial node to resume activity following surgery and direct the propagation of the sinus impulse through both atria. The surgical procedure that was conceived to accomplish these goals is based on the concept of a maze and, as a result, is called the maze procedure [8, 11]. The maze procedure was first applied clinically on September 25, 1987, at the Barnes Hospital in St Louis, Missouri [11]. The maze I procedure caused late incidence of two unacceptable problems: (1) the frequent inability of patients to generate appropriate sinus tachycardia in response to exercise and (2) left atrial dysfunction. Therefore, the maze I was modified twice to the maze III procedure. The maze III procedure was associated with a higher incidence of sinus rhythm, improved long-term sinus node function, fewer pacemaker implantation, and improved long-term atrial transport function. In addition, the maze III procedure is technically less demanding than the maze I and II procedures [12, 13].

The maze III procedure was performed in hundreds of patients and was proven to be highly effective in ablating atrial fibrillation [14–17]. In a recent report Damiano *et al.* showed excellent long-term results in patients having the maze procedure either as an isolated or combined procedure [18, 19]. Another important impact of the maze III procedure is the significant reduction in the rate of cerebrovascular accidents and transient ischemic events. This positive effect is directly related to the high success rate of the procedure in ablating atrial fibrillation and to the amputation of the left atrial appendage [20, 21].

Despite its remarkable success the procedure has not been widely adopted by surgeons, cardiologists, and primary care physicians, in part owing to its complexity and technical difficulty. There was also high incidence of morbidity associated with the procedure such as reoperation for bleeding and 10% of pacemaker implantation. Because of the technical complexity of the maze procedure, it has thus far required a formal median sternotomy with division of the sternum and cardiopulmonary bypass [11, 22]. As a result only few surgeons started to perform the procedure and gained sufficient experience and many were seeking for a less invasive or simpler approach to treat this extremely common arrhythmia.

The maze procedure: modifications for the original procedure and surgical ablation devices

The research of atrial fibrillation continued to evolve and better understanding regarding the pathophysiology of the arrhythmia was obtained. The main focus of the research is atrial remodeling as a result of atrial fibrillation and the electrophysiological basis for the arrhythmia. The research of atrial remodeling and reverse remodeling following successful treatment of atrial fibrillation is evolving and may contribute to our understanding of the mechanism of atrial fibrillation and failure of treatment. Meanwhile the development of new mapping systems led to better understanding of the electrophysiology involved with atrial fibrillation. In 1998, Michael Haissaguerre and his colleagues from Bordeaux, France, published a key work describing the pattern of the arrhythmogenic foci originating atrial fibrillation [23]. They studied patients with paroxysmal atrial fibrillation and found that the pulmonary veins are an important source of ectopic beats, initiating frequent paroxysmal atrial fibrillation and hypothesized that these foci will probably respond to treatment with radiofrequency ablation. Based on these findings a new strategy for nonpharmacological treatment was developed: the pulmonary vein isolation. It is clear now that the pulmonary veins have an important role in the pathophysiology of atrial fibrillation, but some patients would exhibit a much more complex pattern of the arrhythmia and the solution in certain cases is not as simple as sole pulmonary vein isolation [24, 25].

In the late 90s, the first few cases of cryomaze procedure were performed. These were mainly application of cryoablation lines. The objective of the cryoablation is to replace the surgical incision with transmural ablation lines to create conduction block. In 1999, the full maze procedure was performed using cryothermal energy as the only ablation modality. It was later that year when the maze III procedure was modified to the maze IV by isolating the pulmonary veins on each side rather than performing the original box lesion ([26], Figure 8.6). This modification for the maze III procedure was based on the findings published in the work of Haissaguerre [23]. The cryosurgical maze procedure was also performed as a minimally invasive procedure through a right anterior thoracotomy [27].

Most of the surgical modifications to the original maze procedure were based on new surgical ablation devices, utilizing various ablative technologies. The new devices facilitated new surgical procedures to treat atrial fibrillation using different ablation protocols.

Alternative energy sources to treat atrial fibrillation

In the past few years, it is a common approach to replace the surgical incisions with linear lines of ablation. Various ablation devices have been developed using different energy sources to perform the ablation including radiofrequency energy (unipolar and bipolar) [28, 29], microwave [30], laser [31], cryoablation [32], and high-frequency ultrasound [33]. The concept behind these new technologies is to replace the surgical incisions with lines of transmural ablation creating conduction blocks. By using the ablation devices properly the goal of the maze procedure to block reentrant circuits is maintained. Theoretically, the cut and sew maze procedure can be replaced by an easier technique that is much less demanding technically and may be performed using less invasive tools.

1 *Cryoablation*: The use of cryothermal energy in arrhythmia surgery is not new to surgeons [34]. Therefore, it was not surprising that cryoenergy was widely adopted by surgeons while performing the surgical ablation of atrial fibrillation [35, 36]. In the cryosurgical approach the atrial incisions of the standard maze procedure are replaced by linear cryolesions. The cryosurgical procedure results in a shorter and technically less demanding procedure. Whether surgical incisions or cryolesions are used to perform the maze procedure, it is essential to create

transmural atrial lesions to prevent late recurrence of atrial fibrillation. Since the cryolesions actually can be observed as they develop, it is a simple matter to determine when transmural ablation has or has not occurred.

2 *Radiofrequency:* Over the past 15 years, significant advances have been made in radiofrequency ablation devices as a means to ablate cardiac tissue [28, 37]. The energy delivered results in myocardial necrosis and has the ability to electrically isolate myocardial tissue. Radiofrequency is being used as the energy source to treat atrial fibrillation by creating ablation lines in the atrial tissue. Unipolar radiofrequency devices were found to be unreliable in creating transmural lesions, especially when used on beating hearts [38]. These devices produce electrode temperatures of 80–90°C and can cause severe thermal injury to adjacent tissue. One of the most devastating complications with unipolar radiofrequency is left atrial esophageal fistula [39].

The basic physics of radiofrequency energy ablation are based on the rationale that the ablation device and the tissue should be in a close contact. Uneven contact and tissue pressure throughout the catheter increases the energy required and results in incomplete and nontransmural lesion.

As a result of the limitations of the unipolar devices, bipolar devices were developed. These new devices enable the surgeon to perform reproducible transmural lesions. The devices are safe and the risk of perforation or fistula is very low. The bipolar devices are in a form of clamp. There are saline irrigated devices as well as dry devices [40, 41].

3 *Microwave:* Microwaves are electromagnetic waves delivered at a very high frequency. As a result heat is generated in the tissue and myocardial necrosis is detectable [42]. A microwave catheter is a flexible catheter and it includes antenna, either monopolar or helico coil type, mounted on a plastic shaft designed to direct the waves to the targeted site to protect the surrounding tissue.

The clinical experience gained with microwave technology is relatively good; however, most of the reports include left atrial lesions only or pulmonary vein isolation only performed on beating heart with the lesions applied epicardially [43, 44]. A recent report studied cadavers who had epicardial microwave ablation documented nontransmural lesions in all of them [45].

4 *High intensity focused ultrasound:* High intensity focused ultrasound (HIFU) is a technology, which uses focused ultrasound energy to selectively destroy biological tissue at depth without affecting intervening, anatomical structures. The medical ablation system designed to deliver HIFU energy to ablate cardiac tissue. The system consists of the ablation control system (ACS) generator, a family of disposable ablation devices, and a set of accessories. The ACS is a microprocessor-based unit that provides acoustic power to the ultrasound transducers.

The clinical experience with this device is fairly limited, however, promising especially when used epicardially on beating heart inpatients with intermittent atrial fibrillation [33].

5 *Laser:* Laser energy consists in high-energy optical waves delivered through an optical coupling fiber and a radiating tip. The beam emanating from the tip of the probe can be adjusted in power, time, and energy. Although all laser ablation is based on generation of heat, the tissue effects are dependent on the wavelength used. The laser energy commonly used is the Nd:YAG and its tissue effects are caused by combination of direct heating and mechanical damage [42].

The clinical experience is limited and based on epicardial pulmonary vein isolation done using minimally invasive techniques [46].

Surgical alternatives for the treatment of atrial fibrillation

When attempting surgical ablation of atrial fibrillation cardiac surgeons have different options for surgical procedures. Unfortunately, only the full maze procedure is a product of a thorough laboratory and research process and some of the surgical procedures that are performed and published are based on limited experience and technical feasibility rather than true science.

The different surgical approaches for the treatment of atrial fibrillation that have been used and reported are:

1 Procedures confined to the left atrium only; lesions based on the maze procedure or pulmonary vein isolation only.

2 Procedure performed in both atria; maze procedure and its modifications of bi-atrial ablations.

3 Procedure supported with cardiopulmonary bypass and beating heart procedures.

4 Median sternotomy approach versus minimally invasive approach through small thoracotomies and access facilitated by ports.

Clinical factors affecting the modified surgical procedure for atrial fibrillation

Many of the problems that have been encountered several years ago when the maze procedure was developed are now being repeated in patients undergoing these reduced procedures. Therefore, a better classification of the candidates for the procedure may enhance our understanding in the pathophysiology of atrial fibrillation and will improve the results of the modified procedures.

Before modifying the maze procedure there are a few variables that should be discussed and investigated for their possible impact on the results of the surgical treatment in a certain patient:

1 What is the type of atrial fibrillation?
2 How long is the history of atrial fibrillation? In other words, are we expecting a significant atrial tissue remodeling?
3 What is the size of the left and right atria?
4 Are there any other organic heart diseases such as rheumatic heart disease or ischemic heart disease?
5 Are we dealing with an isolated procedure for curing lone atrial fibrillation or combined procedure in which we are expecting the use of CPB?
6 Are there any clots in the left atrial appendage or patent foramen ovale that would limit the ability to perform off-bypass procedures?

It is clear that only a miniscule percentage of the patients with lone atrial fibrillation will ever become candidates for the classical open-heart maze procedures (cut and sew). However, most of us perform device-based ablation procedures, which are less complex and technically demanding. Hence, the entire discussion concerning the complexity of the maze procedure should be shifted from its technical difficulties to the real necessity of the entire lesion set involved with it.

The continuing effort to relieve the invasive downside of the maze procedure is warranted but with caution and no compromises in the success rate.

The surgery for atrial fibrillation should involve a true decision-making process like any other surgical procedure performed by us. Therefore, combining all these variables and the understanding of the importance of each one of them may lead to higher

success of the surgical procedure. There is a clear difference between most of the surgical patients and the patients that are good candidate for percutaneous ablation. Most of the patients that are treated successfully with catheters by the electrophysiologists are those with intermittent atrial fibrillation and smaller left and right atrium.

The maze procedure: current surgical strategies and future development

Modern atrial fibrillation surgery should include different surgical approaches to match the procedure to a given patient. Therefore, a few different surgical options are discussed.

Surgery through midsternotomy

Currently, this type of approach is being offered to patients with atrial fibrillation candidates for a combined surgical procedure, such as mitral valve surgery, aortic valve surgery, and CABG. It is also offered to patients that are candidates for isolated maze procedure that we find high risk for the minimally invasive approach.

The procedure should be performed by incorporating the maze III or IV lesion set. As mentioned, there is no place for the cut and sew technique unless the surgical ablation devices are not available. Any device that satisfied the operator in creating reliable transmural lesions can be used. Surgeons should be familiar with the limitations of each device.

In an effort to reduce the cardiopulmonary bypass and cross-clamp time, different parts of the operation can be performed off bypass and before or after cross-clamping of the aorta.

Right-sided lesions: These can be performed in every case before the patient is connected to cardiopulmonary bypass. One way of doing it is based on applying three purse strings to the right atrial wall through which the ablation device is being introduced (Figures 8.1–8.5; [47]).

Left-sided lesions: There are two possible ways of performing the lesions in the left atrium. The first is using the classical box lesion around all four pulmonary veins as described in the original maze procedure. This approach is usually performed in re-do cases where dissection of the epicardial adhesions around the pulmonary vein may be difficult. The other option is to encircle the right and left

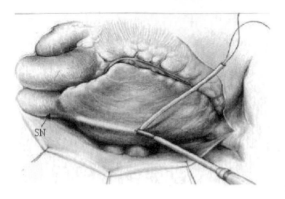

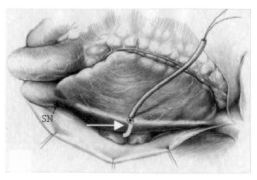

Figure 8.1 A purse-string suture is placed in the posterior–lateral right atrium and a linear cryoprobe is inserted through the purse string into the inside of the right atrium. A cryolesion is placed in a cephalad direction into the postero-lateral aspect of the superior vena cava (SVC) orifice and away from the SA node. Reproduced with permission from [47].

Figure 8.3 Through the same purse string suture, a third lesion is made along the lateral wall of the right atrium down to interatrial septum and the right pulmonary veins (Figure 8.3—closed arrow). Reproduced with permission from [47].

pulmonary veins from the epicardial side, this can be done off-bypass in some cases and with the support of cardiopulmonary bypass but without cross-clamp in others. Following the isolation of the pulmonary veins and the necessary steps the left atrium is opened and a connecting lesion and a mitral valve isthmus lesion to include also the coronary sinus are being created (Figures 8.6–8.9; [47]).

Minimally invasive maze procedure through right anterior mini-thoracotomy

This procedure can be performed for isolated maze procedure or for procedures combining mitral

surgery, tricuspid valve surgery, or repair of an atrial septal defect. The minimally invasive approach can also be performed in re-do surgery, especially when repeated midsternotomy may carry an increased risk.

The procedure also involves groin cannulation to connect the patients to the heart lung machine. When using this approach there are two different options for cross-clamping the aorta. The first is by using a clamp such as the Chitwood clamp and the second option is by the use of one of the aortic balloon endo-clamp.

The right-sided lesions can be performed on a beating heart with or without cardiopulmonary

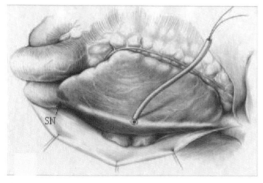

Figure 8.2 Using the same purse-string suture, a second cryolesion is placed into the orifice of the inferior vena cava (IVC) to complete the longitudinal lesion from the SVC to the IVC. Reproduced with permission from [47].

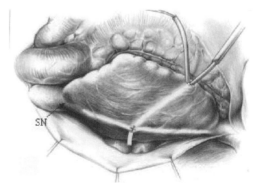

Figure 8.4 The first purse-string suture is tied and a second purse-string suture is placed near the AV groove of the free-wall of the right atrium. The cryoprobe is inserted through this second purse-string suture to create the linear "T" lesion across the lower right atrium. Reproduced with permission from [47].

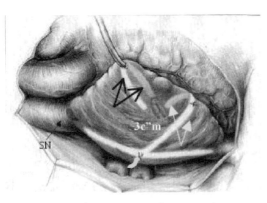

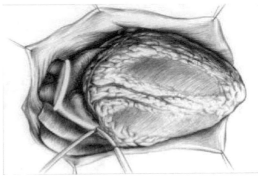

Figure 8.5 Using the same purse-string suture, the cryolesion is extended down to the level of the tricuspid valve annulus at the junction of the anterior and posterior commissures (Figures 8.4 and 8.5—closed white arrows). The second purse-string suture is then tied and a third purse-string suture is placed in the right atrial appendage. A lateral right atrial cryolesion is placed from the tip of the atrial appendage toward the previously placed "T" lesion, leaving at least 3 cm between its tip and the "T" cryolesion. Using the same purse-string suture in the right atrial appendage, a cryolesion is placed from the appendage down to the anteromedial tricuspid valve annulus at the septal commissure (Figure 8.5—open arrows). Reproduced with permission from [47].

Figure 8.7 The ventricular apex is then retracted in a cephalad direction out of the pericardium using the left hand to expose the intrapericardial segments of both left pulmonary veins. After minimal dissection around the left pulmonary veins, the two cryoprobes are "clamped" around both left pulmonary veins as they enter the left atrium posteriorly and cryothermia is applied to both probes. The result is a circumferential, transmural cryolesion around the orifices of the left pulmonary veins. A purse-string suture is then placed in the tip of the left atrial appendage and a linear cryoprobe is inserted inside the atrial appendage with its tip placed into the orifice of the left superior pulmonary vein to create a linear lesion. The cryoprobe is then withdrawn and the left atrial appendage is excluded from the rest of the left atrium by stapling or suturing the base of the appendage from the outside. Reproduced with permission from [47].

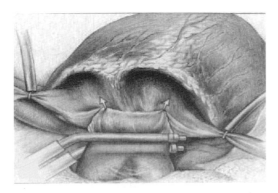

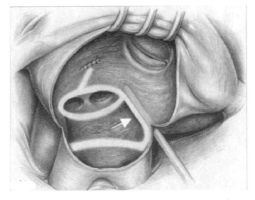

Figure 8.6 The interatrial groove is dissected completely and the right superior and right inferior pulmonary veins are dissected free circumferentially. One linear cryoprobe is placed posterior to the right pulmonary veins as they enter the left atrium. A second identical cryoprobe is placed on the anterior surface of the veins in the same plane. The cryoprobes are then "squeezed" together firmly and 2-minute cryolesion is created by freezing with both probes. This result is a transmural cryolesion around the orifices of the right pulmonary veins. A left ventricular vent is placed via the right superior pulmonary vein. Reproduced with permission from [47].

Figure 8.8 A standard left atriotomy is performed after placement of the aortic cross-clamp and instituting cardioplegic arrest. A lesion connecting the inferior right and left inferior pulmonary veins is performed using the linear cryoprobe. As mentioned, epicardial pulmonary vein isolation can be replaced by endocardial box lesion to isolate all four pulmonary veins, it is then when the left atrial appendage is over sawn from the inside. Reproduced with permission from [47].

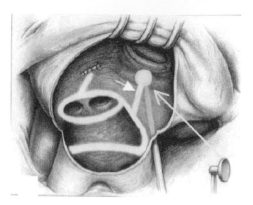

Figure 8.9 Creating a lesion from the pulmonary veins connecting line down to the posterior mitral valve annulus with the linear cryoprobe and ablation of the coronary sinus with the 15 mm right angle probe concludes the procedure (Figure 8.9—arrows). Cryoablation of the coronary sinus is performed on the epicardial surface (open arrow). This technique decreases the aortic cross-clamp time by reducing the number of cryolesions that are necessary after opening the left atrium to three for those that are marked with arrows in Figures 8.8–8.9. Reproduced with permission from [47].

support. This part is performed in a similar way to the midsternotomy approach as was shown in the previous section.

Following cross-clamp a vertical left atriotomy is performed and the left-sided lesions are applied. The left-sided lesions pattern follows the maze III, thus creating a box lesion around all the pulmonary veins that connect it to the left atrial appendage and to the mitral valve isthmus with special attention to the coronary sinus. The left atrial appendage orifice is then over sewn from the endocardial side. Mitral valve procedures should be performed only after completion of the maze procedure to ensure perfect left atrial isthmus ablation. In case of tricuspid valve surgery and repair of an atrial septal defect, double venous cannulation is required and the right atrium is opened so the purse-string approach cannot be applied. When performed properly the results that should be anticipated from the minimally invasive procedure are excellent [35].

Pulmonary vein isolation

Surgery to achieve pulmonary vein isolation only with or without left atrial appendage is now being performed. The procedure can be a totally endoscopic procedure using different ablation devices

[31, 44]. Bilateral limited thoracotomies and or mini-sternotomy can also be used to control and isolate the pulmonary veins [33, 48]. The major advantage of this approach is that it can be performed as a beating heart surgery without the use of cardiopulmonary bypass and in most instances pulmonary vein isolation and left atrial appendage disarticulation can be offered to the patients.

The experiences gathered with this approach is fairly limited and the follow-up in most reports is fairly short in a highly selected group of patients. It is clear that pulmonary vein isolation is not as successful in patients with a more complex atrial fibrillation, such as permanent atrial fibrillation and enlarged left atrium [33].

Map-guided surgery for atrial fibrillation

The traditional model for arrhythmia surgery was based on electrophysiological assessment of the arrhythmia followed by a definitive procedure based on the analysis of each patient. The maze procedure is not a guided procedure and thus theoretically includes some unnecessary lesions for some patients. Data presented in recent months showed that in some patients in a very limited follow-up there is a potential to offer high cure for patients by performing procedures that are confined to the left atrium or include only isolation of the pulmonary veins [33, 48]. However, the success rate for atrial fibrillation by limited procedures is in general less than optimal [49]. The use of epicardial mapping devices showed to be very effective in understanding the pathophysiology of the arrhythmia and guide the surgeons to choose the appropriate procedure with excellent success rate. Map-guided surgery has a lot of potential; however, mapping patients in atrial fibrillation is very complex and the current intraoperative mapping devices would not allow minimally invasive surgery [50].

Hopefully in the future catheter-based mapping devices are going to be incorporated, and the limited surgical ablation procedures will be performed using minimally invasive approach.

References

1 Cox JL, Boineau JP, Schuessler RB *et al.* Electrophysiologic basis, surgical development and clinical results of the maze

procedure for atrial flutter and atrial fibrillation. In: Karp RB & Wechsler AS, eds. *Advances in Cardiac Surgery 1995*, Vol. 6. Mosby-Year book, St Louis, 1996: 1.

2 Queiroga A, Marshall HJ, Clune M, Gammage MD. Ablate and pace revisited: long term survival and predictors of permanent atrial fibrillation. *Heart* September 2003; **89**(9): 1035–1038.

3 Boineau JP, Mooney C, Hudson R *et al*. Observation on re-entrant excitation pathways and refractory period distribution in spontaneous and experimental atrial flutter in dog. In: Kulbertus HE, ed. *Re-Entrant Arrhythmias*. University Park Press, Baltimore, MD, 1977: 79–98.

4 Smith PK, Holman WL, Cox JL. Surgical treatment of supraventricular tachyarrhythmias. *Surg Clin North Am* 1985; **65**: 553–570.

5 Boineau JP, Schuessler RB, Mooney C *et al*. Natural and evoked atrial flutter due to circus movement in dogs. *Am J Cardiol* 1980; **45**: 1167–1181.

6 D'Agostino HJ, Jr, Harada A, Schuessler RB *et al*. Global epicardial mapping of atrial fibrillation in a canine model of chronic mitral regurgitation. *Circulation* 1987; **76**(suppl IV): 165.

7 Yamaguchi S, Sato S, Schuessler RB *et al*. Induced atrial arrhythmias in a canine model of left atrial enlargement. *Pacing Clin Electrophysiol* 1990; **13**: 556.

8 Cox JL, Scussler RB, D'Agostino HJ, Jr *et al*. The surgical treatment of atrial fibrillation: III. Development of a definite surgical procedure. *J Thorac Cardiovasc Surg* 1991; **101**: 569–583.

9 Canavan TE, Schuessler RB, Cain ME *et al*. Computerized global electrophysiological mapping of the atrium in a patient with multiple supraventricular arrhythmias. *Ann Thorac Surg* 1988; **46**: 223–231.

10 Cox JL, Canavan TE, Schuessler RB *et al*. The surgical treatment of atrial fibrillation II. Intraoperative electrophysiologic mapping and description of the electrophysiologic basis of atrial flutter and atrial fibrillation. *J Thorac Cardiovasc Surg* 1991; **101**: 406–426.

11 Cox JL. The surgical treatment of atrial fibrillation: IV. Surgical technique. *J Thorac Cardiovasc Surg* 1991; **101**: 584–592.

12 Cox JL, Boineau JP, Schuessler RB *et al*. Modifications of the maze procedure for atrial flutter and atrial fibrillation. I. Rationale and surgical results. *J Thorac Cardiovasc Surg* 1995; **110**: 473–483.

13 Cox JL, Jaquiss RD, Schuessler RB *et al*. Modifications of the maze procedure for atrial flutter and atrial fibrillation. II. Surgical technique of the maze III procedure. *J Thorac Cardiovasc Surg* 1995; **110**: 485–495.

14 McCarthy PM, Gillinov AM, Castle L, Chung M, Cosgrove D, III. The Cox-maze procedure: the Cleveland clinic experience. *Semin Thorac Cardiovasc Surg* 2000; **12**(1): 25–29.

15 Schaff HV, Dearani JA, Daly RC, Orszulak TA, Danielson GK. Cox-maze procedure for atrial fibrillation: Mayo clinic experience. *Semin Thorac Cardiovasc Surg* 2000; **12**(1): 30–37.

16 Arcidi JM, Jr, Doty DB, Millar RC. The maze procedure: the LDS Hospital experience. *Semin Thorac Cardiovasc Surg* 2000; **12**(1): 38–43.

17 Kosakai Y. Treatment of atrial fibrillation using the maze procedure: the Japanese experience. *Semin Thorac Cardiovasc Surg* January 2000; **12**(1): 44–52.

18 Damiano RJ, Jr, Gaynor SL, Bailey M *et al*. The long-term outcome of patients with coronary disease and atrial fibrillation undergoing the Cox maze procedure. *J Thorac Cardiovasc Surg* 2003; **126**: 2016–2021.

19 Prasad SM, Maniar HS, Camillo CJ *et al*. The Cox maze III procedure for atrial fibrillation: long-term efficacy in patients undergoing lone versus concomitant procedures. *J Thorac Cardiovasc Surg* 2003; **126**: 1822–1828.

20 Bando K, Kobayashi J, Sasako Y, Tagusari O, Niwaya K, Kitamura S. Effect of maze procedure in patients with atrial fibrillation undergoing valve replacement. *J Heart Valve Dis* 2002; **11**(5): 719–724.

21 Ad N, Cox JL, Palazzo TL *et al*. Stroke prevention as an indication for the maze procedure in the treatment of atrial fibrillation. *Semin Thorac Cardiovasc Surg* 2000; **12**: 56–62.

22 Cox JL, Schuessler RB, Lappas DG *et al*. An 8.5 year clinical experience with surgery for atrial fibrillation. *Ann Surg* 1996; **224**(3): 267–275.

23 Haissaguerre M, Jais P, Shah DC *et al*. Spontaneous initiation of atrial fibrillation by ectopic beats originating in the pulmonary veins. *N Engl J Med* September 3, 1998; **339**(10): 659–666.

24 Nademanee K, McKenzie J, Kosar E *et al*. A new approach for catheter ablation of atrial fibrillation: mapping of the electrophysiologic substrate. *J Am Coll Cardiol* 2004; **43**: 2044–2053.

25 Schmitt C, Ndrepepa G, Weber S *et al*. Biatrial multisite mapping of atrial premature complexes triggering onset of atrial fibrillation. *Am J Cardiol* June 15, 2002; **89**(12): 1381–1387.

26 Gaynor SL, Schuessler RB, Bailey MS *et al*. Surgical treatment of atrial fibrillation: predictors of late recurrence. *J Thorac Cardiovasc Surg* January 2005; **129**(1): 104–111.

27 Cox JL, Ad N. New surgical and catheter-based modifications of the maze procedure. *Semin Thorac Cardiovasc Surg* January 2000; **12**(1): 68–73.

28 Khargi K, Deneke T, Haardt H *et al*. Saline-irrigated, cooled-tip radiofrequency ablation is an effective technique to perform the maze procedure. *Ann Thorac Surg* September 2001; **72**(3): S1090–S1095.

29 Gillinov AM, McCarthy PM, Blackstone EH *et al*. Surgical ablation of atrial fibrillation with bipolar radiofrequency

as the primary modality. *J Thorac Cardiovasc Surg* June 2005; **129**(6): 1322–1329.

30 Kabbani SS, Murad G, Jamil H, Sabbagh A, Hamzeh K. Ablation of atrial fibrillation using microwave energy—early experience. *Asian Cardiovasc Thorac Ann* September 2005; **13**(3): 247–250.

31 Garrido MJ, Williams M, Argenziano M. Minimally invasive surgery for atrial fibrillation: toward a totally endoscopic, beating heart approach. *J Card Surg* May–June 2004; **19**(3): 216–220.

32 Mack CA, Milla F, Ko W *et al.* Surgical treatment of atrial fibrillation using argon-based cryoablation during concomitant cardiac procedures. *Circulation* August 30, 2005; **112**(suppl 9): I1–I6.

33 Ninet J, Roques X, Seitelberger R *et al.* Surgical ablation of atrial fibrillation with off-pump, epicardial, high-intensity focused ultrasound: results of a multicenter trial. *J Thorac Cardiovasc Surg* September 2005; **130**(3): 803–809.

34 Ohkawa S, Hackel DB, Mikat EM, Gallagher JJ, Cox JL, Sealy WC. Anatomic effects of cryoablation of the atrioventricular conduction system. *Circulation* 1982; **65**: 1155–1162.

35 Cox JL, Ad N. The minimally invasive maze procedure [Abstract]. *Circulation* 1999; **100**(suppl I): 732.

36 Doll N, Meyer R, Walther T, Mohr FW. A new cryoprobe for intraoperative ablation of atrial fibrillation. *Ann Thorac Surg* 2004; **77**(4): 1460–1462.

37 Jazayeri MR, Hempe SL, Sra JS *et al.* Selective transcatheter ablation of fast and slow pathways using radiofrequency energy in patients with atrioventricular nodal reentrant tachycardia. *Circulation* 1992; **85**: 1318–1328.

38 Hoenicke EM, Strange RG, Jr, Patel H, Prophet GA, Damiano RJ, Jr. Initial experience with epicardial radiofrequency ablation catheter in an ovine model: moving towards an endoscopic maze procedure. *Surg Forum* 2000; **81**: 79–82.

39 Doll N, Borger MA, Fabricius A *et al.* Esophageal perforation during left atrial radiofrequency ablation: is the risk too high? *J Thorac Cardiovasc Surg* 2003; **125**(4): 836–842.

40 Vicol C, Kur F, Eifert S *et al.* Bipolar irrigated radiofrequency ablation of the posterior–inferior left atrium and coronary sinus is feasible and safe. *Heart Surg Forum* 2004; **7**(6): E535–E538.

41 Prasad SM, Maniar HS, Schuessler RB, Damiano RJ, Jr. Chronic transmural ablation by using radiofrequency energy on the beating heart. *J Thorac Cardiovasc Surg* 2002; **124**(4): 708–713.

42 Viola N, Williams MR, Oz MC. The technology in use for the surgical ablation of atrial fibrillation. *Semin Thorac Cardiovasc Surg* 2002; **14**: 198–205.

43 Knaut M, Tugtekin SM, Spitzer S, Gulielmos V. Combined atrial fibrillation and mitral valve surgery using microwave technology. *Semin Thorac Cardiovasc Surg* July 2002; **14**(3): 226–231.

44 Saltman AE, Rosenthal LS, Francalancia NA, Lahey SJ. A completely endoscopic approach to microwave ablation for atrial fibrillation. *Heart Surg Forum* 2003; **6**(3): E38–E41.

45 Accord RE, van Suylen RJ, van Brakel TJ, Maessen JG. Post-mortem histologic evaluation of microwave lesions after epicardial pulmonary vein isolation for atrial fibrillation. *Ann Thorac Surg* September 2005; **80**(3): 881–887.

46 Garrido MJ, Williams M, Argenziano M. Minimally invasive surgery for atrial fibrillation: toward a totally endoscopic, beating heart approach. *J Card Surg* 2004; **19**(3): 216–220.

47 Ad N. The cryosurgical maze procedure. Adult expert technique at CTSNet. Available at: http://www.ctsnet.org/sections/clinicalresources/adultcardiac/expert_tech-5.html.

48 Wolf RK, Schneeberger EW, Osterday R *et al.* Video-assisted bilateral pulmonary vein isolation and left atrial appendage exclusion for atrial fibrillation. *J Thorac Cardiovasc Surg* 2005; **130**: 797–802.

49 Barnett SD, Ad N. Surgical ablation as treatment for the elimination of atrial fibrillation: a meta-analysis. *J Thorac Cardiovasc Surg* 2006; **131**: 1029–1035.

50 Nitta T, Ohmori H, Sakamoto S, Miyagi Y, Kanno S, Shimizu K. Map-guided surgery for atrial fibrillation. *J Thorac Cardiovasc Surg* 2003; **129**: 291–299.

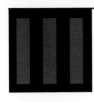

PART III

Modifications of the Cox-maze, use of alternative surgical patterns, and energy sources

CHAPTER 9

The radial procedure for atrial fibrillation: theoretical basis and clinical application

Takashi Nitta

Introduction

The radial procedure was developed as an outgrowth of an alternative to the maze procedure. The atrial incisions are designed to radiate from the sinus node toward the atrioventricular annular margins, parallel to the atrial activation sequence and the atrial coronary arteries. The procedure avoids isolation of any atrial segments except for the left atrial (LA) cuff of the pulmonary veins (PVs). It has been shown that the procedure preserves a physiological atrial activation sequence and recruits more myocardium for atrial transport function. Thus, the procedure is expected to prevent thromboembolism more effectively.

Drawbacks of the maze procedure

Although the maze procedure cures atrial fibrillation (AF) in the majority of patients [1], insufficient LA transport function is occasionally seen after the procedure. A study of postoperative atrial transport function performed approximately 6 months after the maze procedure using Doppler echocardiography or magnetic resonance imaging revealed that 98% of patients had right atrial (RA) transport function but only 86% had LA transport function [2]. Although the presence of atrial mechanical contraction has been demonstrated in most patients after the maze procedure, it is important to consider

Manual of Surgical Treatment of Atrial Fibrillation.
Edited by Hauw T. Sie *et al.* © 2008 Blackwell Publishing,
ISBN: 978-1-4051-4032-4.

whether the amount of atrial mechanical function is enough to provide the level of atrial transport function required to eliminate the risk of systemic thromboembolism. Quantitative analysis of atrial function in patients after the maze procedure revealed that the LA transport function was significantly less than that in normal control subjects, whereas the RA function was comparable [3, 4]. The possible mechanisms underlying the insufficient LA transport function after the maze procedure are the isolated posterior LA between the PV orifices, discordant activation of neighboring atrial segments across the incisions, delayed activation in the lateral LA, and interrupted atrial coronary arteries. The insufficient LA transport function may result in unsatisfactory cardiac function postoperatively in the patients with left ventricular diastolic dysfunction. More importantly, the insufficient LA contraction can permit thrombus formation on the LA endocardium and may cause thromboembolic events even when the heart returns to sinus rhythm.

Concept of the radial procedure

We hypothesized that a procedure with atrial incisions radiating from the sinus node toward the atrioventricular annular margins, running parallel to the activation sequence and atrial coronary arteries, would provide a more physiologic atrial activation–contraction sequence and optimize the atrial contribution to ventricular filling [5]. The concepts of the maze and radial procedures are compared in Figure 9.1. It is hypothesized that the activation

(a)

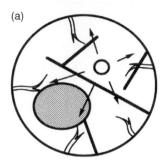

(b)

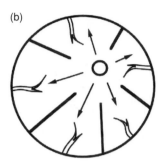

Figure 9.1 Schema of the concepts of the maze procedure (a) and the radial procedure (b). The large outer circle denotes the atria, and its outer limit is bounded by the atrioventricular annular margins. The small circle indicates the sinoatrial node, and the shaded area indicates the isolated portion of the atrium. Arrows indicate the activation wavefront from the sinoatrial node, radiating toward the annular margins. The atrial coronary arteries, arising at the atrioventricular groove, are also schematically drawn. Note that the radial procedure preserves a more physiologic activation sequence and preserves blood supply to most atrial segments, whereas the atrial incisions of the maze procedure desynchronize the activation sequence, and some of the incisions cross the atrial coronary arteries.

wavefront from the sinoatrial node radiates centrifugally toward the atrioventricular annular margins in normal atria and that the atrial coronary arteries, originating at the atrioventricular groove, distribute centripetally toward the sinus node. In the left panel, the atrial incisions of the maze procedure desynchronize this physiologic activation sequence and prolong the total activation time of the atria. Some of the incisions cross the atrial coronary arteries. Also, there is a large electrically isolated region encompassing the PV orifices. In the right panel, the atrial incisions of the radial procedure parallel the direction of the physiologic activation sequence and the direction of the blood supply. Thus, there is no electrically or mechanically isolated region. It is hypothesized that these incisions will better preserve the physiologic activation sequence and blood supply to most atrial segments.

Lesion sets of the radial procedure

Following the concept of the radial procedure, the atrial incisions were designed based on the coronary artery distribution and activation sequence of the atria [6]. Figure 9.2 illustrates the atrial incisions and the subsequent activation sequence during sinus rhythm after the radial and maze procedures. The RA incisions are similar for both procedures, with the exception of the excision of the RA appendage. The RA appendage has been shown to secrete atrial natriuretic peptides [7], and reduced se-

cretion of these peptides has been demonstrated in patients after the maze procedure [8]. To preserve secretion of atrial natriuretic peptides, the RA appendage is not excised in the radial procedure but is incised to prevent reentry in the lateral RA. In addition, major bridging trabeculae in the RA appendage are divided to eliminate reentry in these structures. The other RA incisions are the same as in the maze procedure.

The radial procedure incisions in the LA and interatrial septum are entirely different from those of the maze procedure. One incision, beginning at the anterior limbus of the fossa ovalis, extends inferoposteriorly toward the lower posterior interatrial septum and to the right posteroinferior wall of the LA, passing near the right inferior PV orifice, and continues down to the mitral valve annulus between the middle and posteromedial scallops. The other incision, beginning in the superior LA between the right and left upper PVs, connects with the LA appendage excision line and extends anteromedially further downward to the mitral valve annulus at the anterolateral commissure. These two transverse incisions; which divide the LA into three parts, recruit the posterior LA as a contractile component and preserve both a physiological activation sequence and the atrial coronary arteries. Because these incisions parallel the activation sequence during sinus rhythm, a synchronous LA activation sequence is maintained. In addition, the right and left PVs are isolated using cryoablation. The cryolesions around

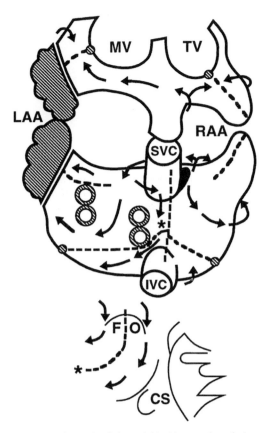

Figure 9.2 Schematic of the atrial incisions and cryolesions in the radial procedure. The upper, middle, and lower panels represent the superior and posterior epicardium and the interatrial septum, respectively. The small dark region of the RA at the junction with the SVC represents the sinus node, and the arrows indicate the activation sequence after the procedure. The broken lines indicate the atrial incisions, and the shaded region represents the excised LA appendage. Unlike the maze procedure, the RA appendage is not excised to preserve the secretion of atrial natriuretic peptide. The small shaded circles indicate the cryolesions at the atrioventricular valve annuli. All the PV orifices are cryoablated circumferentially (shaded). The asterisks in the middle and lower panels are the epicardial and endocardial aspects of the identical sites. MV, mitral valve; TV, tricuspid valve; RAA, right atrial appendage; LAA, left atrial appendage; SVC, superior vena cava; IVC, inferior vena cava; FO, fossa ovalis; CS, coronary sinus.

the right and left PVs are then connected to either the superior or inferior LA transverse incision to prevent reentry around the PVs.

The incision in the interatrial septal was reversed horizontally in order to preserve the blood supply to the posterior septum. A canine study on atrial his-

tology after the maze procedure revealed that a large part of the posterior septum was scarred, suggesting that the septal incision of the maze procedure interrupts the blood supply to the posterior septum from the anterior LA artery. In the radial procedure, the septal incision is placed from the posterior lower septum extending up to the anterior limbus; preventing disruption of blood supply to most areas of the atria and preserving normal septal activation.

Modification of the radial procedure and current surgical technique

The radial procedure with the atrial lesion set as shown in Figure 9.2 was performed in 51 patients with satisfactory clinical results. Recently, with the availability of bipolar radiofrequency (RF) ablation devices [9], the lesion set of the radial procedure has been modified to shorten the procedure time and make the procedure more surgeon-friendly, while maintaining the basic concept of preserving a more physiologic atrial activation–contraction sequence. The lesion set of the current radial procedure is depicted in Figure 9.3. The surgical technique of the current radial procedure [10] is described as follows.

1 *Pulmonary vein isolation*: After the patient is cannulated and placed on cardiopulmonary bypass, the right and left PVs are isolated by means of an RF device. The ablation line should be made on the LA 1 cm medial from the ostia of the PVs to avoid narrowing of the PVs from the RF energy application. It is extremely important to verify complete electrical isolation by demonstrating conduction block during pacing at each PV. This verification is performed using the maximal pacing output while the heart is beating. Patients with permanent AF should be defibrillated before performing this testing.

2 *LA incisions*: The ascending aorta is cross-clamped, cardioplegic solution is infused, and cardiac arrest is obtained. The LA is opened through a right-sided LA incision, which is made on the same region as the ablation line to avoid reentry around the right PV orifice and to allow for placement of Prolene sutures on the nonablated region. The LA incision is extended inferoposteriorly, then medially toward the posterior mitral valve annulus. A marker placed in the middle of the incision assists later closure.

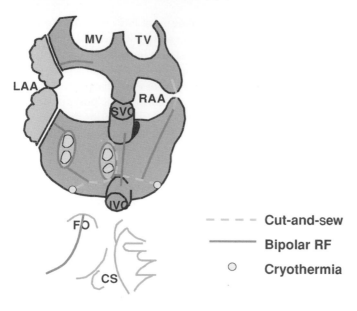

Figure 9.3 Atrial incisions, ablation lines, and sites of cryothermia in the current radial procedure. The schematic symbols are the same as in Figure 9.2. The broken lines indicate cut-and-sew incisions and the full lines indicate the bipolar radiofrequency (RF) linear ablation lines. The small circles indicate the cryothermia at the atrioventricular annuli.

- – – – **Cut-and-sew**
———— **Bipolar RF**
○ **Cryothermia**

The incision ends at the posterior mitral annulus between the middle (P2) and posteromedial scallops (P3) of the posterior mitral leaflet. Since the distal ends of the left circumflex coronary artery and right coronary artery converge at the level of the P2–P3 junction in most patients, the dissection of the atrioventricular fat pad can be safely performed in this area.

The atrial myocardium at the atrioventricular groove is carefully dissected. Then the distal end of the incision to the mitral annulus is cryoablated for 2 minutes at −60°C. The coronary sinus (CS) is also cryoablated endocardially and epicardially. Five-milimeter and fifteen-millimeters cryoprobes are used for the mitral annulus and the CS ablation, respectively. During the CS ablation, the cardioplegia catheter inserted into the CS is pulled back to allow for the creation of a complete circumferential cryolesion on the CS. A linear ablation is made between the left inferior PVs and the posterior LA incision with the bipolar RF device to block the reentrant circuit around the left PVs.

The LA appendage is excised from outside the heart. The bipolar RF device is introduced into the LA through the excised appendage orifice with the tip directed toward the left superior PV. A linear ablation is made between the appendage orifice and the previously made PV ablation line. In patients with a moderate to severely dilated LA, an additional ablation line of 3–5 cm is made on the dome of

the LA in an attempt to prevent atrial reentry. To create this lesion, the bipolar RF device is introduced into the LA through the excised appendage orifice with the tip directed toward the dome of the LA beneath the pulmonary artery trunk. After these lesions are completed, the LA appendage is closed with a 3-0 or 4-0 Prolene continuous suture.

3 *RA incisions*: A horizontal incision is made on the lower RA 2 cm above the insertion of IVC cannula. The incision is extended posteriorly, crossing the crista terminalis, down to the interatrial septum. The intercaval ablation lines are then made using the bipolar RF device. The device is properly placed at the posterior RA between the crista terminalis and the interatrial septum, so that a transmural linear ablation lesion is made along the entire length of this area. Next, a linear lesion between the horizontal incision and the IVC is made with the bipolar RF device.

The incision is then extended anteriorly toward the tricuspid valve annulus. The atrial myocardium in the atrioventricular groove is carefully dissected from inside the RA with a #15 scalpel. It is extremely important to divide all the muscle fibers across this incision. Then the distal end of the atriotomy is cryoablated using a 5-mm cryoprobe, in a similar fashion to the mitral annulus.

A small incision is made at the top of the RA appendage. The appendage is not excised, but all the major trabeculae inside the appendage are

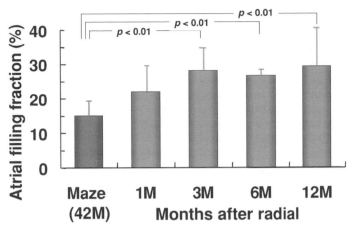

Figure 9.4 Serial change in the LA transport function after the radial procedure, compared with that from long-term follow-up after the maze procedure. The atrial filling fraction (AFF) measured at 1 month after the radial procedure was larger than that at 42 months after the maze procedure (22.0% ± 9.2% versus 15.1% ± 4.0%) but did not reach a statistical significance. The AFF 3, 6, and 12 months after the radial procedure increased to a significantly greater level than those at 42 months after the maze procedure. At 3 months after the radial procedure, the AFF was 28.2% ± 7.9% and was significantly larger than after the maze procedure ($p < 0.01$). The AFF at 6 and 12 months after the radial procedure (26.7% ± 0.7% and 29.4% ± 14.5%, respectively) was also significantly larger than after the maze procedure.

divided to prevent microreentry. A linear ablation line is then made on the lateral RA between the RA appendage incision and the lower RA incision using the bipolar RF device. This line is created by inserting the jaw of the bipolar device from the end of both incisions and performing two overlapping ablations. Another linear ablation line is made at the top of RA, using the bipolar RF device inserted through the RA appendage incision. Care must be taken not to ablate the sinus node artery branching from the proximal right coronary artery. This ablation line prevents the possibility of atrial reentry in this region.

To interrupt the potential of a reentrant circuit developing around the fossa ovalis, a linear ablation line is made on the posteroinferior interatrial septum using the bipolar RF device. Each jaw of the device is inserted into the RA and LA, and the posteroinferior septum is clamped and ablated.

After the completion of the radial incisions, all atrial incisions are closed with a 3-0 or 4-0 Prolene continuous suture. The heart is then deaired and reperfused. A pair of electrodes is usually placed on the epicardium at the top of the interatrial septum for pacing the atria and/or recoding atrial electrograms postoperatively.

Clinical results

Between October 1997 and April 2007, 171 patients underwent the radial procedure. There were 97 male and 74 female patients, and the average patient age was 62 ± 11 years. One hundred thrity-two patients had valvular heart disease (77%), 24 patients were associated with congenital heart disease, 11 patients had coronary artery disease, and 16 patients had no structural heart disease. Permanent AF was seen in 135 patients (79%), while the remaining 36 patients were diagnosed with paroxysmal AF. Twenty-four patients (17%) experienced thromboembolic events prior to surgery. Fifteen patients had LA thrombi present at the time of surgery.

There were four surgical mortalities; none of which were related to the radial procedure. Pacemaker implantation was required in 10 patients. During an average follow-up period of 51 months (1–114 mo, median 45 mo), 151 patients were either in sinus rhythm or had an atrial paced rhythm, resulting in an overall success rate of 90.4%.

Atrial activation during sinus rhythm was examined in 7 patients by intraoperative epicardial mapping after completion of the radial procedure. A 256-channel three-dimensional dynamic mapping system with custom-made epicardial patch electrodes was used for the intraoperative mapping. The maps demonstrated physiologic activation sequence in most atrial regions. The posterior LA between the PVs was viable and activated in a physiological fashion, whereas this region is electrically isolated and thus not activated, after the maze procedure.

In 9 patients, the RA endocardium was mapped during sinus rhythm using a basket catheter that carries 25–32 bipolar electrodes 3–6 weeks after the radial procedure. The maps demonstrated a physiologic activation sequence in the RA endocardium, and no scarred regions were seen. In contrast to these results, in the canine study, it was shown that post-maze scarring resulted in no activation of the posterior septum and nonphysiologic activation sequence in the interatrial septum [6].

The P wave duration, which is the atrial activation time during sinus rhythm, was measured by means of signal averaged ECG in 11 patients after the radial procedure. The data were then compared with that of 5 patients who underwent the maze procedure. The average atrial activation time after the radial procedure was significantly shorter than that after the maze procedure (140 ± 16 ms versus 157 ± 14 ms, $p < 0.05$).

The LA transport function was evaluated by transthoracic Doppler flow spectra measured at the left ventricular inflow in all patients. The atrial transport function was quantified by the peak A/E ratio and the atrial filling fraction. The serial change in the LA transport function was evaluated in 15 patients who received the radial procedure, and compared to that of patients 42 months after undergoing the maze procedure [11]. The atrial filling fraction observed 1 month after the radial procedure was already greater than that seen 42 months after the maze procedure. The difference became significant at 3 months postoperatively, and this excellent transport function was maintained for an extended period of time (Figure 9.4).

All the patients were placed on anticoagulant therapy postoperatively. The therapy was discontinued 3 months postoperatively in patients who did not receive mechanical valves. None of the patients who received the radial procedure had thromboembolic complications up to 9 years after surgery.

Because the radial procedure avoids isolating any segments of the atrium and results in concordant activation of the entire right and LA myocardium it provides greater atrial transport function and prevents thromboembolism. The radial procedure may therefore represent a physiological alternative to the maze as a surgical procedure for AF.

References

1 Cox JL, Schuessler RB, D'Agostino HJ et al. The surgical treatment of atrial fibrillation. III. Development of a definitive surgical procedure. *J Thorac Cardiovasc Surg* 1991; **101**: 569–583.

2 Cox JL, Schuessler RB, Lappas DG, Boineau JP. An 8½-year clinical experience with surgery for atrial fibrillation. *Ann Surg* 1996; **224**: 267–273.

3 Feinberg MS, Waggoner AD, Kater KM, Cox JL, Lindsay BD, Pérez JE. Restoration of atrial function after the maze procedure for patients with atrial fibrillation: assessment by Doppler echocardiography. *Circulation* 1994; **90**(suppl II): II-285–II-292.

4 Itoh T, Okamoto H, Nimi T et al. Left atrial function after Cox's maze operation concomitant with mitral valve operation. *Ann Thorac Surg* 1995; **60**: 354–359.

5 Nitta T, Lee R, Schuessler RB, Boineau JP, Cox JL. Radial approach: a new concept in surgical treatment for atrial fibrillation I. Concept, anatomic and physiologic bases and development of a procedure. *Ann Thorac Surg* 1999; **67**: 27–35.

6 Nitta T, Lee R, Watanabe H et al. Radial approach: a new concept in surgical treatment for atrial fibrillation. II. Electrophysiologic effects and atrial contribution to ventricular filling. *Ann Thorac Surg* 1999; **67**: 36–50.

7 Omari BO, Nelson RJ, Robertson JM. Effect of right atrial appendectomy on the release of atrial natriuretic hormone. *J Thorac Cardiovasc Surg* 1991; **102**: 272–279.

8 Kim KB, Lee CH, Kim CH, Cha YJ. Effect of the Cox maze procedure on the secretion of atrial natriuretic peptide. *J Thorac Cardiovasc Surg* 1998; **115**: 139–146.

9 Gaynor SL, Diodato MD, Prasad SM et al. A prospective, single-center clinical trial of a modified Cox maze procedure with bipolar radiofrequency ablation. *J Thorac Cardiovasc Surg* 2004; **128**: 535–542.

10 Nitta T. The radial procedure for atrial fibrillation. *Oper Tech Thorac Cardiovasc Surg* 2004; **9**: 83–95.

11 Ishii Y, Nitta T, Fujii M et al. Serial change in the atrial transport function after the radial incision approach. *Ann Thorac Surg* 2001; **71**: 572–576.

CHAPTER 10

The mini-maze operation

Z.A. Szalay

Introduction

Atrial fibrillation (AF) is one of the most prevalent arrhythmias [1], associated with significant morbidity and mortality and therefore a major health care problem. Electrophysiologic studies have demonstrated, that AF is a reentry arrhythmia, which is characterized by macro-reentry loops [2]. However, the precise electrophysiologic mechanism of AF is still not well understood [3, 4]. It is associated with significant morbidity and mortality and is frequently resistant to medical therapy. Its incidence increases with each decade of life, functional class, duration of mitral valve disease, and left atrial size [5]. AF may be associated with two major complications: firstly, loss of atrial contraction results in formation of intracardiac thrombus with significant risk of systemic embolism. Secondly, irregularity of cardiac rhythm and high ventricular rate may impair left ventricular function [6]. AF requires treatment in order to prevent these potential complications, such as antiarrhythmic medications and anticoagulation. However, these drugs have well-known adverse effects. In 1980, Cox *et al.* described left atrial isolation procedure [7] and in 1982, Scheinman *et al.* introduced catheter fulguration of His bundle [8]. In 1985, Guiraudon *et al.* described the corridor procedure for treatment of AF [9]. However, none of these techniques could eliminate all detrimental sequelae of AF. Because of absence or insufficient atrial contraction hemodynamic parameters were not improved, and danger of thromboembolism persisted. After accomplishing various electrophysiological animal experiments Cox *et al.* performed the maze I procedure in 1987 [10]. Thereafter he modified the technique and currently the maze III procedure is the technique of choice for the management of AF resistant to medical therapy [11]. The aim of the maze III operation is to interrupt all potential macro-reentry loops by multiple left and right atrial incisions, but with preservation of atrial transport function and sinus node function. In at least 90% of the patients AF can be converted into sinus rhythm early and late after this operation [12]. However, the maze III operation is a complex and time-consuming procedure with long cardiopulmonary and aortic cross-clamp times, limiting its applicability to patients undergoing concomitant complex cardiac surgery or to those with severely reduced left ventricular function [13]. To simplify this procedure several variants of the Cox-maze III operation have been developed [3, 14, 15]. Furthermore, new technologies such as radiofrequency ablation, cryotherapy, and microwave therapy have been introduced to the market [16–18]. Early results of these procedures are promising but little is known about long-term results. In 1995, we developed a variant of the Cox-maze procedure based on several publications [19–22], with the aim to reduce cross-clamp time, which is of great value especially in polymorbid patients and patients with concomitant heart disease. This variant includes all Cox-maze III incisions except the endocardial incision to tricuspid and mitral annulus combined with cryoablation and incision of interatrial septum (Figure 10.1).

Patients and methods

Between November 1995 and May 2001, a mini-maze procedure was performed upon 77 patients with chronic symptomatic AF. There were 38 men

Manual of Surgical Treatment of Atrial Fibrillation.
Edited by Hauw T. Sie *et al.* © 2008 Blackwell Publishing,
ISBN: 978-1-4051-4032-4.

Table 10.1 Baseline data and preoperative characteristics.

Variable	N = 77
Sex (male)	38
Age (years)	64 ± 8.07 (40–83)
MR (yes)	38/77
MS or combined MVD (yes)	20/77
TI (yes)	21/77
CAD (yes)	26/77
LBBB (yes)	5/77
LAD_{max} (mm)	64 ± 0.9 (49–83)
RAD_{max} (mm)	57 ± 0.8 (33–74)
LVEDD (mm)	54 ± 0.9 (39–71)

CAD, coronary artery disease; LAD_{max}, maximal left atrial diameter; LBBB, left bundle branch block; LVEDD, left ventricular end-diastolic diameter; MR, mitral regurgitation; MS, mitral stenosis; MVD, mitral valve disease; RAD_{max}, maximal right atrial diameter; TI, tricuspid insufficiency.

and 39 women with a mean age of 64 ± 8.7 years (range, 40–83). Patient characteristics and baseline data are depicted in Table 10.1. Permanent chronic AF was found in 67 patients (87%), and symp-

tomatic intermittent AF in 10 (13%). The mean duration of preoperative AF was 7 ± 6 years (range, 1–35 yr). The primary indication for operation was mitral valve disease in 58 patients (75%), while chronic AF was the only indication for surgery in two patients (2.6%). The mean left ventricular ejection fraction was 49 ± 9% (range, 20–66%), and less than 40% in nine patients (12%). Baseline data and preoperative patient characteristics are given in Table 10.1. AF persisted in all patients despite antiarrhythmic therapy. All patients complained of severe unpleasant sensations related to tachycardia. Concomitant procedures were carried out in 75 of 77 patients (97.5%), Table 10.2.

Surgical procedure and intraoperative data

The aim of the mini-maze procedure was to reduce aortic cross-clamp time, to minimize injury of structures at risk, e.g. circumflex coronary artery and coronary sinus, and yet interrupt the most frequent reentry circuits. All procedures were

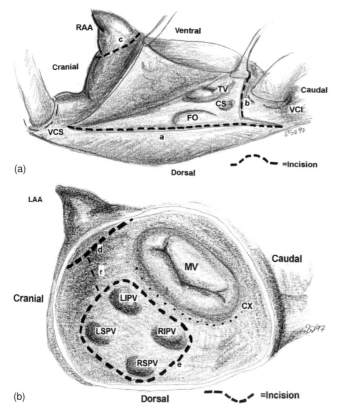

Figure 10.1 Surgical technique of the mini-maze operation: (a) right atrial view and (b) left atrial view.

Table 10.2 Concomitant surgical procedures.

Variable	N = 77
ECC time (min)	139 ± 5.3
Cross-clamp time (min)	86 ± 2.6
Isolated mini-maze procedure	2/77
MV repair	8
+ TV repair	8
+ TV repair + CABG	2
+ CABG	12
+ AV replacement + CABG	1
MV replacement	15
+ TV repair	6
+ CABG	2
+ AV replacement	2
+ AV replacement + TV repair	2
AV replacement	5
+ CABG	1
CABG	7
+ TV repair	1
TV repair + ASD closure	2
ASD closure	1

ASD, atrial septal defect; AV, aortic valve; CABG, coronary artery bypass grafting; ECC, extracorporal circulation; MV, mitral valve; TV, tricuspid valve.

performed through median sternotomy, using standard cardiopulmonary bypass (CPB) under moderate hypothermia and ante- and retrograde cold blood cardioplegia. When performing a valve operation, the valve was excised first, then the maze incisions were performed, followed by valve replacement or reconstruction. In case of coronary artery surgery, the distal anastomoses were performed first. Left and right atrial incisions used in the mini-maze procedure are shown in Figure 10.1. All right atrial incisions were performed on the beating heart. Compared to the maze III procedure, the following incisions were not performed: endocardial incision to tricuspid and mitral annulus, incision of interatrial septum, and cryoablation. Informed consent was obtained from all patients. Concomitant surgery performed with the mini-maze operation is listed in Table 10.2.

Early postoperative treatment
Patients who showed persistent AF postoperatively were treated with antiarrhythmic agents. If patients did not respond to medical therapy, electrical cardioversion was done before discharge and antiarrhythmic medication was continued. If a patient showed bradycardia 3 weeks postoperatively, an electrophysiological evaluation was performed and a permanent pacemaker was implanted as indicated. All patients were anticoagulated with warfarin for at least 3 months. If significant atrial transport function was demonstrated by echocardiography and/or magnetic resonance imaging (MRI) in the absence of an implanted mechanical device, anticoagulation was discontinued at this point.

Follow-up
After 3 and 12 months, patients were hospitalized and the following diagnostic procedures were performed: stress ECG and 24-hour ECG to detect episodes of bradycardia and to assess the increase of the heart rate during exercise; echocardiography and MRI to classify atrial transport function and to determine if anticoagulation could be discontinued. Patients with a permanent pacemaker had echocardiography only. Electrophysiological evaluation was carried out in all patients after 3 and 12 months to measure sinus node recovery time and to provoke AF or atrial flutter. The following pre- and intraoperative data were collected and analyzed by uni- and multivariate analysis: age, sex, duration of AF, preoperative presence of left bundle branch block (LBBB), New York Heart Association functional class, left ventricular ejection fraction, and any preoperative cardiac valve or coronary artery pathology. In addition, maximum left atrial diameter, maximum right atrial diameter, end-diastolic left ventricular diameter, end-systolic left ventricular diameter as well as aortic cross-clamp and cardiopulmonary bypass times were included in the analysis. In May 2003, a standard questionnaire was sent to all patients operated on between November 1995 and May 2001 to evaluate their New York Heart Association (NYHA) functional class, heart rhythm disturbances, pacemaker implantation, number of rehospitalizations, occurrence of stroke, and actual medication. Furthermore, a 12-lead electrocardiogram with long DII derivation was requested from the referring physicians. Mean follow-up time was 50 ± 22.2 months and was completed in 92% (71 of 77 patients).

Echocardiography

Two-dimensional and Doppler transthoracic echocardiography was performed using a Hewlett-Packard Sonos 4500 or 5500 (Hewlett-Packard, Andover, MA, USA) machine. Left atrial size was assessed by measuring the two-diagonal dimensions (mediolateral and superior inferior by the apical long axis). The right atrial dimension was measured in the apical four-chamber imaging plane. Standard parasternal and apical images were obtained and left ventricular function was assessed visually. Atrial mechanical function was assessed by pulsed Doppler examination of the mitral inflow, using the apical four-chamber view. The Doppler sample volume was positioned between the tips of the mitral leaflets. All measurements were made during quiet respiration with the patient in the left lateral position. Peak velocities of the early filling (E) wave and atrial filling (A) wave were measured, as well as their velocity time integrals and percentage A filling. Atrial mechanical activity was considered present if an atrial filling (A) wave was detected in late diastolic after the ECG P-wave.

Magnetic resonance imaging

MRI examination was carried out with a 1.5T unit (Vision or Sonata; Siemens Corp, Erlangen, Germany). Flow measurement was performed with an ECG-triggered segmented velocity encoded (VENC) gradient-echo (GE) sequence in breath-hold (fast low-angle shot (FLASH), repetition time (TR) 28 ms, echo time (TE) 5.5 ms, VENC 150 cm). The slice for flow measurement was placed across mitral valve area. Acquisition was repeated three times to calculate a velocity–time curve on 18 points during the entire cardiac cycle. The E and A waves were identified and the quotation of A_{max} to E_{max} was assessed.

When echo showed an A-wave greater than 70 cm/s and MRI moderate or good atrial contraction at follow-up, anticoagulation was discontinued except in patients with mechanical valve prostheses.

Electrophysiological assessment

Interatrial conduction time and sinus node recovery time were measured during electrophysiological control after 3 and 12 months. Furthermore, high-frequency stimulation was applied to prove if AF could be induced.

Results

Intraoperative data

The overall cardiopulmonary bypass time was 138 ± 42 minutes (range, 70–284 min), whereas the mean aortic cross-clamp time was 87 ± 22 minutes (range, 29–132 min). The mean additional aortic cross-clamp time to perform the mini-maze incisions was 27 ± 6 minutes (range, 19–33 min).

Mortality and morbidity

The average intensive care unit stay was 2.5 ± 1.5 days (range, 1–5 days). Postoperative morbidity was as follows: reexploration for postoperative bleeding had to be performed in one patient (1.3%). Another patient suffered from transient postoperative pancreatitis but fully recovered.

One of 77 patients (1.3%) died within 30 days after operation. A 65-year-old man who underwent coronary artery bypass grafting, mitral valve reconstruction, and the mini-maze operation died suddenly due to acute cardiac tamponade from rupture of the ascending aorta on the 11th postoperative day. Autopsy revealed plaque rupture of a calcified ascending aorta. Late death occurred in 7 of 76 (9.2%). Actuarial survival was 91%, 90%, and 87% after 1, 3, and 5 years, respectively. Sudden death was the cause of late mortality in six patients and one patient died of subphrenic abscess after an abdominal surgical procedure in another hospital. One of the six patients had coronary artery disease combined with mitral insufficiency and the other five patients did not have ischemic heart disease. Multivariate logistic regression analysis revealed that the only independent risk factors for late death was presence of preoperative total left bundle branch block ($p = 0.02$). Patients who were in sinus rhythm or were paced by atrial stimulation had a significantly better overall survival than patients with persistent AF, although there were no differences between both groups with regard to age and preoperative risk factors (Figure 10.2).

NYHA functional class

Fifty-six of 61 contacted survivors (92%) were in NYHA class I or II, whereas 5 of 61 (8%) patients were in NYHA class III at the time of follow-up. Three of the NYHA class III patients suffered from AF at follow-up. Judgment of NYHA class was not

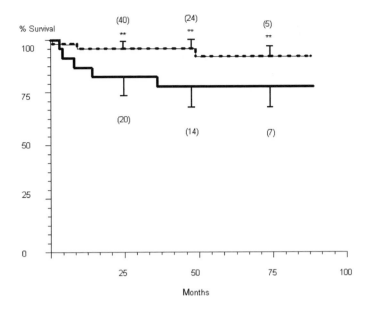

Figure 10.2 Long-term survival after mini-maze procedure: patients with sinus rhythm (dashed line) versus patients with persistent AF (straight line).

possible in one patient owing to a metastatic rectum cancer. There was no independent predictor for higher NYHA classification after the mini-maze operation.

Postoperative cardiac rhythm and pacemaker implantation

In the early postoperative period, most patients showed junctional rhythm and had atrial pacing by temporary pacemakers. Postoperative atrial arrhythmias developed in 18/77 patients (23%), occurring within the first 12 postoperative days. Electrical cardioversion was performed in 7/77 patients (9%) for treatment of refractory postoperative AF.

Pacemaker implantation

Postoperative pacemaker implantation was necessary in 15 of 77 patients (19%): 8 of 15 owing to postoperative sick sinus syndrome (SSS) and 7 of 15 owing to bradytachycardia syndrome. During follow-up another five patients required pacemaker implantation: 3 of 5 owing to bradytachycardia syndrome and 2 of 5 because of SSS. There were no surgical complications due to pacemaker implantation of which 10 were single chamber atrium mode programmed and 10 dual-chamber pacing mode programmed. Multivariate analysis showed that presence of preoperative tricuspid insufficiency ($p = 0.03$) and larger right atrium ($p = 0.017$) were in-

dependent predictors for postoperative pacemaker implantation.

Forty-four of 62 (71%) contacted survivors were in sinus rhythm or paced by an atrial pacemaker at long-term follow-up. Nine patients who were in stable sinus rhythm or were paced by an atrial pacemaker at 1-year follow-up converted to AF at late follow-up. Patients converting to AF were not different from patients who did not, especially with regard to duration of AF (9.1 ± 7.4 versus 4.8 ± 4.0 months; $p = 0.078$) and preoperative left atrial diameter (64 ± 5.8 versus 62 ± 7.3 mm). One patient with AF at 1-year follow-up converted to stable sinus rhythm at late follow-up. Independent predictors for failed restoration of sinus rhythm or regular heart rhythm with atrial pacemaker stimulation were presence of preoperative mitral regurgitation ($p = 0.03$) and larger left atrial diameter ($p = 0.04$) at long-term follow-up. Longer duration of preoperative AF was not a predictor for failure in this study ($p = 0.57$).

Medication

At follow-up six patients were still under anticoagulation therapy with warfarin owing to incomplete atrial transport function or persistent AF. Thirty-nine of 62 patients (63%) still had antiarrhythmic medication. The reason why a high number of

Table 10.3 Successful versus unsuccessful mini-maze operation (after 12 mo).

Variable	Univariate analysis	Multivariate analysis	
Preoperative duration of AF (longer)	$p = 0.03$	$p = 0.01$	OR = 1.33
LA diameter preoperatively (larger)	$p < 0.01$		
EF preoperatively (lower)	$p = 0.03$		
LVESD preoperatively (bigger)	$p = 0.05$	$p = 0.02$	OR = 1.2
Preoperative mitral valve stenosis (yes)	$p = 0.006$	$p = 0.005$	OR = 117.5

patients still had antiarrhythmic therapy could not be evaluated through the questionnaire.

Cerebral stroke

In one patient intraoperative cerebral stroke with hemiplegia occurred. Another patient suffered from cerebral stroke during follow-up. This patient had to stop anticoagulation therapy owing to roentgenographically documented proctitis and gastrointestinal bleeding although he suffered from persistent AF.

Rehospitalization

Nine of 62 patients (14%) contacted were rehospitalized during the follow-up period. Rhythm disturbances were the main cause for rehospitalization. Five of these patients were in AF. The others were rehospitalized due to hyperglycemia [1], stroke [1], gastrointestinal bleeding [1], and heart failure [1].

Echocardiography

After 3 months transthoracic echocardiography revealed active left atrial systolic contraction in 46 out of 68 patients (68%). Whereas 38/54 (70%) showed active left atrial systolic contraction after 1 year. A total of 87% of the patients with SR showed atrial transport function after 3 and 12 months.

Magnetic resonance imaging

Echocardiography and MRI showed excellent correlation as MRI proved active systolic atrial transport function in 82% of the patients after 3 and in 78% after 12 months [23].

Electrophysiology

Postoperative pacemaker implantation was necessary in 15 patients (19%), in eight because of an SSS. After 3 months, the sinus node recovery function was found to have normalized in one of these patients, whereas asymptomatic prolongation of the sinus node recovery time was identified in three, from which sinus node recovery time normalized within 12 months in two. In four of the patients with SR, AF was inducible, but self-limited. Residual postoperative atrial flutter was identified in two patients; it was successfully ablated in both patients.

Predictors for failure of the mini-maze procedure after 12 months

Table 10.3 compares patients with successful and those with unsuccessful mini-maze operation.

Univariate analysis after 12 months identified the following preoperative predictors for failure of the mini-maze operation: longer duration of preoperative AF ($p = 0.05$); increased left atrial diameter ($p < 0.001$); reduced left ventricular function ($p = 0.03$); increased left ventricular end-diastolic diameter ($p = 0.05$); and the presence of preoperative mitral valve stenosis ($p = 0.006$).

Independent predictors for failure of the mini-maze operation after 12 months were longer preoperative duration of AF ($p = 0.001$; OR = 1.33); increased left ventricular end-diastolic diameter ($p = 0.02$; OR = 1.2), and the presence of preoperative mitral valve stenosis ($p = 0.005$; OR = 117.5). After these results we did not perform the mini-maze operation in patients with mitral valve stenosis and presence of AF, and so in the analysis of the long-term follow-up only preoperative presence of mitral insufficiency and preoperative larger left atrium were detected for independent predictors for nonrestoration of sinus rhythm.

Discussion

AF is the most common arrhythmia and is associated with significant morbidity and mortality. In the United States, 2.2 million people are currently affected by this arrhythmia and this number increases by 120,000 cases annually [1].

In patients with chronic AF and mitral valve regurgitation, AF mostly persists despite successful mitral valve reconstruction. Even in patients with a history of intermittent AF, presenting sinus rhythm immediately prior to surgery, AF may develop early or late postoperatively and may persist despite an apparently normally functioning mitral valve. Long duration of preoperative AF, the size of the left atrium, preoperative valve-related pulmonary artery hypertension, and a history of prior antiarrhythmic drug treatment have been found to be predictors for persistence or recurrence of AF after successful mitral surgery [24, 25], but definitive information in regard to this is unavailable in literature. The true mechanism underlying idiopathic AF associated with mitral valve disease is still unknown.

The Cox-maze procedure has proven to be extraordinarily effective in treating AF [12]. However, this procedure is very complex and not many surgeons perform it on a regular basis. For this reason several mini-variants have been developed in order to simplify the procedure and to reduce cross-clamp time and cardiopulmonary bypass time [3, 14, 15]. With our mini-variant we could significantly reduce mean cross-clamp time from 127 ± 40 minutes (full maze III and comparable cases) to 87 ± 21 minutes [26].

Similarly, the mini-maze operation modifies and even omits some of the maze III incisions, resulting in a shorter aortic cross-clamp and cardiopulmonary bypass time. The mini-maze operation as performed in our patients mainly consisted of the circumferential incision around the pulmonary veins as well as in the amputation of both atrial appendages. Time-consuming incisions toward the mitral and tricuspid valve annulus were omitted. With this partial maze operation we had success rates of over 70% in recovering sinus rhythm and atrial transport function [23]. Kosakai *et al.* showed almost similar results. In their study a larger left atrial dimension and a longer duration of preoperative AF failed to restore SR after successful mitral valve repair with the maze procedure [22].

Hence, the mini-maze operation is designed to be performed in patients with either severely decreased left ventricular function or in those with other complex and time-consuming procedures to be concomitantly performed including mitral valve reconstruction. In these patients, the results achieved with this mini-maze modification compare favorably with those achieved with the original maze III operation. However, even the mini-maze operation may have a potential risk in complex patients.

Other less invasive techniques with new devices have been developed in order to motivate more surgeons performing AF ablation surgery. These include cryoablation, unipolar and bipolar radiofrequency energy, microwave energy, laser energy, and ultrasound [16–18]. The initial results are promising although not comparable with the results achieved by the Cox-maze procedure [12].

Survival

In our series, the early mortality rate was 1.3% and the late mortality rate, 9.2%. Cause of late mortality was sudden death in most patients. Other authors performing mini-maze operations describe early mortality rates between 0% and 2.7% [3, 14, 15, 27]. Actuarial survival after the mini-maze operation was 91% after 1 year, 90% after 3 years, and 87% after 5 years. Izumoto and associates [28] found 1- and 5-year survival rates of 95.1% and 87.8% after a modified maze procedure, which concurs with our results. The only independent predictor for overall mortality was presence of left bundle branch block in our study. This is not surprising since others confirmed that complete left bundle branch block affects overall mortality indeed [29]. One of the reasons is that left bundle branch block is known to adversely influence ventricular function owing to nonsynchronized contractions of left and right ventricle. Biventricular pacing is able to resynchronize contraction of both ventricles leading to improvement of left ventricular ejection fraction. This is even true in patients with AF as stated by Leon and colleagues [30]. Since left bundle branch block was an independent predictor for increased overall mortality in our population one may suggest that biventricular pacing may improve long-term survival. We found that actuarial survival in patients with sinus rhythm or regular rhythm due to AAI pacing had a better long-term survival compared with the group of patients still suffering from AF (Figure 10.2). This result is not surprising, as it is well known that patients with AF have increased risk for late death [31].

NYHA classification

Most of our patients were in good clinical conditions at follow-up. Only five patients or 8% were in NYHA class III or IV. Three of these patients had unsuccessful operation concerning AF. We could not find any independent predictor for higher NYHA classification. This is confirmative as NYHA classification is a subjective variable seldom correlating with objective hemodynamic measurement. In the study published by Izumoto and colleagues [28], the NYHA class at follow-up was 1.5 ± 0.5.

Sinus rhythm

At follow-up 71% of patients were in sinus rhythm or had regular heart rhythm due to AAI pacing. The results published by Cox et al., as stated by Damiano at the 2003 AATS meeting, showed a higher success rate than this with freedom from recurrent AF at 93%. However, others performing mini-variants of the Cox-maze III procedure found similar results. Izumoto and associates [28] reported that 64.8% of patients undergoing a modified maze operation were in sinus rhythm whereas Raanani and colleagues [32] reported a 75% success rate at 3 years. We are fully aware that our 71% success rate is significantly below Cox's 93% success rate. However, since we combined rather complex operations with the mini-maze procedure we were cautious of the fact that longer cross-clamp time would impair the survival rate of the patients. If the main purpose for the operation would be restoration of sinus rhythm we would also perform the full Cox-maze III procedure to achieve a better success rate. Interestingly, nine patients in our series in sinus rhythm after 1 year showed AF at follow-up. In the series of Izumoto and associates [28], only 72% of 104 patients in sinus rhythm immediately after operation showed stable sinus rhythm at follow-up. Sixteen patients (22%) converted to AF and four patients (6%) developed SSS [28]. The authors think that underlying heart disease could have an impact on recurrent AF. Another factor for this high recurrence rate might be selective use of cryoablation lines. In our study, one patient having AF after 1 year converted to sinus rhythm during follow-up.

This has also been shown by Izumoto and associates [28] who observed two patients converting from AF to sinus rhythm during follow-up. There is no explanation for this interesting observation. In our study, independent predictors for nonrestoration of sinus rhythm and regular heart rhythm with AAI stimulation mode at long-term follow-up were presence of preoperative mitral insufficiency and larger left atrium. This concurs with the Katamatas group [33] who also found a larger diameter of left atrium to be a predictor for unsuccessful sinus rhythm restoration after the original Cox-maze III procedure. Furthermore, they found that amplitude of atrial fibrillatory wave was also predictive for unsuccessful sinus rhythm restoration. In a previous analysis (follow-up after 12 mo), we found that presence of mitral valve stenosis, longer duration of AF, and increased preoperative LVESD were predictors for failure after the mini-maze operation [34]. After this analysis we did not perform the mini-maze operation in patients with mitral valve stenosis and presence of AF for more than 8 years. This may explain the different results after 12 months and at long-term follow-up.

Pacemaker implantation

Early postoperative pacemaker implantation was necessary in 19% of our patients and another five patients needed a pacemaker during follow-up. SSS and bradytachycardia syndrome were indications in 10 patients each. Cox and associates [12] reported pacemaker requirement in 15% of patients early after operation. In Izumoto's series, 6% of patients underwent early postoperative pacemaker implantation owing to SSS. During follow-up four patients developed SSS and required pacemaker implantation. There is no statement in this paper regarding DDD pacemaker implantation owing to the bradytachycardia syndrome. In our study, independent predictors for postoperative pacemaker implantation were preoperative tricuspid insufficiency and larger right atrium. Indeed secondary tricuspid insufficiency due to mitral valve disease was frequently observed in our study group. As a consequence the right atrium was enlarged in several cases and this might be the reason why the frequency of pacemaker implantation was higher compared to other studies mentioned.

Medication

At follow-up, six patients were still under antico-agulation therapy with warfarin due to nonrestora-tion of atrial transport function. However, Cox and colleagues [35] stated that even if atrial transport function is not adequate, anticoagulation may be stopped. More than 50% of patients were still under antiarrhythmic medication at follow-up although most of them were in sinus rhythm or had regu-lar heart rhythm in AAI pacing mode. We could not evaluate why so many patients were still treated with antiarrhythmic drugs. Although we informed the family doctors and cardiologists that medica-tion may be stopped when heart rhythm gets regular and atrial transport function sufficient, we assume that they either were afraid of complying or simply ignored our advice.

Cerebral stroke

Cerebral stroke is the most disastrous complica-tion for patients with AF. In the Framingham study there was a more than fivefold increase of strokes in the presence of AF compared with patients hav-ing sinus rhythm [36]. One of our patients suffered intraoperative stroke and another one after cessa-tion of warfarin medication. Cox and coworkers [35] observed only two perioperative strokes in a study group of 340 patients and there was only one minor stroke during the follow-up period. As a re-sult of this large study Cox suggests discontinuing anticoagulation therapy for all patients 3 months postoperatively even if there is no or minor atrial transport function.

Rehospitalization

Nine patients (14%) were readmitted to hospital during follow-up period. Five of them were in AF and one of the patients had congestive heart failure. Four patients were rehospitalized for cardioversion during the follow-up period: in one patient car-dioversion was successful. The other reasons for re-hospitalization were not cardiac related. It is well known that frequency of hospitalization in patients with AF is significantly higher compared with pa-tients with sinus rhythm. Therefore, the health care costs for patients with this dysrhythmia increase dramatically [37]. For this reason it is of signifi-cant socioeconomic importance to reduce the total number of patients suffering from AF.

In our patients, preoperative diagnosis of a mitral valve stenosis, a longer preoperative duration of AF and an increased left ventricular end-systolic diam-eter were found to be incremental risk factors for failure of the mini-maze operation at 12 months follow-up. In patients without these incremental risk factors for failure (duration of AF shorter than 10 years preoperatively, LVESD <50 mm, no pre-operative mitral valve stenosis), the mini-maze op-eration achieved a stable sinus rhythm in 100% of those patients 12 months after surgery. Contrarily, in those with the incremental risk factors mentioned above, the mini-maze operation failed to achieve a stable sinus rhythm, thus only adding to the pe-rioperative risk by prolonging aortic cross-clamp and cardiopulmonary bypass time in those already undergoing high-risk or complex cardiac surgery. Therefore, the mini-maze procedure should be rec-ommended in patients with complex combined procedures and in those with poor left ventricu-lar function, in which the maze III procedure may not be suitable due to the prolongation of the aor-tic cross-clamp and cardiopulmonary bypass time. In our patients, a mean aortic cross-clamp time of 27 minutes (range 19–33 min) had to be added to the original surgical procedure, whereas the classical maze procedure has reported to prolong the aortic cross-clamp time up to 70 minutes [38]. The mini-maze procedure was found to be a safe procedure even in higher risk patients with severely decreased left ventricular function and in those undergoing combined valve and coronary artery surgery. How-ever, the mini-maze operation may probably fail in patients with preoperative mitral valve stenosis, an increased preoperative left ventricular end-systolic diameter and a long preoperative duration of AF. Surprisingly, similar findings have been reported in patients with normal left ventricular function undergoing isolated maze—or only maze and mi-tral valve surgery. The indication to combine AF surgery with valve surgery and/or coronary artery bypass grafting should be based on careful identifi-cation of patients who will likely benefit from a more extended surgical approach. In patients with pre-served left ventricular function undergoing surgery for highly symptomatic AF, the maze III procedure remains our technique of choice clearly offering the best success rate available. However, the easier to perform mini-maze operation probably may help to extend the successful AF surgery to higher risk patients with severely decreased left ventricular function and to those patients with chronic or intermittent atrial surgery undergoing complex combined cardiac surgical procedures.

In conclusion, the mini-maze procedure can be carried out for achieving good early and long-term results in terms of early and late mortality. Left bundle branch block was an independent risk factor for late death. Prophylactic implantation of a biventricular pacemaker could probably reduce mortality in patients with left bundle branch block. Restoration of SR can be achieved in 71% of patients. Predictors for restoration of sinus rhythm were absence of mitral insufficiency and larger left atrium at long-term follow-up. Modifications of the maze III operation or catheter techniques might be available in the near future and patients with poor left ventricular function and combined operations could be treated at a higher success rate, and lower risk.

References

1 Kannel WB, Abbott RD, Savage DD et al. Epidemiologic features of chronic atrial fibrillation: the Framingham study. N Engl J Med 1982; **306**: 1018–1022.

2 Cox J, Sundt T. The surgical treatment of atrial fibrillation. Annu Rev Med 1997: 511–523.

3 Sueda T, Nagata H, Orihashi K et al. Efficacy of a simple left atrial procedure for chronic atrial fibrillation in mitral valve operations. Ann Thorac Surg 1997; **63**: 1070–1075.

4 Cosio FG, Palacios J, Vidal JM et al. Electrophysiologic studies in atrial fibrillation. Slow conduction of premature impulse: a possible manifestation of the background for reentry. AM J Cardiol 1983; **51**: 122–130.

5 Levy S. Factors predisposing to the development of atrial fibrillation. PACE 1997; **20**: 2670–2674.

6 Capucci A, Villani GQ, Aschieri D. Risk of complications of atrial fibrillation. PACE 1997; **20**: 2684–2691.

7 Williams JM, Ungerleider RM, Lofland GK, Cox JL. Left atrial isolation: new technique for the treatment of supraventricular arrhythmias. J Thorac Cardiovasc Surg 1980; **80**: 373–380.

8 Scheinman MM, Morady F, Hess DS et al. Catheter-induced ablation of the atrioventricular junction to control refractory supraventricular arrhythmias. JAMA 1982; **248**: 851.

9 Guiraudon GM, Campbell CS, Jones DL et al. Combined sino-atrial node atrio-ventricular node isolation: a surgical alternative to His bundle ablation in patients with atrial fibrillation. Circulation 1985; **72**: 220.

10 Cox JL, Schuessler RB, D'Agostino HJ et al. The surgical treatment of atrial fibrillation (development of a definitive surgical procedure). J Thorac Cardiovasc Surg 1991; **101**: 569–583.

11 Cox JL, Boineau JP, Schuessler RB et al. Modification of the maze procedure for atrial flutter and atrial fibrillation. J Thorac Cardiovasc Surg 1995; **110**: 473–484.

12 Cox JL, Ad N, Palazzo T et al. Current status of the maze procedure for the treatment of atrial fibrillation. Semin Thorac Cardiovasc Surg 2000; **12**: 15–19.

13 Cox JL, Scheussler RB, Lappas DG, Boineau IP. An 8.5 year clinical experience with surgery for atrial fibrillation. Ann Surg 1996; **224**: 267–275.

14 Takami Y, Yasuura K, Takagi Y et al. Partial maze procedure is effective treatment for chronic atrial fibrillation associated with valve disease. J Card Surg 1999; **14**: 103–108.

15 Tuinenburg AE, Van Gelder IC, Tieleman RG et al. Mini-maze suffices as adjunct to mitral valve surgery in patients with preoperative atrial fibrillation. J Cardiovasc Electrophysiol 2000; **11**: 960–967.

16 Sie HT, Beukema WP, Ramdat Misier AR, Elvan A, Ennema JJ, Wellens HJ. The radiofrequency modified maze procedure. A less invasive surgical approach to atrial fibrillation during open-heart surgery. Eur J Cardiothorac Surg 2001; **19**: 443–447.

17 Gaita F, Gallotti R, Calo L et al. Limited posterior left atrial cryoablation in patients with chronic atrial fibrillation undergoing valvular heart surgery. J Am Coll Cardiol 2000; **36**: 159–166.

18 Knaut M, Spitzer SG, Karolyi L et al. Intraoperative microwave ablation for curative treatment of atrial fibrillation in open heart surgery—the MICRO-STAF and MICRO-PASS pilot trial. Microwave application in surgical treatment of atrial fibrillation. Microwave application for the treatment of atrial fibrillation in bypass surgery. Thorac Cardiovasc Surg 1999; **47**(suppl 3): 379–384.

19 Johnson DC. Early experience with the modified maze operation for atrial fibrillation with and without mitral valve surgery. Aust Assoc J Cardiac Thorac Surg 1992; **1**: 13–16.

20 McCarthy PM, Cosgrove DM, Castle LW et al. Combined treatment of mitral regurgitation and atrial fibrillation with valvuloplasty and the maze procedure. Am J Cardiol 1993; **71**: 483–486.

21 Kawaguchi A, Kosakai Y, Isobe F et al. Factors affecting rhythm after the maze procedure for atrial fibrillation. Circulation 1996; **94**: II-139–II-142.

22 Kosakai Y, Kawaguchi AT, Isobe F et al. Cox maze procedure for chronic atrial fibrillation associated with mitral valve disease. J Thorac Cardiovasc Surg 1994; **108**: 1049–1055.

23 Bauer EP, Szalay ZA. Predictors for atrial transport function after mini-maze operation. *Ann Thorac Surg* 2001; **72**: 1251–1255.

24 Vogt PR, Turina MI. Preoperative predictors of recurrent atrial fibrillation late after successful mitral valve reconstruction. *Eur J Cardiothorac Surg* 1998; **13**: 619–624.

25 Kalil, RAK, Maratia, CB, D'Ávila, A, Ludwig, FB. Predictive factors for persistence of atrial fibrillation after mitral valve operation. *Ann Thorac Surg* 1999; **67**: 614–617.

26 Szalay ZA, Skwara W, Pitschner HF, Faude I, Klovekorn WP, Bauer EP. Midterm results after the mini-maze procedure. *Eur J Cardiothorac Surg* 1999; **16**: 306–311.

27 Izumoto H, Kawazoe K, Kitahara H, Kamata J. Operative results after the Cox/maze procedure combined with a mitral valve operation. *Ann Thorac Surg* 1998; **66**: 800–804.

28 Izumoto H, Kawazoe K, Eishi K, Kamata J. Medium-term results after the modified Cox/maze procedure combined with other cardiac surgery. *Eur J Cardiothorac Surg* 2000; **17**: 25–29.

29 Hesse B, Diaz LA, Snader CE, Blackstone EH, Lauer MS. Complete bundle branch block as an independent predictor of all-cause mortality: report of 7073 patients referred for nuclear exercise testing. *Am J Med* 2001; **110**: 253–259.

30 Leon AR, Greenberg JM, Kanuru N *et al*. Cardiac resynchronization in patients with congestive heart failure and chronic atrial fibrillation: effect of upgrading to biventricular pacing after chronic right ventricular pacing. *J Am Coll Cardiol* 2002; **39**: 1258–1263.

31 Benjamin EJ, Wolf PA, D'Agostino RB, Silbershatz H, Kannel WB, Levy D. Impact of atrial fibrillation on the risk of death. *Circulation* 1998; **98**: 946–952.

32 Raanani E, Albage A, David TE, Yau TM, Armstrong S. The efficacy of the Cox/maze procedure combined with mitral valve surgery: a matched control study. *Eur J Cardiothorac Surg* 2001; **19**: 438–442.

33 Kamata J, Kawazoe K, Izumoto H *et al*. Predictors of sinus rhythm restoration after Cox maze procedure concomitant with other cardiac operations. *Ann Thorac Surg* 1997; **64**: 394–398.

34 Szalay ZA, Skwara W, Kloevekorn WP *et al*. Predictors for failure to cure atrial fibrillation with the mini maze operation. *J Cardiac Surg* 2004; **19**: 1–6.

35 Cox JL, Ad N, Palazzo T. Impact of the maze procedure on the stroke rate in patients with atrial fibrillation. *J Thorac Cardiovasc Surg* 1999; **118**: 833–840.

36 Wolf PA, Abbott RD, Kannel WB. Atrial fibrillation as an independent risk factor for stroke: the Framingham study. *Stroke* 1991; **22**: 983–988.

37 Wolf PA, Mitchell JB, Baker CX, Kannel WB, D'Agostino RB. Impact of atrial fibrillation on mortality, stroke and medical costs. *Arch Intern Med* 1998; **158**: 229–234.

38 Cox JL, Boineau JP, Schuessler RB, Kater KM, Lappas DG. Five-year experience with the maze procedure for atrial fibrillation. *Ann Thorac Surg* 1993; **56**: 814–824.

CHAPTER 11

Alternative energy sources for the surgical treatment of atrial fibrillation

Mark J. Russo & Mathew R. Williams

Introduction

Since Cox first described the maze in 1989, many have sought faster and less invasive approaches to the procedure [1]. In 1994, Kosakai *et al.* described a simplified maze procedure using cryoablation [2]. Cox had long used cryoablation to create spot lesions during the maze [3], and he later described a "cryo-maze" exclusively using cryo to create its lesion set [4]. Shortly after, a number of groups described a modified maze III procedure using a hyperthermic energy source, radiofrequency (RF), to ablate atrial tissue [5]. More recently, the use of other energy sources, including microwave [6–9], laser [10, 11], and ultrasound [12, 13], have been described.

The application of energy as an alternative to the scalpel resulted in the resurgence of surgical treatment for arrhythmias, especially atrial fibrillation (AF). The "cut-and-sew" method initially described by Cox required additional aortic cross-clamp and cardiopulmonary bypass (CPB) times of 1 and 3 hours, respectively; by applying energy to induce conduction block, the additional operative time can instead be measured in minutes. Moreover, these modalities decreased the technical demands of the operation thus limiting the potential risks to the patient and reducing the learning curve for the surgeon.

Manual of Surgical Treatment of Atrial Fibrillation.
Edited by Hauw T. Sie *et al.* © 2008 Blackwell Publishing,
ISBN: 978-1-4051-4032-4.

Mechanism of tissue injury

The majority of energy sources in clinical use create lesions via hyperthermic energy (e.g., RF, microwave, laser, and ultrasound). These energy sources span the electromagnetic spectrum from large RF waves to small—near infrared—laser energy. Though these modalities ablate tissue by generating heat, each works by a slightly different mechanism (Table 11.1).

Radiofrequency energy, unmodulated alternating current at frequencies ranging between 500 and 1000 kHz, acts by resistive or ohmic heating. Because the tissue acts as a resistor, heat is generated. True resistive heating occurs only to a tissue depth of approximately 1 mm, therefore the remainder of the tissue is ablated by conductive heat from the area of resistive heating. Though inefficient, this heating process provides for well-controlled and generally safe ablation.

Microwave energy is high-frequency electromagnetic radiation that causes the oscillation of polar molecules, primarily water molecules. This process, called dielectric heating, creates frictional heat. In addition, to the dielectric heating, the device delivers a small amount of conductive heat. Microwave ablation can be performed at either 915 MHz or 2450 MHz, which are the frequencies allowed by the Federal Communications Commission for medical microwave use. The currently marketed microwave devices use 2450 MHz.

With *laser* ablation, a laser energy is absorbed by water and, like microwave energy, causes dielectric heating. It produces harmonic oscillation of

Table 11.1 Hyperthermic energy sources.

Energy source	Frequency	Mechanism of heating
Radiofrequency	500–1000 kHz	Resistive or ohmic
Microwave	2450 MHz	Dielectric
Laser	1000 GHz	Dielectric
Ultrasound	3.8–6.4 MHz	Mechanical

Table 11.2 Measures for comparison of energy sources.

- Effects of tissue
    - Preservation of the tissue architecture (charring)
    - Width-to-depth ratio
- Lesion transmurality and continuity
- Applicability to epicardial approach

water. This leads to the production of kinetic energy and subsequent heat that causes tissue to coagulate. While RF and microwave energy focus energy at the device–tissue interface and rely in large part on conductive heating to ablate tissue, a theoretical advantage of laser energy is that light energy penetrates deep into the tissue allowing for more equal and controlled ablation of tissue. The only available device using laser energy, the Optiwave 980 by Edwards Lifesciences (Irvine, CA), utilizes a 980-nm diode laser.

In *ultrasound* ablation, ultrasound waves travel through the tissue causing compression, refraction, and particle movement, resulting in kinetic energy and heat. Like laser energy, ultrasound waves penetrate the tissue surface. Ultrasound energy exists in two forms: focused, called high-intensity focused ultrasound (HIFU), and nonfocused. The FDA-approved Epicor device uses HIFU energy at a frequency range between 3.8 and 6.4 MHz.

Cryoablation uses hypothermic energy to freeze tissue. At the cellular level, tissue disruption occurs in three phases. First, mitochondrial and organelle dysfunction occurs that is likely due to intracellular ice crystal formation. Next, edema and subsequent necrosis occur upon thawing. Finally, during the remodeling phase, the resultant lesion is replaced with fibrous scar tissue. Early systems used nitric oxide. However, in an effort to decrease ablation time, newer systems using argon- and helium-based cooling mechanisms have been developed that achieve much colder temperatures and therefore faster ablating times.

Characteristics of energy sources

With numerous energy sources available, it is necessary to understand the advantages and disadvantages of each. Important measures for comparison include: (1) local effects on ablated tissue; (2) success achieving contiguous and transmural lesions; and (3) applicability to endocardial and epicardial approaches (Table 11.2).

Tissue ablation

Atrial ablation using hyperthermic energy at temperatures greater than 50 °C has been shown to be sufficient to cause electrophysiological disruption of tissue. However, the tissue temperature should not exceed 100 °C, the boiling point of water. At this temperature tissue architecture may be disrupted leading to carbonization and charring [14]. Char may serve as an insulator that prevents coagulation of tissue and thus the creation of an optimal lesion. In addition, on the endocardial surface it may serve as a nidus for thrombus. Different energy sources have varying propensities for the formation of char.

The ratio of width to depth of the lesion should also be considered. By creating narrow lesions, more functional myocardium is preserved. Preservation of myocardium may be particularly important in patients with elements of heart failure. Theoretically, modalities less reliant on conductive heating will produce narrower lesions.

Transmurality and continuity

With the classic "cut-and-sew" method, transmurality and lesion continuity were easily accomplished and observed. However, when using energy, the ability to achieve transmurality is dependent on a number of factors including the energy source; its application, epicardial versus endocardial; atrial thickness, which may vary by as much as 10 times in a single patient; and the presence of epicardial fat [15]. As a result, the success in achieving continuous, transmural lesions is variable.

Though it should be noted that there are instances where nontransmural, noncontiguous lesions are effective and similarly (albeit rare) times when they are not effective, achieving transmural and contiguous lesions should remain the surgeon's goal. Santiago and colleagues [16] demonstrated this among 10 patients requiring mitral valve repair or replacement who underwent a maze procedure using RF; at 6 months follow-up only two of five patients with endocardial lesions converted to sinus rhythm (SR) while four of five patients with more extensive lesions ranging from myocardial to transmural converted to SR. Likewise, in a canine model undergoing pulmonary vein isolation, van Brakel *et al.* [17] demonstrated complete electrophysiological isolation in four dogs with contiguous lesions, conversely isolation was complete in only 9 of 12 dogs with noncontiguous lesions.

Epicardial versus endocardial approach

Early in the development of energy sources, ablation was performed primarily by an endocardial approach. Endocardial ablation is easier to perform than epicardial. During endocardial ablation the field is stationary, empty, and in direct contact with the energy probe. There are several factors that may limit the effectiveness of epicardial ablation including epicardial fat and convective cooling. Most energy sources work by direct heating from the energy source and via conductive heating from the focus of direct energy. However, epicardial fat limits direct heating by separating the energy source from the atrial tissue and acting as an insulator of the underlying tissue. When creating lesions, different energy sources have varying degrees of success overcoming epicardial fat. In addition, to these limitations in direct heating from the epicardial surface, conductive heating is limited by the heat sink effect of flowing atrial and myocardial blood; this leads to wide lesions with a rim of spared atrial tissue near the endocardium, where the heat sink is the greatest. A final concern remains that not all desired lesions can be safely created from the epicardium. For example, there is widespread concern that, the circumflex artery will be injured when creating the "connecting lesion" to the mitral valve annulus [15].

Nevertheless, the full potential of tissue ablation by energy sources can only be realized with the refinement of epicardial ablation. First, epicardial ablation is inherently safer. In epicardial ablation, the energy source is directed only toward

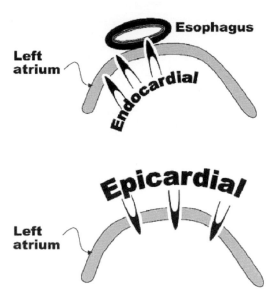

Figure 11.1 Endocardial and epicardial directional energy. Top: any energy source applied from the endocardium of the left atrium has several inherent problems and risks. Energy is directed extracardially toward surrounding structures, therefore, over-penetration of the left atrial wall can cause injury to nearby structures, such as the esophagus. Bottom: any energy source applied from the epicardium can be directed so that it affects only the atrial blood pool once it has penetrated the atrial wall. Therefore, epicardial ablation is inherently safer than endocardial ablation. (Reprinted with permission.)

atrial blood; while with endocardial ablation, energy is directed extracardially toward surrounding structures, and over-penetration may cause damage to adjacent structures, such as the esophagus [18] (Figure 11.1). Moreover, epicardial ablation makes closed, beating heart procedures possible, thereby decreasing bypass times during open cases and increasing potential for use of minimally invasive approaches.

Modalities

In this section, each of the five different energy modalities will be discussed. Expanded sections on RF, microwave, and cyro can be found in later chapters.

Radiofrequency

Among all energy sources, the greatest experience, as well as the greatest number of devices, lies with RF.

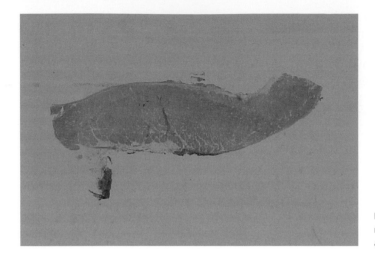

Figure 11.2 Trichome-stained myocardium following epicardial RF ablation.

There are three types of RF devices: unipolar (standard), irrigated (cooled tip), and bipolar. *Unipolar RF ablation* is the simplest way to apply the energy; with unipolar ablation, the energy is focused at the ablating surface and disperses throughout the body exiting through a grounding pad, which acts as the second pole. Because energy disperses from a single element, it is slow and inefficient relative to other modalities—though it remains faster than the Cox approach with left-sided ablation sets requiring 10–20 minutes compared with approximately 1 hour for the Cox procedure. In addition, as heat disperses throughout the body from a single pole, there is a greater possibility to injure an adjacent noncardiac tissue such as the esophagus—a known complication. Charring and carbonization also appear to be more prevalent in RF ablations [15].

To overcome these limitations irrigated or "cooled tip" RF ablation was developed. Under this design the active electrode is irrigated with cold saline. The saline creates a cooling effect on the surface of the tissue and actually drives the focus (hottest point) of energy deeper into the tissue, providing for both faster and deeper ablation. The irrigation also helps prevent the accumulation of char on the ablating surface.

Bipolar RF, a further improvement, has the ability to make faster and more controlled lesions (Figure 11.2). It relies on having a pole on each side of the target tissue. This arrangement enables lesions to be made in less than 10 seconds, as all of the energy is focused between two closely approximated poles. The bipolar devices have impedance sensors designed to detect when transmural ablation has occurred; however clinical experience has shown the sensors to be unreliable. Even if repeated ablations are needed to achieve electrophysiologically effective lesions, lesions can still be created rapidly. These lesions can be created from the epicardium on a closed heart, provided the lesion is in an area of the heart that can be opposed to itself. Thick areas of tissue between the poles can make it more difficult to achieve transmurality. Alternatively, one of the poles can be inserted into the heart. Since both poles must be perfectly opposed to each other, there is somewhat limited flexibility with these devices. In addition, fat poses a significant barrier to transmural lesions. Nevertheless, bipolar RF has been applied successfully both endo- and epicardially. Bugge *et al.* [19] demonstrated that bipolar RF ablation more often achieved transmural lesions and produced narrower lesions than the unipolar device in an epicardial approach on closed, beating ovine hearts.

Microwave

In both animal models and clinical experience, microwave energy rapidly and reliably produces effective lesions with minimal to no risk of tissue surface charring (Figure 11.3). Moreover, microwave has proven to be safe; during the first

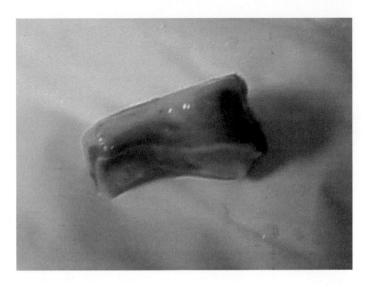

Figure 11.3 Gross specimen following microwave ablation.

1500 procedures using microwave energy, there were no reported procedure-related complications [20].

Two probes—the FLEX-4 and FLEX-10—are currently marketed by the Guidant Corp (Indianapolis, IN) (Figure 11.4). The FLEX-4 may be used for both endocardial and epicardial ablation. The FLEX-10 with its flexible ablating element was designed for epicardial use via a min-

imally invasive approach. The FLEX-10 device is composed of an ablating antenna within a teflon sheath. The antenna is withdrawn in 2-cm increments until the ablation is completed, and each 2-cm burn is performed for 90–120 seconds at 65 W. Thicker atria may require more wattage. This technique ensures that the lesions are overlapping and the ablation device does not require repositioning.

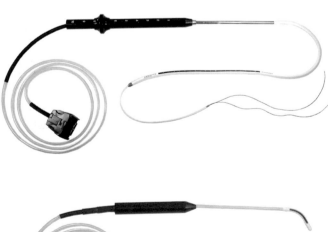

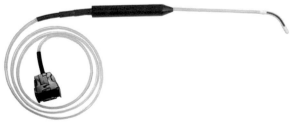

Figure 11.4 The FLEX-4 and 10 microwave devices, Guidant Corp (Indianapolis, IN). The FLEX-4 may be used for both endocardial and epicardial ablation. The FLEX-10 with its flexible ablating element was designed for epicardial use via a minimally invasive approach. (Photo courtesy of Guidant Corporation. Reprinted with permission.)

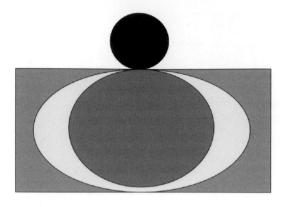

■ Direct heating

□ Conductive heating

Figure 11.5 Laser ablation: contribution of direct versus conductive heating. The Optiwave device (Edwards, CA) utilizes a 980-nm diode laser. This wavelength was chosen due it its effective penetration of cardiac tissue. It reliably ablates tissue with absorption of actual laser energy as deep as 4 mm into the tissue. Only a small contribution is made by conductive heating mechanisms.

Laser

Laser ablation is wavelength dependent. The FDA-approved Optiwave 980 device by Edwards Lifesciences (Irvine, CA) utilizes a 980-nm diode laser. This wavelength was chosen due to its effective penetration of cardiac tissue. It reliably ablates tissue with absorption of actual laser energy as deep as 4 mm into the tissue. Only a small contribution is made by conductive heating mechanisms (Figure 11.5). This compares with RF where resistive heating is limited to 1 mm below the device tissue interface. Therefore, one theoretical advantage of laser is that while other modalities focus energy at the device–tissue interface and rely primarily on conductive heating to achieve ablation, the laser's more uniform penetration of light energy through tissue allows for more equal and controlled ablation of tissue.

Laser technology may also help overcome the barrier of epicardial fat. With an extinction coefficient that is much lower in fat than myocardium, very little energy is absorbed by the fat as compared to the myocardium. As a result, the 980-nm laser energy is far less susceptible to the attenuated efficacy experienced by other modalities when fat is present. This has been supported by simulated benchtop models

in our laboratory. In fact, laser appeared to achieve transmurality almost uniformly on all specimens 7 cm or less regardless of proportion of fat (unpublished data).

Also, because laser energy does not rely on conductive heating, tissue architecture is not disrupted, endocardial structure is preserved, and char is unlikely to form. Collectively, these characteristics benefit the patient by reducing the risk of a thromboembolic event. However, as a result there may be little superficial evidence that a lesion was created. To ensure that the lesions are created contiguously, it may be advisable for the surgeon to mark the end of the lesion with a suture or marking pen.

Laser energy is delivered to the tissue via a fiber optic cable. A gold foil is positioned around 180° of the fiber acts as a mirror and reflects the energy back in the opposite direction, thus focusing energy in only one direction. The fiber optic table is coupled to a diffusing tip. The diffusing tip contains scattering particles in a silicone matrix that directs the energy radially and perpendicular to the fiber direction. The particles have a concentration gradient along the length of the fiber such that the energy distribution is uniform along the entire ablating surface. This allows for linear ablation of the energy rather than focusing energy on a single spot—as with a laser pointer (Figure 11.6).

An epicardial device (Figure 11.7) has been developed by Edwards that possesses a diffusing tip contained within a semioval-shaped sheath made of expandable polytetrafluorethylene (ePTFE). The diffusing tip, which is 4 cm in length, lies behind a clear window on the ablating surface. The handle of the device is indexed so the tip can be withdrawn to specific, preset stations. There are seven total stations that permit ablation of up to 28 cm (4 cm/station) without the need to reposition the device. This design assures overlap of each subsequent lesion [11] (Figure 11.8).

Both animal studies and clinical experience at our institution suggest that this is a promising technology [10]. In a study of canine models, the laser was successfully applied to both the endocardial and epicardial approaches. The device achieved transmural lesions in 100% of subjects from an endocardial approach. In each of the cases, these lesions were found to be electrophysiologically effective when subjected to bipolar pacing. Moreover, tissue architecture was

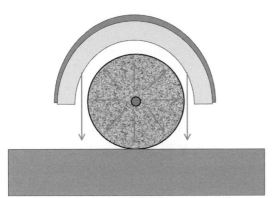

Figure 11.6 Optiwave design. Using the Optiwave device (Edwards, CA), laser energy is delivered to the tissue via a fiber optic cable. A gold foil, positioned around 180° of the fiber, acts as a mirror and reflects the energy back in the opposite direction, thus focusing energy in only one direction. The fiber optic table is coupled to a diffusing tip. The diffusing tip contains scattering particles in a silicone matrix that directs the energy radially and perpendicular to the fiber direction. The particles have a concentration gradient along the length of the fiber such that the energy distribution is uniform along the entire ablating surface. This allows for linear ablation of the energy rather than focusing energy on a single spot (as with a laser pointer).

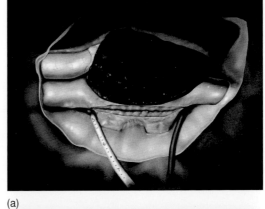

(a)

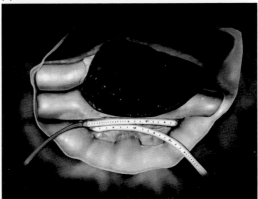

(b)

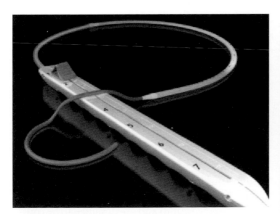

Figure 11.7 Optiwave epicardial device. An epicardial device has been developed by Edwards that possesses a diffusing tip contained within a semioval-shaped sheath made of expandable polytetrafluorethylene (ePTFE). The diffusing tip, which is 4 cm in length, lies behind a clear window on the ablating surface. The handle of the device is indexed so the tip can be withdrawn to specific, preset stations. There are seven total stations that permit ablation of up to 28 cm (4 cm/station) without the need to relocate the device. (Reprinted with permission from Edwards.)

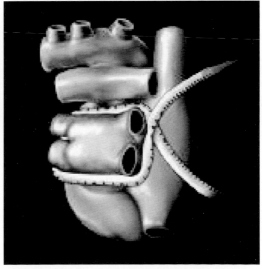

(c)

Figure 11.8 Pulmonary vein isolation with Optiwave epicardial device. After placing the probe, the ablations are performed according to the indexed stations visible on the probe surface. (Reprinted with permission from Edwards.)

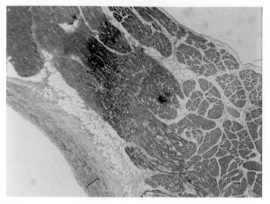

(a)

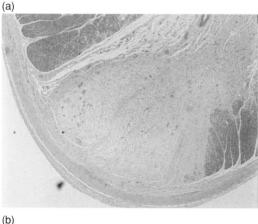

(b)

Figure 11.9 Myocardium following laser ablation in the acute phase (a) and in the chronic phase (b).

preserved (Figure 11.9). Similar results were seen with the epicardial device with transmural lesions seen in >90% of subjects using an epicardial approach. Moreover, in early clinical experience at our institution we have observed success in achieving freedom from AF in short-term follow-up with no complications or deaths related to laser ablation.

Ultrasound

Ultrasound has been used extensively in partial maze procedures to isolate pulmonary veins via catheters in the electrophysiology lab [21]. In this setting tubular transducers deliver cylindrical zones of ultrasonic waves producing circumferential lesions around individual pulmonary veins. Nevertheless, clinical experience with ultrasound in the surgical treatment of AF is limited.

Early use ultrasound suggests a number of important advantages. First, in our experience, HIFU allows for rapid, high-concentration energy in a confined space and produces transmural epicardial lesions through epicardial fat in less than 2 seconds (Figure 11.10a). In addition, the potential exists for the development of transducers to both image and ablate tissue. By imaging tissue in advance, atrial wall thickness can be measured; ablation parameters can be adjusted; and later reimaging can assess transmurality following ablation (Figure 11.10b). Finally, it has been proposed that due to the absence of acoustic heating of the blood, ultrasound energy, unlike the other energy modalities, can safely create the left atrial isthmus lesion from the epicardial surface without damaging the circumflex coronary artery. The blood flowing through the coronaries cools the endothelial lining, protecting the artery from thermal damage [22].

St Jude Medical currently markets the FDA-approved Epicor Medical Ablation System. This system includes a generator and a group of disposable ablation devices, including the UltraWand (Figure 11.11a), a handheld ablation device, and the UltraCinch device (Figure 11.11b), which creates lesions circumferentially around the pulmonary vein orifices via an array of multiple ultrasound transducers. The transducers of the UltraCinch are positioned around the epicardium. A thin perforated membrane covering the transducers circulates normal saline during ablation to enhance acoustic coupling and cooling.

The transducers are designed to deliver energy at a depth of up to 10 mm from their surface (Figure 11.12). The generator functions via three sequential stages of ablation using a range of frequencies (3.8–6.4 MHz), powers (15–130 W), and ablating times determined by a proprietary algorithm. These stages ablate tissue from endocardium back to the epicardium and are designed to be completed within 10 minutes.

Overall HIFU technology appears to be promising. In a series of 27 patients, Guffi and colleagues [13] applied ultrasound during a limited maze procedure on a closed, beating heart. This group reported a success rate of 74% at 29 months follow-up with one device related (nonfatal) complication— a left atrial wall rupture. More recently, a multicenter trial, including 103 patients who underwent

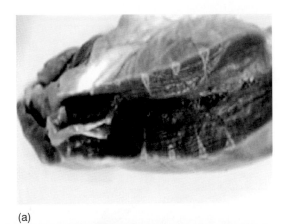

(a)

(b)

3 second, 2 second, and 1 second 50W lesions

4 second, 3 second, 2 second, and 1 second 50W lesions

4 second, 3 second, and 2 second 50W lesions

Two half-second, 50 W lesions

Figure 11.10 (a) Appearance of HIFU lesions created in pig ventricle; (b) Lesions visualization after creation.

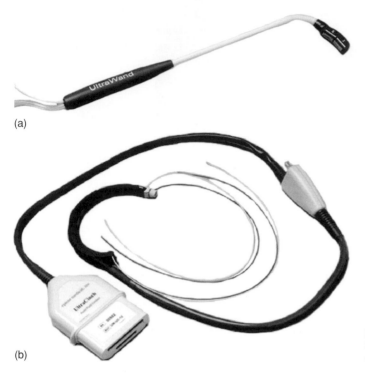

(a)

(b)

Figure 11.11 (a) UltraWand and (b) UltraCinch. (Reprinted with permission from St Jude Medical.)

epicardial, beating heart ablation, reported an 85% freedom from AF at 6-month visit with no reported complications or deaths related to the device or procedure [12].

Cryoablation
Cryoablation has the longest history in surgical atrial ablation [23]. It has two important advantages. First, cyroablation does not disrupt tissue architecture and has limited potential for endocardial damage, therefore it does not cause tissue vaporization or charring. In addition, depth of the lesion can be visually monitored. Moreover, cryo is able to achieve transmurality in a relatively short ablation time; application of a nitrous oxide-based cryoprobe to atrial tissue for 2 minutes at 60°C reliably produces a transmural lesion that can be confirmed visually.

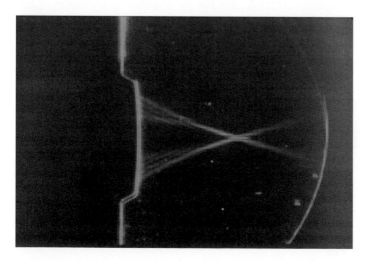

Figure 11.12 Laser representation of the acoustic field.

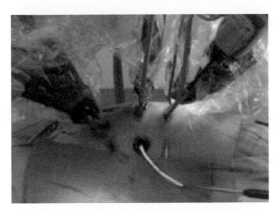

Figure 11.13 Totally endoscopic, off-pump surgical atrial fibrillation ablation.

Initially, it appeared that its bulky nature may limit its use, however, modifications allowed for creating flexible linear probes for use in epicardial and endocardial ablation. While early systems used nitric oxide, in an effort to decrease ablation time, newer systems using argon- and helium-based cooling mechanisms have been developed that achieve much colder temperatures and therefore faster ablating times. Though a few cases of coronary artery stenosis [24] have been reported while using cyroablation to create spot lesions over the tricuspid and mitral valve annuli; in general, cyroablation has had an excellent clinical safety record.

Minimally invasive approaches

At present, the maze procedure remains primarily an adjunct performed in conjunction with another open-heart surgery. However, patients with AF who have structural heart abnormalities requiring surgical repair comprise a small proportion of the entire population affected by AF. Therefore, the ultimate objective of ablation surgery remains the development of an effective, minimally invasive approach that can be applied as an isolated procedure on a closed heart without sternotomy or CPB (Figure 11.13). Such an approach could dramatically increase the number of patients who benefit from this treatment.

While tissue ablation using energy has made this procedure possible, application of this technology must be further optimized in order to ensure that electrophysiologically effective lesions can be cre-

ated reliably and reproducibility on a closed, beating heart without disrupting the tissue architecture or injuring adjacent structures. A number of centers have reported great progress moving toward this goal. And in fact some, including our center, have successfully performed an isolated, totally endoscopic, off-pump procedure [25–28].

Our approach has been pulmonary vein isolation with left atrial appendage excision [25]. We have used both microwave and laser sources during this endoscopic approach. These devices have similar designs, including an ablating probe within a sheath, as previously described. During the procedure, the sheath is passed into the transverse sinus and out under the inferior vena cava, staying posterior to the left atrial appendage, but away from the atrioventricular groove. The probe is withdrawn in short increments until the ablation is completed. This technique ensures that the lesions are overlapping, and the ablation device does not require repeated repositioning. The left atrial appendage may then be amputated via left thoracoscopy using an endoscopic stapler.

Conclusion

The maze, as Cox first described it in 1989, was highly invasive and required significant increases in operative time. Therefore, despite its impressive results, it was not widely adopted. By decreasing the time demands and technical difficulty of the procedure, the development of energy as an alternative has resulted in the resurgence of surgical treatment of AF. Experience has been accumulating with a number of energy sources including RF, microwave, cryo, laser, and ultrasound. Each has advantages and disadvantages, nevertheless use of energy in ablation remains a significant advance in the surgical treatment of AF. Refinement of these modalities will ultimately lead to widespread application of minimally invasive surgical ablative procedures.

References

1 Cox JL, Boineau JP, Schuessler RB *et al.* Successful surgical treatment of atrial fibrillation: review and clinical update. *JAMA* 1991; **266**: 1976–1980.

2 Kosakai Y, Kawaguchi AT, Isobe F *et al.* Cox maze procedure for chronic atrial fibrillation associated with mitral

valve disease. *J Thorac Cardiovasc Surg* 1994; **108**: 1049–1054.

3 Cox JL, Ferguson TB, Jr, Lindsay BD, Cain ME. Perinodal cryosurgery for atrioventricular node reentry tachycardia in 23 patients. *J Thorac Cardiovasc Surg* 1990; **99**: 440–449.

4 Cox JL, Ad N, Palazzzo T *et al*. Current status of the maze procedure for the treatment of atrial fibrillation. *Semin Thorac Cardiovasc Surg* 2000; **12**: 15–19.

5 Patwardhan AM, Dave HH, Tamhane AA *et al*. Intraoperative radiofrequency microbipolar coagulation to replace incisions of maze III procedure for correcting atrial fibrillation in patients with rheumatic valvular disease. *Eur J Cardiothorac Surg* 1997; **12**: 627–633.

6 Williams MR, Knaut M, Berube D, Oz MC. Application of microwave energy in cardiac tissue ablation: from in vitro analyses to clinical use. *Ann Thorac Surg* 2002; **74**: 1500–1505.

7 Spitzer SG, Richter P, Knaut M, Schuler S. Treatment of atrial fibrillation in open heart surgery—the potential role of microwave energy. *Thorac Cardiovasc Surg* 1999; **47**: 374–378.

8 Williams MR, Argenziano M, Oz MC. Microwave ablation for surgical treatment of atrial fibrillation. *Semin Thorac Cardiovasc Surg* 2002; **14**: 232–237.

9 Knaut M, Spitzer SG, Karolyi L *et al*. Intraoperative microwave ablation for curative treatment of atrial fibrillation in open heart surgery—the MICRO-STAF and MICROtrial. MICROwave application in surgical treatment of atrial fibrillation. MICROwave for the treatment of atrial fibrillation in bypass-surgery. *Thorac Cardiovasc Surg* 1999; **47**: 379–384.

10 Williams MR, Casher J, Russo MJ, Hong KH, Oz MC, Argenziano M. Laser energy source in surgical atrial fibrillation ablation: preclinical experience. *Ann Thorac Surg* 2006; **82**: 2260–2264.

11 Williams MR, Russo MJ, Oz MC, Argenziano M. Epicardial cardiac ablation using laser energy *Heart Surg Forum* 2006; **9**: E598–E600.

12 Ninet J, Roques X, Seitelberger R *et al*. Surgical ablation of atrial fibrillation with off-pump, epicardial, high-intensity focused ultrasound: results of a multicenter trial. *J Thorac Cardiovasc Surg* 2005; **130**: 803–809.

13 Guffi M, Visconti Brick A, Seixas T *et al*. Intraoperative treatment of chronic atrial fibrillation with ultrasound. *J Cardiovasc Surg (Torino)* 2005; **46**: 69–75.

14 Nath S, Lynch C, Whayne JG *et al*. Cellular electrophysiological effects of hyperthermia on isolated guinea pig papillary muscle. Implications for catheter ablation. *Circulation* 1993; **88**: 1826–1831.

15 Williams MR, Garrido M, Oz MC, Argenziano M. Alternative energy sources for surgical atrial ablation. *J Card Surg* 2004; **19**: 201–206.

16 Santiago T, Melo J, Gouveia RH *et al*. Epicardial radiofrequency applications: in vitro and in vivo studies on human atrial myocardium. *Eur J Cardiothorac Surg* 2003; **24**: 481–486.

17 van Brakel TJ, Bolotin G, Salleng KJ *et al*. Evaluation of epicardial microwave ablation lesions: histology versus electrophysiology. *Ann Thorac Surg* 2004; **78**: 1397–1402.

18 Cox JL. Surgical treatment of atrial fibrillation: a review. *Europace* 2004; **5**: S20–S29.

19 Bugge E, Nicholson IA, Thomas SP. Comparison of bipolar and unipolar radiofrequency ablation in an in vivo experimental model. *Eur J Cardiothorac Surg* 2005; **28**: 76–80.

20 Schuetz A, Schulze CJ, Sarvanakis KK *et al*. Surgical treatment of permanent atrial fibrillation using microwave energy ablation: a prospective randomized clinical trial. *Eur J Cardiothorac Surg* 2003; **24**: 475–480.

21 Saliba W, Wilber D, Packer D *et al*. Circumferential ultrasound ablation for pulmonary vein isolation: analysis of acute and chronic failures [Comment]. *J Cardiovasc Electrophysiol* 2002; **13**: 957–961.

22 Curra F, Mourad P, Crum LA. High intensity focused ultrasound and tissue heating: the effect of nonlinear sound propagation and vessel presence. *Proc IEEE Ultrason Symp* 1998; **2**: 1419–1422.

23 Cox JL. The surgical treatment of atrial fibrillation: IV. Surgical technique. *J Thorac Cardiovasc Surg* 1991; **101**: 584–592.

24 Holman WL, Ikeshita M, Ungerleider RM *et al*. Cryosurgery for cardiac arrhythmias: acute and chronic effects on coronary arteries. *Am J Card* 1983; **51**: 149–155.

25 Argenziano M, Williams MR. Robotic atrial septal defect repair and endoscopic treatment of atrial fibrillation. *Semin Thorac Cardiovasc Surg* 2003; **15**: 130–140.

26 Saltman AE, Rosenthal LS, Francalancia NA, Lahey SJ. A completely endoscopic approach to microwave ablation for atrial fibrillation. *Heart Surg Forum* 2003; **6**: E38–E41.

27 Reade CC, Johnson JO, Bolotin G *et al*. Combining robotic mitral valve repair and microwave atrial fibrillation ablation: techniques and initial results. *Ann Thorac Surg* 2005; **79**: 480–484.

28 Loulmet DF, Patel NC, Patel NU *et al*. First robotic endoscopic epicardial isolation of the pulmonary veins with microwave energy in a patient in chronic atrial fibrillation. *Ann Thorac Surg* 2004; **78**: e24–e25.

CHAPTER 12

Radiofrequency modified maze surgery for chronic atrial fibrillation and concomitant cardiac surgery: Zwolle experience

Hauw T. Sie, Willem P. Beukema, Arif Elvan, Hacer Sen, Anand Ramdat Misier, Giuseppe D'Ancona & Fabio Bartolozzi

Introduction

Atrial fibrillation (AF) is a common arrhythmia, present in 0.4% of the general population and in more than 1% of the population older than 60 years of age [1, 2]. About 40–60% of patients undergoing mitral valve (MV) operations have AF at the time of the operation [3–7]. Although cardiac contractile function usually improves after MV surgery, in many patients long-standing AF will persist after valve surgery [3–7]. Pharmacological and electrical cardioversion in this setting is often ineffective, and attempts to establish sinus rhythm by serial cardioversions are disappointing; therefore, this arrhythmia is usually considered to be permanent. During the past decades several surgical methods have been designed to treat AF. The most effective one seems to be the maze procedure developed by Cox and associates [8–10]. The maze procedure restores sinus rhythm and atrioventricular (AV) synchrony with demonstrable atrial transport function. In patients undergoing complex cardiac procedures, surgeons are reluctant to expose their patients to the risks of the "cut-and-sew" maze procedure. Radiofrequency (RF) catheter ablation has become an important mode of treatment in patients

with supraventricular and ventricular tachycardias. In patients with atrial flutter (AFL) or atrial reentrant tachycardias, RF energy is used to create continuous linear lesions in the atrium, interrupting a critical part of the reentrant circuit. The RF modified maze based on Cox's maze III is a simple and effective alternative to eliminate AF during cardiac surgery [11–18]. We describe our experience with RF modified maze procedure in Zwolle.

Methods

Patient characteristics

All 300 patients included in this study had an indication for cardiac surgery irrespective of AF. Inclusion criterion for AF surgery was AF lasting for more than 1 year. The decision to perform cardiac surgery was made by the patient's cardiologist and cardiothoracic surgeon. Conventional clinical and hemodynamic criteria were applied to assess the indication for surgery. Before the surgical intervention, clinical characteristics of each patient including New York Heart Association (NYHA) classification and medication were assessed by one investigator. Rhythm characteristics (presence and duration of AF) were assessed by using the patient's history and previous electrocardiograms. Echocardiographic data were obtained within 3 months before cardiac surgery. Patients who needed urgent cardiac surgery were excluded from this study. All

Manual of Surgical Treatment of Atrial Fibrillation.
Edited by Hauw T. Sie *et al.* © 2008 Blackwell Publishing,
ISBN: 978-1-4051-4032-4.

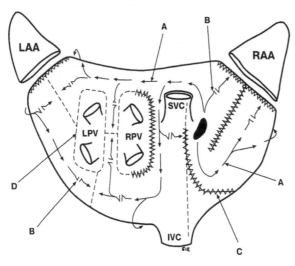

Dorsal aspect

Figure 12.1 RF modified maze schematic view of the dorsal aspect of the heart. A/B—lines of electrical activation; C—zigzaglines depicting the incisions in the atria; D—dotted lines depicting the ablation lines. IVC, inferior vena cava; LAA, left atrial appendage; LPV, left pulmonary veins; RAA, right atrial appendage; RPV, right pulmonary veins; SVC, superior vena cava.

patients consented to their data being registered and used for publication as did the Board of Hospital Administrators. All patients underwent an RF modified maze procedure as an adjunct to the open-heart operation. Patients were followed in the outpatient clinic or follow-up data were obtained from attending or referring physicians.

The data were obtained from two registries, i.e., the unipolar RF maze registry and the bipolar RF maze registry.

Unipolar RF maze group

From November 1995 to June 2003, 200 patients were included in the "unipolar" RF maze registry. These 200 patients with structural heart disease and permanent AF were scheduled for elective cardiac surgery. RF modified maze procedure was performed using a unipolar RF ablation device. RF energy was used to create long continuous endocardial lesions under direct vision with a hand-held cooled tip probe. The RF energy was administered by using a continuous sinusoidal unmodulated waveform of 500 kHz and delivered in a unipolar mode between the 4-mm tip electrode of a specially designed probe and a 106-cm external backplate electrode that was underneath the back of the patient. The ablation procedure was done in a bloodless operating field, and temperature-guided energy applications were performed with a preselected catheter tip temperature of 60°C. The tip was irrigated with saline

solution at a flow rate of 4 mL/min. In the first 173 patients a custom-made RF probe with a saline irrigation system incorporated to cool the tip of the probe was used along with an HAT 200S generator (Sulzer-Osypka GmbH, Grenzach-Wyhlen, Germany). In 85 patients who had undergone surgery after November 2000 the Medtronic cooled tip Cardioblate pen was used. The tip of both types of RF probe was irrigated with saline at room temperature at a flow rate of 4–6 mL/min.

Application of energy was done by oscillating the probe back and forth at a speed of 1 cm/sec for approximately 20 seconds with a standard power setting of 25–30 W and saline irrigation flow rate of 5 mL/min.

Surgical procedure

The heart was exposed through a median sternotomy and suspended in a pericardial cradle. Cardiopulmonary bypass was instituted by using standard aortic and bicaval cannulation and moderate hypothermia (28°C). All atrial incisions currently used in the Cox-maze procedure were replaced in our RF modification by endocardial linear ablation lines as illustrated in Figures 12.1 through 12.4 except for the incisions to enter the left and right atrial cavity. According to the original maze III both appendages were excised as well. There was no need for additional cryosurgical applications. Concomitant procedures (e.g., aortic valve replacement and

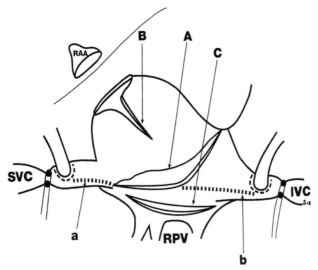

Right lateral view

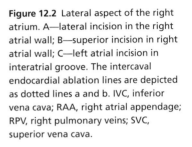

Figure 12.2 Lateral aspect of the right atrium. A—lateral incision in the right atrial wall; B—superior incision in right atrial wall; C—left atrial incision in interatrial groove. The intercaval endocardial ablation lines are depicted as dotted lines a and b. IVC, inferior vena cava; RAA, right atrial appendage; RPV, right pulmonary veins; SVC, superior vena cava.

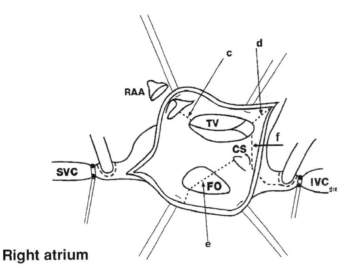

Right atrium

Figure 12.3 View inside the right atrium. The right atrium is exposed by stay sutures. The endocardial ablation lines are presented as dotted lines c, d, e, and f. CS, coronary sinus; FO, foramen ovale; IVC, inferior vena cava; RAA, right atrial appendage; SVC, superior vena cava; TV, tricuspid valve.

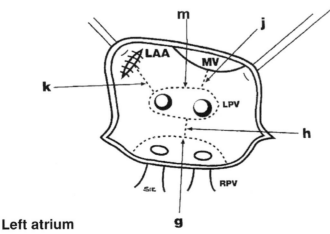

Left atrium

Figure 12.4 View inside the left atrium. The left atrium is exposed by stay sutures. The endocardial ablation lines are presented as dotted lines g, h, j, k, and m. LAA, left appendage; LPV, left pulmonary veins; MV, mitral valve; RPV, right pulmonary veins.

coronary bypass grafting) were performed immediately after aortic cross-clamping and before completing the left-sided maze and the MV procedure.

Right-sided maze procedure. After both caval cannulas were snared, the right atrium was opened through a posterior longitudinal incision starting caudally of the superior caval cannulation site at the dorsolateral aspect of the right atrium (Figures 12.1 and 12.2). This incision was extended along the border of the interatrial septum, slightly curved and finally ending at the AV groove opposite the inferior caval cannulation site (Figure 12.2A). The right atrial appendage was excised, and an anterior incision (Figure 12.2B) of approximately 4 cm was made from the middle of the anterolateral aspect of the base of the amputated auricle toward the inferior caval vein orifice. RF energy was then used to extend the electrical block caused by the first surgical incision (Figure 12.2A) cranially as far as possible toward the superior caval cannulation site (Figure 12.2, dotted line a) and caudally toward the inferior caval cannulation site (Figure 12.2, dotted line b). Additional RF ablation lines (Figure 12.3) were drawn from the medial aspect of the base of the excised right atrial appendage into the anulus of the tricuspid valve (Figure 12.3, dotted line c) and from the caudal end of the first surgical incision at the AV groove (Figure 12.2A) to the posterior part of the anulus of the tricuspid valve (Figure 12.3, dotted line d). This part of the maze procedure was performed on the beating heart without a cross-clamp. The septal part of the procedure was performed in a later stage of the operation, just before closing the left atrium to prevent tearing of the septum.

Left-sided maze procedure. The aorta was cross-clamped, and the heart was arrested with cold cardioplegic solution. Access to the inside of the left atrium was gained via a standard atriotomy in the interatrial groove, as for an MV procedure (Figure 12.2C). After excision of the left atrial appendage and resuturing of the amputation site, the left-sided maze was performed by linear ablation lines as illustrated in Figure 12.4. In addition to the incision in the interatrial groove (Figure 12.2C), isolation of the right pulmonary veins was completed by a unilateral ablation line (Figure 12.4, dotted line g). The left pulmonary veins were encircled (Figure 12.4, dotted line f), and a connecting line (Figure 12.4, dotted line h) was drawn between both islands of pulmonary veins. Ablation lines were also performed from the ablation line isolating the left pulmonary vein to the base of the left atrial appendage amputation site (Figure 12.4, dotted line k) and to the posterior MV anulus (Figure 12.4, dotted line j). Subsequently, the MV procedure was carried out. The maze procedure was then completed with an ablation line drawn on the right-sided aspect of the interatrial septum starting from the middle of the posterior longitudinal right atriotomy (Figure 12.2A) across the interatrial septum up to the caudal aspect of the os of the coronary sinus extended to the inferior vena cava cannulation site (Figure 12.3, dotted line e). After rewarming the left atrium was closed and the cross-clamp released. The heart was then deaired extensively before defibrillation and to closing of the right atrium. Occasionally atrial pacing or AV pacing was needed to wean the patient from bypass.

Bipolar RF maze group

From October 2003 to May 2005, 100 patients were included in the "bipolar" RF maze registry. We evaluated the medium-term results of a novel ablation technique to eliminate AF by means of an irrigated bipolar RF ablation device. We produced lines of conduction block using the Cardioblate irrigated RF ablation clamp (Medtronic Inc., Minneapolis). The biatrial lesion pattern used was similar to the modified maze including isolation of the coronary sinus and isolation of the right cavotricuspid and left mitral isthmus. All lesions were made with this bipolar RF ablation device, which has a self-regulating ablation protocol based on an impedance feedback system. Transmurality feedback is indicated based on a steady-state plateau in tissue impedance.

This biatrial procedure can safely be performed partially on a beating heart.

Preoperative management

In the 300 patients enrolled in the study, ventricular rate control medication, i.e., calcium channel blockers and/or digoxin, was allowed to continue until the day before surgery. Oral anticoagulant therapy (warfarin) for the prevention of thromboembolism secondary to chronic AF was discontinued 2 days before surgery. B-Adrenergic blockers were continued.

Postoperative management and follow-up

Early postoperative care, including anticoagulant management, was similar as for routine cardiac surgery. Cardiac rhythm was continuously monitored after surgery until stable rhythm returned. Temporary epicardial wires attached to the right ventricle as well as to the right atrium were used to pace the patient, to monitor the rhythm, or to overdrive the atrium. Postoperative atrial arrhythmias were treated with sotalol 80–120 mg or amiodarone 200 mg and combined with direct-current cardioversion if necessary. All patients were operated in one institution and by the same surgeon (H.T.S.). After discharge, patients were seen in the outpatient clinic within 4 weeks, at 3 months and at 6 months after operation, or earlier when necessary. Antiarrhythmic drugs were tapered gradually after cardiac rhythm was considered stable. The presence of atrial contraction as documented by transthoracic and transesophageal Doppler echocardiography was performed at 3 and 6 months after surgery and related to the presence of electrical activity in the surface electrocardiogram. After 6 months and up to 3 years, patient status was determined by screening records of outpatient visits and correspondence with referring physicians.

Statistical analysis

All data are reported as mean and standard deviation. Analysis of variance was applied to compare effects over time and effects per time point. The arrhythmia-free survival curves were constructed by using the Kaplan–Meier method, differences between groups were investigated with the log-rank test. A confidence level of 95% was considered statistically significant.

Results

Unipolar RF maze group

The unipolar RF maze group included 200 patients with a mean age of 68 ± 9.5 years and median age of 70 years with permanent AF, i.e., AF with a duration of ≥ 12 months (Table 12.1). Mean duration of permanent AF was 66 ± 70 months (median

Table 12.1 Demographics.

	Bipolar RF maze (n = 100 patients)	Unipolar RF maze (n = 200 patients)
Gender		
Male	67/100 (67%)	92 (46%)
Female	33/100 (33%)	108 (54%)
Age		
Mean ± SD (yr)	68.1 ± 10.9	68.2 ± 11.3
Median (Q1–Q3)	70.9 (60.5–75.9)	71.2 (59.1–76.5)
Min–max	32–87	30–88
Age distribution		
30–40	3/100 (3%)	3/200 (1.5%)
40–50	4/100 (4%)	11/200 (10.5%)
50–60	17/100 (17%)	31/200 (15.5%)
60–70	20/100 (20%)	71/200 (35.5%)
70–80	45/100 (45%)	82/200 (41%)
80–90	11/100 (11%)	2/200 (1%)

35 mo, range 12–396 mo). Preoperatively, 82.9% of patients were in functional NYHA class 3 and 5.0% in functional NYHA class 4. Left ventricular (LV) ejection fraction (EF) was normal (LVEF 50–60%) in 49.3%, moderately decreased (LVEF 30–50%) in 37.3%, and poor (LVEF <30%) in 13.4% of patients. The etiology of AF was MV disease in the great majority of patients (Tables 12.2 and 12.3).

Cardiac rhythm at follow-up after unipolar RF maze

The long-term follow-up period ranged from 12 to 80 months (mean 40). Complete data were available for 158 patients at the latest follow-up. Eight of 166 long-term surviving patients were excluded from the analysis because they were lost to follow-up. The arrhythmia-free survival in the study patient is shown in Figure 12.5. Sinus or atrial rhythm (AR) was present in 116 of 158 patients (73.4%) and AV sequential pacing was documented in 10 of 158 long-term survivors (6.3%). Thirty-two patients (20.3%) remained in AF or flutter (Table 12.2). Successful elimination of AF in patients with MV-related procedures ranged from 72 to 87% in contrast to 62.5% of patients (20 of 32) in whom non-MV surgery was performed. The lowest percentage of sinus rhythm, 42% (5 of 13), occurred in the patients who underwent CABG (Table 12.3). In six patients with sick sinus syndrome (3%) and one patient with postoperative complete AV block

Table 12.2 Etiology AF.

	Bipolar RF maze (n = 100 patients)	Unipolar RF maze (n = 200 patients)
Mitral valve	80/100 (80%)	173/200 (87%)
Prolapse	8	35
Annulus dilatation	35	33
Degenerative MI	20	53
Ruptured chordae	4	9
Rheumatic	11	42
Ischemic and/or hypertension	34	57
Other	6	11
Aortic valve disease	25/100 (25%)	31/200 (15.5%)
NYHA class		
II	1/100 (1%)	22 (11%)
III	91/100 (91%)	166 (83%)
IV	8/100 (8%)	6 (3%)
Euroscore		
Mean ± SD	6.29 ± 2.78	5.3 ± 2.1
Median (Q1–Q3)	6 (4–8)	5 (4–6)
Min–max	2–16	1–13

Table 12.3 Preoperative echocardiography.

LV ejection fraction		
<25%	3	10
25–35%	10	49
35–45%	18	35
45–55%	24	54
>55%	37	52
LVEF mean ± SD (%)	43 ± 9.1	40 ± 8.3
LA (pslax, mean ± SD in mm)	47.80 ± 7.55e	50.9 ± 9.1
LA (pslax, range in mm)	43–50	33–80

pslax, parasternal longaxis view.

a pacemaker was implanted. In 60 of 121 patients (49%) who underwent MV surgery antiarrhythmic drugs (AAD), predominantly sotalol (80 mg daily) or amiodarone (200 mg daily), were maintained, in the majority of cases because of paroxysmal atypical AFL. The lowest incidence of AAD use (37%) was in patients with MV repair (23 of 61) whereas the highest use of AAD (65%) was in the group of patients who had had a mechanical MV prosthesis implanted (25 of 38). Fifty-four percent of patients (12 of 22)

with a biological MV prosthesis were treated with antiarrhythmic drugs. Restoration of sinus or AR, absence of spontaneous left atrial echocontrast, and documented left-sided atrial transport (presence of an A wave) by transesophageal Doppler echocardiography were reasons to consider discontinuation of Coumadin during follow-up. Anticoagulation therapy was discontinued in 59% of patients (36 of 61) who underwent MV repair and in 32% of patients (7 of 22) with a biological MV prosthesis.

Mortality and morbidity after unipolar RF maze

Among the 200 patients, there were seven inhospital deaths (3.5%). Three patients died of multiorgan failure, two patients died of low cardiac output. One late tamponade and one mitral annulus rupture were the cause of death in another two patients. Postoperative inhospital complications were

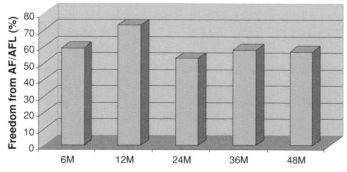

Figure 12.5 Cardiac rhythm after unipolar RF maze and concomitant cardiac surgery. Freedom from AF/AFL includes all patients with sinus rhythm, atrial rhythm, or atrial-based paced rhythm. Postop, postoperative rhythm. 6M, 12M, 24M, 36M, and 48M mean 6, 12, 24, 36, and 48 months after RF maze, respectively. See text for details.

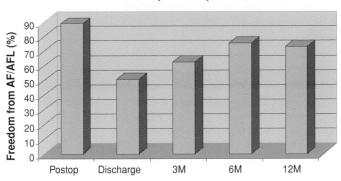

Follow-up after bipolar RF maze

Figure 12.6 Cardiac rhythm after bipolar RF maze and concomitant cardiac surgery. Freedom from AF/AFL includes all patients with sinus rhythm, atrial rhythm, or atrial-based paced rhythm. Postop, postoperative rhythm. Discharge means cardiac rhythm at the time of discharge from the hospital. 3M, 6M, and 12M mean 3, 6, and 12 months after RF maze, respectively. See text for details.

rethoracotomy in 16 patients, use of an intraaortic balloon pump in eight patients, and sternal wound infection in three patients. Endocarditis, stroke, and AV conduction block occurred in one patient each. There were no complications related to the RF maze procedure such as collateral damage to adjacent structures. Constrictive pericarditis occurred late in two patients. During follow-up 27 patients (13.5%) died because of end-stage heart failure (8 patients), hemorrhagic stroke (4 patients, all but 1 patient using Coumadin), cancer (2 patients), gastrointestinal ischemia/infarction (1 patient on Coumadin therapy), and miscellaneous causes (13 patients). The overall proportion of patients surviving in this series is shown in Figure 12.3.

Bipolar RF maze

The baseline patient characteristics are summarized in Table 12.1. MV disease was the etiology of AF in the majority of the patients (Table 12.2). Most of the patients were in functional NYHA class III at the time of operation (Table 12.2). The mean euroscore was 6.3 ± 2.8. Left atrium was enlarged with an echocardiographic left atrial dimension of 48 ± 7.5 mm measured using the parasternal long axis view. The duration of AF 57.1 ± 57.8 months (range 4–360 mo). Mean cardiopulmonary bypass (CPB) and cross-clamp durations were 238.7 ± 85.3 minutes and 119.3 ± 50 minutes, respectively. Mean ablation time was 236.9 ± 64.4 seconds. Concomitant procedures included MV plasty ($n = 54$), MV replacement ($n = 13$), aortic valve replacement ($n = 19$), aortic root replacement ($n = 2$),

tricuspid valve plasty ($n = 86$), and coronary bypass grafting ($n = 42$).

The inhospital mortality was 6% (n = 6, 4 noncardiac and 2 cardiac causes). During the mean follow-up of $19 + / - 11$ months (range 1–40 months) late mortality was 3% (2 cardiac causes, 1 noncardiac cause). One patient (1.0%) was lost from follow-up and complete data were available of 90 survivors. SR, AR, or atrial-based paced rhythm (ABPR) was present in 75.6% at 6 months, in 73.2% at 12 months, and in 73.8% at 18 months (Figure 12.6). Antiarrhythmic drugs were used in 49% of survivors who were free of AF or flutter.

Discussion

Main findings

We describe the intermediate to long-term results of a large cohort of patients with long-lasting AF who underwent the RF modified maze procedure as a concomitant procedure as reported previously [11, 12]. The study group consists of an unselected population of patients with a variety of cardiac diseases who underwent intraoperative RF ablation mainly in combination with additional cardiac procedures. Inhospital mortality in our total patient group was comparable with mortality rates in previous reports of patients who underwent mainly isolated MV surgery with or without AF [2–7, 19–21].

Comparison with previous studies

The maze procedure was pioneered by Cox et al., who designed the procedure in the laboratory as an open-heart operation through a median sternotomy (maze I) and subsequently made two modifications culminating in the maze III procedure [8–10, 22]. The cut-and-sew Cox-maze procedure abolishes AF in 74–97% of patients. Some investigators report a significantly lower stroke rate in maze versus non-maze patients in matched cohorts [23–32]. None of these studies however was randomized controlled trials.

Variant maze procedures, i.e., modifications of the lesion set of the Cox-maze III and the use of energy sources like RF, cryoablation, and microwave have not been able to completely mimic the results of the cut-and-sew maze with return of sustained SR between 44 and 92%, with the exception of a study of Raman and coworkers, who in a multi-center trial studied 132 patients with AF (75% permanent), who underwent an RF maze procedure (70% endocardial lesion set and 30% epicardial lesion set) as an adjunct to elective open-heart surgery [11, 12, 15–18, 30–34]. Preoperative LA size was 54 ± 3 mm and 45 ± 4 mm for the endocardial and epicardial groups, respectively. Inhospital mortality was 6.8%. At 6 months follow-up with 50 patients at risk SR was present in 90% of patients and at 12 months all 15 patients at risk had SR [35].

A recent meta-analysis [36] of clinical outcomes of randomized maze-related surgical procedures for medically refractory AF finds successful restoration of SR in the maze group (80.7% versus 17.3%, $p < 0.000001$). A consistent and highly significant finding, however it suffers from small sample sizes and except for the successful restoration of SR all other significant findings [less stroke in the maze group (0% versus 5.8%, $p = 0.008$), increased need for pacemaker therapy in the maze group (3.9% versus 1.5%), and increased postoperative bleeding in the "cut-and-sew" maze (4.3% versus 0%, $p = 0.007$)] were overturned by sensitivity analyses (omitting 1 study renders the p value insignificant). Mortality did not differ between groups. Mean LVEF was normal in all randomized studies with the exception of the study of Jessurun et al. [37] in which it was slightly depressed at 45%. Since a low EF is a risk factor for stroke, AF and mortality, the incidence of stroke and AF may be higher in a cohort with low EFs. Follow-up was relatively short (12–18 mo). Mean duration of AF was between 6 months and 3.7 years and an unknown number of patients may have had AF for not more than 12 months, which favors "spontaneous" restoration of sinus rhythm after surgical correction of the underlying defect (only 1 study mentions median duration of AF).

A prospectively randomized study by Doukas et al. [38] compared an RF modification of the maze procedure in 49 patients referred for MV surgery with at least 6 months of continuous AF with single MV surgery in 48 patients (control group). Preoperative LVEF was 57% in the RF maze group and 58% in the control group. At 12 months SR was present in 44.4% of the RF maze group and in 4.5% of control group patients ($p < 0.001$; 95% CI, 2.4–86.3). At 12 months patients in SR had a significantly better LVEF (59% versus 54.2%, $p = 0.004$), LV end-diastolic volume was lower (3.93 cm versus 4.26 cm, $p = 0.03$) and exercised significantly longer. Filho et al. used cooled-tip RF ablation in patients with permanent AF (duration 66.1 ± 57.4 mo and 43.8 ± 2 8.5 mo for the maze group and non-maze group, respectively) and rheumatic MV disease that were randomly assigned to undergo MV surgery with a maze procedure ($n = 35$) or MV surgery alone ($n = 35$). Mean age and mean LVEF in the maze group was 55.4 ± 12.8 years and 62.8 ± 9.2%, respectively, and in the non-maze group 50.7 ± 9.7 years and 66.1 ± 10.5%. After a mean follow-up of 12 months mortality in both groups was not different. SR was present in 79.4% of the maze group and in 26.9% of the non-maze group ($p = 0.001$).

One may conclude that in the majority of reported maze studies patients are between 50 and 60 years of age, have normal or moderately decreased LVEFs, permanent AF > 12 months, and 75% or more have structural heart disease, AF not being the primary reason for surgery. Short-term and intermediate term SR postclassical maze or variant maze varies widely and is reported between 44 and 95%. Mortality benefit for maze over non-maze has not yet been proven and in the six trials that have randomized patients to maze or non-maze stroke rate is not significantly lower in the maze group compared with the non-maze group. Part of almost all surgical procedures is amputation of the left atrial appendage (LAA) [39–42].

Stroke and RF modified maze procedure

AF is an independent risk factor for stroke and may play a role in 15–20% of all ischemic strokes. Annual stroke rate in nonrheumatic AF patients without oral anticoagulation is 4.5% [43–48]. The stroke rate in this registry was low. Only six strokes (5 ischemic and 1 hemorrhagic) occurred after discharge. This may be explained by the fact that the great majority of patients were taking oral anticoagulants, whether in SR or AF and by the fact that in all patients the LAA was obliterated or amputated.

Warfarin reduces the risk of stroke by 62%, albeit at the cost of intracranial hemorrhage incidence of 0.5% per year [43–48]. In a recent subanalysis of the RACE study, a randomized study comparing long-term effects of rhythm and rate control strategies on morbidity and mortality in patients with persistent AF, thromboembolic complications occurred equally in the SR group and AF group, despite the use of oral anticoagulation in both groups [49].

Surgical obliteration or amputation of the LAA may be a potentially valuable (additional) strategy for stroke prophylaxis and may be a (partial) explanation for the extremely low stroke rate in some studies of maze surgery [39–42, 50].

Limitations

A major limitation of all studies or registries of treatment of AF is the fact that the burden of atrial arrhythmia cannot reliably be determined unless a device with a specific algorithm to detect atrial arrhythmia is in situ. Quality of life issues need to be addressed. There is the issue of silent AF: how sure can we be about sinus rhythm being present most of the time and does maze induced SR translate in a reduction of stroke. At the present time there is not enough available evidence for clinicians to answer the question who is to profit from maze surgery and who will not. Careful individual patient assessment will guide us, until new randomized studies and longer follow-up of current studies will provide the answers to the key questions.

Limitations with using monopolar RF, microwave, or cryoenergy to treat AF is that it is not possible to verify transmurality of the linear lesions at the time of energy delivery. Electrical activity may still traverse nontransmural lesions created endo-cardially on the epicardial surface of the atrium or through gaps in the ablation lines. However, given that there is no real-time method to document complete conduction block one may speculate on the importance of functional block in these ablation lesions on clinical outcome. The RF modified maze, however, simplifies the classic cut-and-sew maze operation with long-term results similar to other reports as discussed in the previous chapter. The results of this observational study with a relatively large number of patients are from a single center performed by one same surgeon and multicenter studies are needed. Almost half of the patients are still on antiarrhythmic drugs at latest follow-up because the decision to cease medication was at the discretion of referring physicians. With regard to patients who underwent non-MV surgery and RF ablation of AF the limited number of patients do not allow us to draw definitive conclusions on the efficacy of this treatment to eliminate the arrhythmia in this particular group of patients.

References

1 Ostrander LD, Jr, Brandt RL, Kjeldsberg MO. Electrocardiographic findings among the adult population of a total natural community, Tecumseh, Michigan. *Circulation* 1965; **31**: 888–898.

2 Chua LY, Schaff HV, Orszulak TA, Morris JJ. Outcome of mitral valve repair in patients with preoperative atrial fibrillation. *J Thorac Cardiovasc Surg* 1994; **107**: 408–411.

3 Handa N, Schaff HV, Morris JJ, Anderson BJ, Kopecky SL, Enriquez-Sarano M. Outcome of valve repair and the Cox maze procedure for mitral regurgitation and associated atrial fibrillation. *J Thorac Cardiovasc Surg* 1999; **118**: 626–635.

4 Hansen JF, Andersen ED, Olesen KH *et al.* DC-conversion of atrial fibrillation after mitral valve operation. An analysis of the long-term results. *Scand J Thorac Cardiovasc Surg* 1979; **13**: 267–270.

5 Sato S, Kawashima Y, Hirose H, Nakano S, Matsuda H, Shirakura R. Long-term results of direct-cardioversion after open commissurotomy for mitral stenosis. *Am J Cardiol* 1986; **57**: 629–633.

6 Skoularigis J, Rothlisberger C, Skudicky D, Essop MR, Wisenbaugh T, Sareli P. Effectiveness of amiodarone after mitral valve surgery. *Am J Cardiol* 1993; **72**: 423–427.

7 Obaida JF, El Farra M, Bastien OH, Lie'vre M, Martelloni Y, Chassignolle JF. Outcome of atrial fibrillation after mitral valve repair. *J Thorac Cardiovasc Surg* 1997; **114**: 179–185.

8 Cox JL, Schuessler RB, D'Agostino HJ, Jr, Stone CM, Chang BC, Caine ME. The surgical treatment of atrial fibrillation. III. Development of a definitive surgical procedure. *J Thorac Cardiovasc Surg* 1991; **101**: 569–583.

9 Cox JL, Jaquiss RDB, Schuessler RB, Boineau JP. Modification of the maze procedure for atrial flutter and atrial fibrillation. II. Surgical technique of the maze III procedure. *J Thorac Cardiovasc Surg* 1995; **110**: 485–495.

10 Kosakai Y, Kawaguchi AT, Isobe F *et al.* Cox maze procedure for chronic atrial fibrillation associated with mitral valve disease. *J Thorac Cardiovasc Surg* 1994; **108**: 1049–1055.

11 Sie HT, Beukema WP, Elvan A, Ramdat Misier AR. Long-term results of irrigated radiofrequency modified maze procedure in 200 patients with concomitant cardiac surgery: six years experience. *Ann Thorac Surg* 2004; **77**: 512–517.

12 Sie HT, Beukema WP, Ramdat Misier AR *et al.* Radiofrequency modified maze in patients with atrial fibrillation undergoing concomitant cardiac surgery. *J Thorac Cardiovasc Surg* 2001; **122**: 249–256.

13 Pasic M, Bergs P, Muller P *et al.* Intraoperative radiofrequency maze ablation for atrial fibrillation: the Berlin modification. *Ann Thorac Surg* 2001; **72**: 1484–1491.

14 Mohr FW, Fabricius AM, Falk V *et al.* Curative treatment of atrial fibrillation with intraoperative radiofrequency ablation: short-term and midterm results. *J Thorac Cardiovasc Surg* 2002; **123**: 919–927.

15 Khargi K, Deneke T, Haardt H *et al.* Saline-irrigated cooled tip radiofrequency ablation is an effective technique to perform the maze procedure. *Ann Thorac Surg* 2001; **72**(suppl): S1090–S1095.

16 Melo JQ, Neves J, Adragao P *et al.* Surgery for atrial fibrillation using radiofrequency catheter ablation: assessment of results at one year. *Eur J Cardiothorac Surg* 1999; **15**: 851–855.

17 Williams MR, Stewart JR, Bolling SF *et al.* Surgical treatment of atrial fibrillation using radiofrequency energy. *Ann Thorac Surg* 2001; **71**: 1939–1944.

18 Raman JS, Seevanayagam S, Storer M, Power JM. Combined endocardial and epicardial radiofrequency ablation of right and left atria in the treatment of atrial fibrillation. *Ann Thorac Surg* 2000; **72**(suppl): S1096–S1099.

19 Yuda S, Nakatani S, Kosakai Y, Yamagishi M, Miyatake K. Long-term follow-up of atrial contraction after the maze procedure in patients with mitral valve disease. *J Am Coll Cardiol* 2001; **37**: 1622–1627.

20 Kim KB, Cho KR, Sohn DW, Ahn A, Rho JR. The Cox-maze III procedure for atrial fibrillation associated with rheumatic mitral valve disease. *Ann Thorac Surg* 1999; **68**: 799–804.

21 Handa N, Schaff HV, Morris JJ, Anderson BJ, Kopecky SL, Enriquez-Sarano M. Outcome of valve repair and the Cox maze procedure for mitral regurgitation and associated atrial fibrillation. *J Thorac Cardiovasc Surg* 1999; **118**: 628–635.

22 Cox JL, Ad N, Palazzo T *et al.* Current status of the maze procedure for the treatment of atrial fibrillation. *Semin Thorac Cardiovasc Surg* 2000; **12**: 15–19.

23 Schaff HV, Dearani JA, Daly RC, Orszulak TA, Danielson GK. Cox-maze procedure for atrial fibrillation: Mayo Clinic experience. *Semin Thorac Cardiovasc Surg* 2000; **12**: 30–37.

24 Millar RC, Arcidi JM, Alison PJM. The maze III procedure: should the indications be expanded? *Ann Thorac Surg* 2000; **70**: 1580–1586.

25 Kosakai Y. Treatment of atrial fibrillation using the maze procedure: the Japanese experience. *Semin Thorac Cardiovasc Surg* 2000; **12**: 44–52.

26 Raanani E, Albage A, David T, Yau T, Armstrong S. The efficacy of the Cox/maze procedure combined with mitral surgery: a matched control study. *Eur J Cardiothorac Surg* 2001; **19**: 438–442.

27 Prasad SM, Maniar HS, Camillo CJ *et al.* The Cox maze III procedure for lone atrial fibrillation: long-term efficacy in patients undergoing lone versus concomitant procedures. *J Thorac Cardiovasc Surg* 2003; **126**: 1822–1828.

28 Gillinov AM, Sirak J, Blackstone EH *et al.* The Cox maze procedure in mitral valve disease: predictors of recurrent atrial fibrillation. *J Thorac Cardiovasc Surg* 2005; **130**: 1653–1660.

29 Jatene MB, Marcial MB, Tarasoutchi F, Cardoso RA, Pomerantzeff P, Jatene AD. Influence of the maze procedure on the treatment of rheumatic atrial fibrillation-evaluation of rhythm control and clinical outcome in a comparative study. *Eur J Cardiothorac Surg* 2000; **17**: 117–124.

30 Pasic M, Bergs P, Müller P *et al.* Intraoperative radiofrequency maze ablation for atrial fibrillation: the Berlin modification. *Ann Thorac Surg* 2001; **72**: 1484–1491.

31 Melo J, Andragão P, Neves J *et al.* Endocardial and epicardial radiofrequency ablation in the treatment of atrial fibrillation with a new intra-operative device. *Eur J Cardiothorac Surg* 2000; **18**: 182–186.

32 Chen M, Chang J, Chang H *et al.* Clinical determinant of sinus conversion by radiofrequency maze procedure for persistent atrial fibrillation in patients undergoing concomitant mitral valve surgery. *Am J Cardiol* 2005; **96**: 1553–1557.

33 Manasse E, Gaita F, Ghiselli S *et al.* Cryoablation of the left posterior atrial wall: 95 patients and 3 years of mean follow-up. *Eur J Cardiothorac Surg* 2003; **24**: 731–740.

34 Knaut M, Tugtekin SM, Matschke K. Pulmonary vein isolation by microwave energy ablation in patients with permanent atrial fibrillation. *J Cardiac Surg* 2004; **19**: 211–215.

35 Raman JS, Ishikawa S, Storer MM, Power JM. Surgical radiofrequency ablation of both atria for atrial fibrillation: results of a multicenter trial. *J Thorac Cardiovasc Surg* 2003; **126**: 1357–1366.

36 Reston JT, Shuhaiber JH. Meta-analysis of clinical outcomes of maze-related surgical procedures for medically refractory atrial fibrillation? *Eur J Cardiothorac Surg* 2005; **28**: 724–730.

37 Jessurun ER, van Hemel NM, Kelder JC *et al.* Mitral valve surgery and atrial fibrillation: is atrial fibrillation surgery also needed? *Eur J Cardiothorac Surg* 2000; **17**: 530–537.

38 Doukas G, Samani NJ, Alexiou C *et al.* Left atrial radiofrequency ablation during mitral valve surgery for continuous atrial fibrillation. *JAMA* 2005; **294**: 2323–2329.

39 Filho CAC, Lisboa LAF, Dallan L *et al.* Effectiveness of the maze procedure using cooled-tip radiofrequency ablation in patients with permanent atrial fibrillation and rheumatic mitral valve disease. *Circulation* 2005; **112**(suppl I): I-20–I-25.

40 Akpinar B, Guden M, Sagbas E *et al.* Combined radiofrequency modified maze and mitral valve procedure through a port access approach: early and mid-term results. *Eur J Cardiothorac Surg* 2003; **24**: 223–230.

41 Deneke T, Khargi K, Grewe PH *et al.* Efficacy of an additional maze procedure using cooled-tip radiofrequency ablation in patients with chronic atrial fibrillation and mitral valve disease. A randomized, prospective trial. *Eur Heart J* 2002; **23**: 558–566.

42 de Lima G, Kalil RA, Leiria TLL *et al.* Randomized study of surgery for patients with permanent atrial fibrillation as a result of mitral valve disease. *Ann Thorac Surg* 2004; **77**: 2089–2095.

43 Ruel M, Masters RG, Rubens FD *et al.* Late incidence and determinants of stroke after aortic and mitral valve replacement. *Ann Thorac Surg* 2004; **78**: 77–84.

44 Blackshear JL, Odell JA. Appendage obliteration to reduce stroke in cardiac surgical patients with atrial fibrillation. *Ann Thorac Surg* 1996; **61**: 755–759.

45 Hart RG, Benavente O, McBride R, Pearce LA. Antithrombotic therapy to prevent stroke in patients with atrial fibrillation. *Ann Intern Med* 1999; **131**: 492–501.

46 Johnson WD, Ganjoo AK, Stone CD, Srivyas RC, Howard M. The left atrial appendage: our most lethal human attachment. Surgical implications. *Eur J Cardiothorac Surg* 2000; **17**: 718–722.

47 Halperin JL, Gomberg-Maitland M. Obliteration of the left atrial appendage for prevention of thromboembolism. *J Am Coll Cardiol* 2003; **42**: 1259–1261.

48 García-Fernández MA, Pérez-David E, Quiles J *et al.* Role of left atrial appendage obliteration in stroke reduction in patients with mitral valve prosthesis: a transesophageal echocardiographic study. *J Am Coll Cardiol* 2003; **42**: 1253–1258.

49 Rienstra M, van Gelder IC, Hagens VE, Veeger NJGM, van Veldhuisen DJ, Crijns HJGM. Mending the rhythm does not improve prognosis in patients with persistent atrial fibrillation: a subanalysis of the RACE study. *Eur Heart J* 2006; **27**: 357–364.

50 Cox JL, Ad N, Palazzo T. Impact of the maze procedure on the stroke rate in patients with atrial fibrillation. *J Thorac Cardiovasc Surg* 1999; **118**: 833–840.

CHAPTER 13

Bipolar radiofrequency ablation of atrial fibrillation

A. Marc Gillinov

Introduction

Surgical treatment of atrial fibrillation (AF) is the most effective means of curing this arrhythmia. Developed by Dr James Cox, the classic maze procedure eliminates AF in more than 90% of patients [1–3]. Although the maze procedure is highly effective, the complexity and time associated with the operation prevented widespread application by surgeons. The maze procedure includes a biatrial lesion set; the most important lesions are those in the left atrium (Figure 13.1). The left atrial lesion set of the maze procedure serves as an important starting point for the development of new surgical approaches to AF.

Recently, there has been a resurgence of interest in direct surgical ablation of AF, fueled by technological advances and demonstration that the pulmonary veins and left atrium are the sites of triggers and drivers of AF in most patients [4–7]. Advances in the understanding of the pathogenesis of AF and development of new ablation technologies enable surgeons to perform pulmonary vein isolation and create strategically placed, linear left atrial lesions rapidly and safely [8–14]. Alternate energy sources used to create lines of conduction block and replace surgical incisions of the maze procedure include radiofrequency (RF), microwave, ultrasound, cryothermy, and laser [14–16]. Excellent early and intermediate-term results have been reported with a variety of energy sources and lesion sets [8–16]. Each of the surgical ablation tools has unique fea-

Manual of Surgical Treatment of Atrial Fibrillation.
Edited by Hauw T. Sie *et al.* © 2008 Blackwell Publishing, ISBN: 978-1-4051-4032-4.

tures that influence patient selection and the surgical procedure. At the Cleveland Clinic Foundation, we have extensive experience with the use of bipolar RF for intraoperative ablation of AF [9, 17–20]. The objectives of this report are to (1) describe available bipolar RF technology, (2) review preclinical and clinical results, (3) address use of bipolar RF for ablation of lone AF, and (4) discuss remaining challenges related to AF ablation with bipolar RF.

Bipolar RF technology

RF ablation uses alternating current to heat tissue, creating thermal injury that results in a line of conduction block. In unipolar systems, grounding is achieved by an indifferent electrode applied to the skin (usually the back), and current flows from the tip of the RF catheter and resistively heats tissue in tip contact [9]. With bipolar RF systems, the electrodes reside in the jaws of a surgical instrument that is configured as a clamp. The operator depresses a foot pedal, and RF energy is delivered to the tissue between the jaws of the clamp. Potential advantages of bipolar energy delivery over unipolar systems include enhanced safety profiles, creation of continuous lesions, and the ability to assess transmurality at the time of ablation. Because discrete lesions are created only on the tissue contained between the jaws of the clamp, collateral damage to adjacent structures (e.g., coronary arteries, esophagus) is extremely unlikely [21–24]. Creation of lesions with unipolar RF systems may result in partial thickness lesions and gaps, and conduction through such regions is the most common cause of recurrent postablation AF and atrial flutter [25, 26]. Finally, with bipolar RF, positioning of electrodes on either

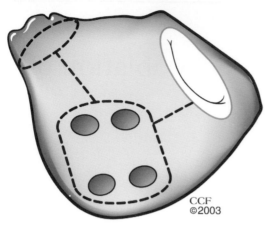

Figure 13.1 Left atrial lesion set of the maze III procedure. There is a pulmonary vein encircling lesion and connections to the mitral annulus and to the base of the left atrial appendage. The left atrial appendage is removed. Reprinted with the permission of the Cleveland Clinic Foundation.

side of the tissue to be ablated facilitates assessment of lesion integrity; this is not possible with current unipolar ablation systems. Of the three commercially available bipolar RF systems (Figure 13.2), two employ algorithms based upon tissue conductance or impedance to ensure transmural ablation and conduction block.

Released in November 2001, the Atricure Isolator (West Chester, OH) was the first bipolar RF system on the market in the United States. With the Atricure system, RF energy is delivered between two electrodes (5-cm length, 0.12-in width) mounted on the jaws of a specially designed clamp. When the clamp is closed on the target tissue, the electrodes are brought into close contact and energy is delivered (75 volts, 750 milliamps) in a focused and defined manner. The RF generator monitors voltage, current, temperature, time, and tissue conductance. Energy delivery is continued until tissue conductance between electrodes in the jaws of the clamp decreases and reaches a steady state for 2 seconds. Lesion creation generally requires 5–15 seconds. Discrete, visible lesions are created with little lateral spread of thermal injury [27–30].

Configured as a clamp, the bipolar Cardioblate system from Medtronic (Minneapolis, MN) incorporates saline irrigation during ablation that cools the electrode–tissue interface in order to reduce production of microbubbles, which could have a theoretical impact upon measures of tissue impedance.

With this bipolar RF system, a proprietary algorithm based upon tissue impedance is used to ensure acute lesion transmurality [31].

The Cobra Bipolar system (Boston Scientific, San Jose, CA) consists of two 64-mm long ablation inserts, which may be mounted on the opposing jaws of a stainless steel surgical clamp. Each insert has two RF electrodes embedded in a polyester covering, and the electrodes have a thermocouple mounted on each end. Clamps of different shape and configuration may be employed depending upon patient anatomy and surgeon preference. With this system, RF current is delivered for 45 seconds at 40 W, with a preset temperature of 90 °C. There is no mechanism for assessment of lesion transmurality.

Bipolar RF preclinical results

Each of these bipolar systems was subjected to rigorous preclinical testing before market release. While these preclinical animal studies do not exactly duplicate clinical conditions, they provide cause for optimism concerning the use of bipolar RF. Working at Washington University, Gaynor and colleagues [28] and Prasad and colleagues [27, 29, 30] demonstrated both acute and chronic conduction block after single applications of the Atricure bipolar RF device; histologic examination confirmed that lesions were always transmural. Lesions were discrete, and there was no damage to adjacent organs or pulmonary vein stenosis [27]. This group subsequently demonstrated the feasibility of an off-pump procedure that uses bipolar RF to create virtually all the lesions of the maze procedure [28].

Preclinical experience with the Medtronic irrigated bipolar RF system is similarly encouraging. In an ex vivo porcine preparation, Hamner and colleagues observed 100% transmurality when examining lesions created with irrigated bipolar RF [32]. Using the same technology, Bonanomi and colleagues confirmed the efficacy of irrigated bipolar RF in vivo [31]. Such preclinical results documenting transmurality and conduction block have not been observed consistently with unipolar energy delivery [33, 34].

Bipolar RF clinical experience

Although bipolar RF has been available for clinical use for only a short time, early clinical results

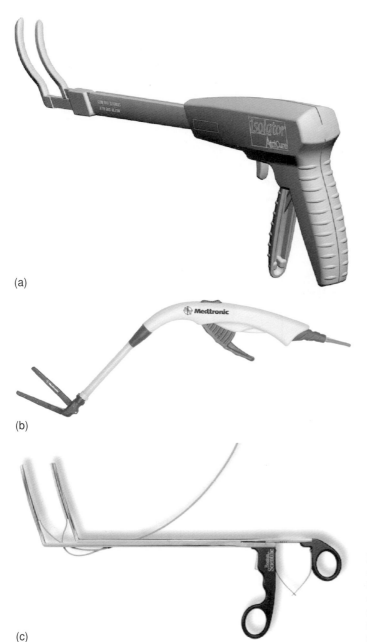

(a)

(b)

(c)

Figure 13.2 Bipolar radiofrequency devices used for ablation. (a) Atricure Isolator (Atricure Inc, West Chester, OH). (b) Medtronic Cardioblate Bipolar (Medtronic Inc, Minneapolis, MN). (c) Cobra Bipolar System (Boston Scientific, San Jose, CA).

in patients with AF undergoing concomitant heart surgery (usually valvular heart surgery) are encouraging. In contrast to findings reported from preclinical studies, human experience indicates that each lesion should be created at least three times with bipolar RF to ensure transmurality [35]. Use of pacing or electrogram protocols might also be indicated to assess lesions. Potential reasons for this trans-murality difference between preclinical and clinical application may relate to human atrial tissue thickness and structure [35]. Pitfalls identified in clinical practice include bunching of tissue in the jaws of the clamp creating uneven folds of atrium with inconsistent electrode contact and extrusion of tissue beyond the tips of the clamp when the jaws are brought together, limiting the extent of the ablation.

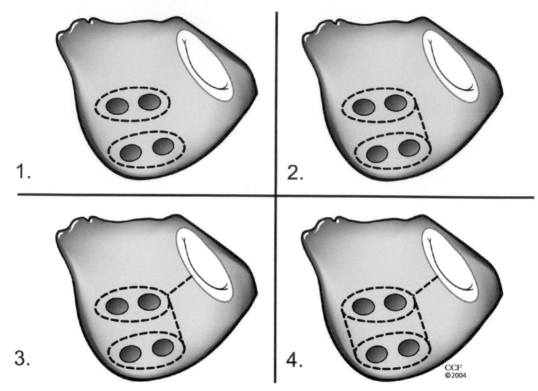

Figure 13.3 Left atrial lesion sets for ablation of atrial fibrillation created with bipolar radiofrequency. White ovals represent the mitral valve, sets of four black ovals represent pulmonary veins, and dashed lines represent sites of ablation. All ablation lesions are performed with bipolar radiofrequency except in lesions 3 and 4, in which the lesion connecting the left pulmonary veins to the mitral annulus is created with cryothermy. (Reproduced from [20] and reprinted with permission from The Cleveland Clinic Foundation.)

Either of these occurrences might result in lesions that are not transmural.

In humans, a variety of left atrial lesions can be created with bipolar RF, both on and off pump. Pulmonary vein isolation is easily achieved from the epicardial surface of the heart. Left atrial connecting lesions require placement of one jaw on the endocardium and one jaw on the epicardium; this is achieved safely after cardiac arrest and construction of a left atriotomy. Lesions at the mitral and tricuspid annuli and on the right atrial isthmus are most easily created with unipolar energy sources; we favor cryothermy to create these lesions in order to minimize the risk of damage to adjacent structures. However, recently bipolar RF has been used to create a lesion at the coronary sinus without adverse events [36].

There is not yet a consensus concerning choice of left atrial lesion set for ablation of AF in cardiac surgical patients. Reports include several different lesion sets created primarily with bipolar RF (Figure 13.3). Most resemble the maze procedure and include bilateral pulmonary vein isolation and at least one left atrial connecting lesion; the most common left atrial connecting lesions include a connection between the left and right pulmonary veins and a connection between the pulmonary veins and the mitral annulus, the latter lesion usually created with cryothermy. There is considerable controversy concerning the necessity of this lesion on the left atrial isthmus, which extends from the mitral annulus to the region of the left pulmonary veins. This isthmus may serve as a site for postablation left atrial flutter [37–39]. However, an incomplete lesion in this region may actually potentiate the development of atrial tachyarrhythmias [39]. Therefore, when this lesion is included in the ablation, it must be transmural

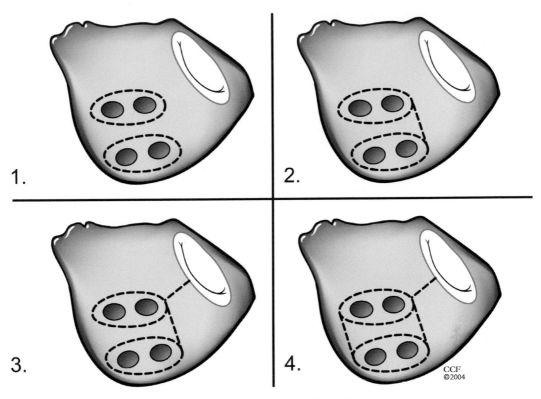

Figure 13.4 Prevalence of AF after ablation in 332 patients with mitral valve disease. Note high early prevalence, which levels off at 3–6 months. Reprinted with permission from The Cleveland Clinic Foundation.

and include a full thickness lesion on the coronary sinus.

Early results from single center and multicenter studies of AF ablation with bipolar RF suggest 80–96% freedom from AF at 6 months to 1 year [17, 20, 35, 40–42]. Factors that influence the return of AF include preoperative duration of AF, left atrial diameter, presence of permanent AF, and choice of lesion set in permanent AF [20, 41]. Analysis of more than 500 ablation procedures at the Cleveland Clinic Foundation suggests that a mitral isthmus lesion should be included in patients with permanent AF [20]. While it is possible that a simplified lesion set will cure AF in many patients with paroxysmal AF, there is general agreement that patients with permanent AF require a lesion set that closely parallels that of the maze III procedure [20, 41]. There is increasing evidence that the addition of right atrial lesions is unnecessary in the majority of patients with AF [42, 43].

Although early results in patients having combined valvular heart surgery and bipolar RF ablation of AF are encouraging, further work is necessary to confirm long-term efficacy. Close, long-term follow-up of heart rhythm is necessary before declaring patients cured [44]. More uniform analysis and reporting of results is essential to facilitate interpretation and comparison of reports from different groups [8]. In particular, all postoperative documentations of heart rhythm must be included in analysis, rather than reporting only "ECG rhythm at last follow-up."

Early postablation AF requires special comment. After any AF ablation, including those performed with bipolar RF, early postablation AF is common [17, 20, 45]. The etiology of postablation AF has not been elucidated. After application of bipolar RF, postoperative AF occurs in 50–60% of patients. However, this AF is usually transient, resolving by 6 months (Figure 13.4). Our current policy is to

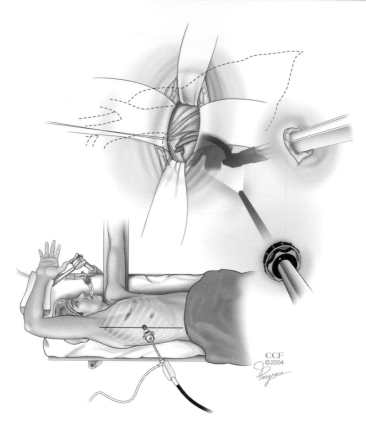

Figure 13.5 Video-assisted isolation of the right pulmonary veins using bipolar radiofrequency. Access is obtained via the third intercostal space. A similar approach on the left facilitates pulmonary vein isolation and excision of the left atrial appendage. Reprinted with permission from The Cleveland Clinic Foundation.

treat postablation AF with a course of antiarrhythmic therapy of 3 months' intended duration. If a patient remains in AF at 1 month postdischarge, we recommend electrical cardioversion. If the patient is in sinus rhythm at 3 months, we recommend withdrawal of antiarrhythmic agents. Patients are maintained on warfarin for 3 months. If a patient has no documented AF at this time, warfarin is discontinued; however, this approach to anticoagulation management has not been validated. If a patient has AF 6 months or more after ablation, we consider the ablation to have been a failure.

Bipolar RF and ablation of isolated AF

There is great interest in the development of minimally invasive surgical approaches to perform ablation in patients with isolated AF who do not require other cardiac surgery. With more than 2.4 million Americans suffering from AF and the consequent increased risks of stroke and mortality,

adverse events associated with anticoagulation and antiarrhythmic medications, and rising medical costs, there is a clear need for development of new treatment strategies [46–48]. While catheter-based AF ablation continues to advance, risks of pulmonary vein stenosis, esophageal injury, and thromboembolism, coupled with long procedure times and operator dependence, have limited its widespread adoption [49, 50]. The challenge to surgeons is to develop truly minimally invasive, epicardial approaches to AF ablation that are safe, effective, and simple.

Recent experience suggests that bipolar RF may be used to facilitate such an approach [51]. With endoscopic assistance, a bipolar RF device may be introduced through a small, non-rib-spreading thoracotomy (keyhole incision) to perform pulmonary vein isolation (Figure 13.5). In addition, the left atrial appendage can be excised using endoscopic stapling techniques. This procedure, which is performed from the epicardial surface of the heart, enables safe pulmonary vein isolation without the risks of pulmonary vein stenosis or esophageal injury. Refinements in technology will soon enable a completely endoscopic approach that uses bipolar RF and can be completed in 1–2 hours.

The left atrial appendage

Surgical procedures used to treat AF should almost always include excision or exclusion of the left atrial appendage. While arrhythmias rarely arise from the left atrial appendage and ablation of its base is of uncertain value, this structure is a source of morbidity and mortality in AF patients. Ten to fifteen percent of patients with AF develop intracardiac thrombus, and this thrombus is usually located in the left atrial appendage [52]. This thrombus is an important cause of stroke in patients with AF [52].

Because ablation does not cure AF in all patients and because atrial contractility may never return to normal in some patients after ablation, we recommend management of the left atrial appendage at the time of surgical ablation [53]. In patients having concomitant cardiac surgery, this is simple and safe and may consist of excision or exclusion with suture or a stapler. In patients undergoing minimally invasive surgical AF ablation, epicardial excision or exclusion of the left atrial appendage is usually performed with a stapler [51]. In the near future it is likely that new devices designed specifically for management of the appendage will facilitate surgical treatment.

Remaining challenges

As surgeons and industry partners pursue AF ablation with bipolar RF in patients having concomitant heart surgery and in those with isolated AF, they will need to proceed with greater knowledge and application of electrophysiologic principles and procedures. Current surgical approaches are anatomically based and limited by ablation instrumentation. Improved ablation tools are required to create left atrial connecting lesions, particularly in the beating heart, minimally invasive approaches. Imaging advances are required to facilitate approaches that require only 2 or 3 ports, eliminating the need for small incisions. Real-time mapping systems are necessary to characterize the AF before ablation, and, more importantly, to assess the integrity of lesions created from the epicardial surface of the heart after ablation. Finally, intense long-term follow-up is a prerequisite to the development of surgical "cures" for AF.

Acknowledgments

Dr Gillinov serves as a consultant to Atricure, Inc, and to Edwards Lifesciences, LLC.

References

1 Cox JL, Schuessler RB, D'Agostino HJ, Jr *et al.* The surgical treatment of atrial fibrillation. III. Development of a definitive surgical procedure. *J Thorac Cardiovasc Surg* 1991; **101**: 569–583.

2 Cox JL, Schuessler RB, Boineau JP. The development of the maze procedure for the treatment of atrial fibrillation. *Semin Thorac Cardiovasc Surg* 2000; **12**: 2–14.

3 Cox JL, Ad N, Palazzo T *et al.* Current status of the maze procedure for the treatment of atrial fibrillation. *Semin Thorac Cardiovasc Surg* 2000; **12**: 15–19.

4 Haissaguerre M, Jais P, Shah DC *et al.* Right and left atrial radiofrequency catheter therapy of paroxysmal atrial fibrillation. *J Cardiovasc Electrophysiol* 1996; **7**: 1132–1144.

5 Haissaguerre M, Jais P, Shah DC *et al.* Spontaneous initiation of atrial fibrillation by ectopic beats originating in the pulmonary veins. *N Eng J Med* 1998; **339**: 659–666.

6 Harada A, Sasaki K, Fukushima T *et al.* Atrial activation during chronic atrial fibrillation in patients with isolated mitral valve disease. *Ann Thorac Surg* 1996; **61**: 104–112.

7 Sueda T, Nagata H, Orihashi K *et al.* Efficacy of a simple left atrial procedure for chronic atrial fibrillation in mitral valve operations. *Ann Thorac Surg* 1997; **63**: 1070–1075.

8 Gillinov AM, Blackstone EH, McCarthy PM. Atrial fibrillation: current surgical options and their assessment. *Ann Thorac Surg* 2002; **74**: 2210–2217.

9 Gillinov AM, McCarthy PM. Atricure bipolar radiofrequency clamp for intraoperative ablation of atrial fibrillation. *Ann Thorac Surg* 2002; **74**: 2165–2168.

10 Gillinov AM, Smedira NG, Cosgrove DM, III. Microwave ablation of atrial fibrillation during mitral valve operations. *Ann Thorac Surg* 2002; **74**: 1259–1261.

11 Gillinov AM, McCarthy PM, Marrouche N, Natale A. Contemporary surgical treatment for atrial fibrillation. *PACE* 2003; **26**: 1–4.

12 Sie HT, Beukema WP, Ramdat Misier AR, Elvan A, Ennema JJ, Wellens HJ. The radiofrequency modified maze procedure. A less invasive approach to atrial fibrillation during open-heart surgery. *Eur J Cardiothorac* 2001; **19**: 443–447.

13 Mohr FW, Fabricius AM, Falk V *et al.* Curative treatment of atrial fibrillation with intraoperative radiofrequency ablation: short-term and midterm results. *J Thorac Cardiovasc Surg* 2002; **123**: 919–927.

14 Williams MR, Stewart JR, Bolling SF *et al.* Surgical treatment of atrial fibrillation using radiofrequency energy. *Ann Thorac Surg* 2001; **71**: 1939–1944.

15 Cox JL, Ad N. New surgical and catheter-based modifications of the maze procedure. *Semin Thorac Cardiovasc Surg* 2000; **12**: 68–73.

16 Damiano RJ, Jr. Alternative energy sources for atrial ablation: judging the new technology. *Ann Thorac Surg* 2003; **75**: 329–330.

17 Gillinov AM, McCarthy PM, Blackstone EH *et al.* Bipolar radiofrequency to ablate atrial fibrillation in patients undergoing mitral valve surgery. *Heart Surg Forum* 2004; **7**: 63–68.

18 Gillinov AM. Ablation of atrial fibrillation with mitral valve surgery. *Curr Opin Cardiol* 2005; **20**: 107–114.

19 Gillinov AM, McCarthy PM. Advances in the surgical treatment of atrial fibrillation. *Cardiol Clin* 2004; **22**: 147–157.

20 Gillinov AM, McCarthy PM, Blackstone EH *et al.* Surgical ablation of atrial fibrillation with bipolar radiofrequency as the primary modality. *J Thorac Cardiovasc Surg* 2005 129:1322–1329.

21 Gillinov AM, Pettersson G, Rice TW. Esophageal injury during radiofrequency ablation for atrial fibrillation. *J Thorac Cardiovasc Surg* 2001; **122**: 1239–1240.

22 Doll N, Borger MA, Fabricius A *et al.* Esophageal perforation during left atrial radiofrequency ablation: is the risk too high? *J Thorac Cardiovasc Surg* 2003; **125**: 836–842.

23 Berreklouw E, Bracke F, Meijer A, Peels KH, Relik D. Cardiogenic shock due to coronary narrowings one day after a maze III procedure. *Ann Thorac Surg* 1999; **68**: 1065–1066.

24 Fayad G, Modine T, Le Tourneau T *et al.* Circumflex artery stenosis induced by intraoperative radiofrequency ablation. *Ann Thorac Surg* 2003; **76**: 1291–1293.

25 Gaita F, Riccardi R, Caponi D *et al.* Linear cryoablation of the left atrium versus pulmonary vein cryoisolation in patients with permanent atrial fibrillation and valvular heart disease. *Circulation* 2005; **111**: 136–142.

26 Ouyang F, Antz M, Ernst S *et al.* Recovered pulmonary vein conduction as a dominant factor for recurrent atrial tachyarrhythmias after complete circular isolation of the pulmonary veins. *Circulation* 2005; **111**: 127–135.

27 Prasad SM, Maniar HS, Diodata MD, Schuessler RB, Damiano RJ, Jr. Physiological consequences of bipolar radiofrequency energy on the atria and pulmonary veins: a chronic animal study. *Ann Thorac Surg* 2003; **76**: 836–842.

28 Gaynor SL, Ishii Y, Diodata MD *et al.* Successful performance of Cox-maze procedure on beating heart using bipolar radiofrequency ablation: a feasibility study in animals. *Ann Thorac Surg* 2004; **78**: 1671–1677.

29 Prasad SM, Maniar HS, Schuessler RB, Damiano RJ. Chronic transmural atrial ablation by using bipolar radiofrequency energy on the beating heart. *J Thorac Cardiovasc Surg* 2002; **124**: 708–713.

30 Prasad SM, Maniar HS, Moustakidis P, Schuessler RB, Damiano RJ. Epicardial ablation on the beating heart: progress towards an off-pump maze procedure. *Heart Surg Forum* 2002; **5**: 100–104.

31 Bonanomi G, Schwartzman D, Francischelli D, Hebsgaard K, Zenati MA. A new device for beating bipolar radiofrequency atrial ablation. *J Thorac Cardiovasc Surg* 2003; **126**: 1859–1866.

32 Hamner CD, Lutterman A, Potter DD, Sundt TM, III, Schaff HV, Francischelli D. Irrigated bipolar radiofrequency ablation with transmurality feedback for the surgical Cox-maze procedure. *Heart Surg Forum* 2003; **6**: 418–423.

33 Santiago T, Melo JQ, Gouveia RH, Martins AP. Intra-atrial temperatures in radiofrequency endocardial ablation: histologic evaluation of lesions. *Ann Thorac Surg* 2003; **75**: 1495–1501.

34 Thomas SP, Guy DJR, Boyd AC, Eipper VE, Ross DL, Chard RB. Comparison of epicardial and endocardial linear ablation using handheld probes. *Ann Thorac Surg* 2003; **75**: 543–548.

35 Gaynor SL, Diodata MD, Prasad SM *et al.* A prospective, single-center clinical trial of a modified Cox maze procedure with bipolar radiofrequency ablation. *J Thorac Cardiovasc Surg* 2004; **128**: 535–542.

36 Vicol C, Kur F, Eifert S *et al.* Bipolar irrigated radiofrequency ablation of the posterior–inferior left atrium and coronary sinus is feasible and safe. *Heart Surg Forum* 2004; **7**: 499–502.

37 Oral H, Ozaydin M, Chugh A *et al.* Role of the coronary sinus in maintenance of atrial fibrillation. *J Cardiovasc Electrophysiol* 2003; **14**: 1329–1336.

38 Luria DM, Nemec J, Etheridge SP *et al.* Intra-atrial conduction block along the mitral valve annulus during accessory pathway ablation: evidence for a left atrial "isthmus". *J Cardiovasc Electrophysiol* 2001; **12**: 744–749.

39 Cox JL, Ad N. The importance of cryoablation on the coronary sinus during the maze procedure. *Semin Thorac Cardiovasc Surg* 2000; **12**: 20–24.

40 Mokadam NA, McCarthy PM, Gillinov AM *et al.* A prospective multicenter trial of bipolar radiofrequency ablation for atrial fibrillation: early results. *Ann Thorac Surg* 2004; **78**: 1665–1670.

41 Gaynor SL, Schuessler RB, Bailey MS *et al.* Surgical treatment of atrial fibrillation: predictors of late recurrence. *J Thorac Cardiovasc Surg* 2005; **129**: 104–111.

42 Ryan WH, Prince HG, Wheatley GH *et al.* Experience with various surgical options for the treatment of atrial fibrillation. *Heart Surg Forum* 2004; **7**: 195–198.

43 Deneke T, Khargi K, Grewe PH *et al.* Left atrial versus bi-atrial maze operation using intraoperatively cooled-tip radiofrequency ablation in patients undergoing open-heart surgery. *J Am Coll Cardiol* 2002; **39**: 1644–1650.

44 Pacifico A, Henry PD. Ablation for atrial fibrillation: are cures really achieved? *J Am Coll Cardiol* 2004; **43**: 1940–1942.

45 Ishii Y, Gleva MJ, Gamache C *et al.* Atrial tachyarrhythmias after the maze procedure. *Circulation* 2004; **110**(suppl II): II-164–II-168.

46 Wolf PA, Mitchell JB, Baker CS, Kannel WB, D'Agostino RB. Impact of atrial fibrillation on mortality, stroke, and medical costs. *Arch Intern Med* 1998; **158**: 229–234.

47 Lloyd-Jones DM, Wang TJ, Leip EP *et al.* Lifetime risk for development of atrial fibrillation. The Framingham Heart Study. *Circulation* 2004; **110**: 1042–1046.

48 Stewart S, Murphy N, Walker A, McGuire A, McMurray JJV. Cost of an emerging epidemic: an economic analysis of atrial fibrillation in the UK. *Heart* 2004; **90**: 286–292.

49 Pappone C, Oral H, Santinelli V *et al.* Atrio-esophageal fistula as a complication of percutaneous transcatheter ablation of atrial fibrillation. *Circulation* 2004; **109**: 2724–2726.

50 Pappone C. Pulmonary vein stenosis after catheter ablation for atrial fibrillation. *J Cardiovasc Electrophysiol* 2003; **14**: 165–167.

51 Wolf RK, Schneeberger EW, Osterday R *et al.* Video assisted bilateral pulmonary vein isolation and left atrial appendage exclusion for atrial fibrillation. *J Thorac Cardiovasc Surg* 2005130:797–802.

52 Johnson WD, Ganjoo AK, Stone CD, Srivyas RC, Howard M. The left atrial appendage: our most lethal human attachment! Surgical implications. *Eur J Cardiothorac* 2000; **17**: 718–722.

53 Gillinov AM, Petterson GP, Cosgrove DM. Stapled version of the left atrial appendage. *J Thorac Cardiovasc Surg* 2005 129:679–680.

CHAPTER 14

Surgical ablation therapy using microwave energy: endo- and epicardial approach

Michael Knaut & Stefan Brose

Introduction

Worldwide the maze procedure is recognized to be the "Gold Standard" in the surgical therapy of atrial fibrillation (AF) [1–3]. Because of its complexity this procedure could not generally be established as a routine cardiosurgical therapy.

The spontaneous conversion rate to sinus rhythm after cardiac surgery is lower than 10%. Therefore, Raine *et al.* [4] concluded that an additional ablation procedure should be performed in order to achieve postoperative sinus rhythm in all mitral valve surgery (MVS) cases. There are similar opinions regarding coronary bypass surgery [5, 6]. The introduction of less invasive ablation procedures has led to a renewed interest in the surgical therapy of AF.

Currently, more and more study groups are performing intraoperative ablation of permanent AF [7]. Until now, the most frequently used ablation method is radiofrequency that was introduced into clinical treatment in 1986 [8]. Other surgical ablation therapies are based on cryotherapy or laser technologies.

One possible alternative to these methods is the use of microwave energy for ablation. Until now, approximately 10,000 patients have been treated with this therapy worldwide. In Dresden, this technology was introduced in 1998 and meanwhile 470 patients have been treated with microwave ablation. While severe complications (e.g., lesions of the left

Manual of Surgical Treatment of Atrial Fibrillation.
Edited by Hauw T. Sie *et al.* © 2008 Blackwell Publishing,
ISBN: 978-1-4051-4032-4.

coronary artery) were reported with incorrect epicardial placement of the device [9], there have been no reports of complications with endocardial use of microwave ablation. Therefore, the procedure seems to be very safe and associated with low complication rates. The results regarding the restoration of sinus rhythm and atrial transport function are comparable to other ablation methods [10].

Technical description of the microwave probes, generator

The Microwave Ablation System (Guidant Corporation, Santa Clara, CA) is composed of two ablation probes (Model FLEX 4® and Model FLEX 10®) and a Microwave Generator (1000 Series) from Guidant, Santa Clara, CA, USA. The ablation probes are sterile, single-use, hand-held surgical devices that contain a microwave antenna that emits microwave energy in a controlled fashion. The FLEX 4 has a 4-cm shapeable ablating tip shielded on one side. The ablating tip is attached to a malleable shaft and a handle. The cable extending from the end of the handle is connected to the generator output cable. The ablating tip creates lesions of approximately 4 cm length.

The FLEX 10 ablation probe is a sterile, hand-held, single-use, surgical ablation device. The system has a flexible 2-m long insulated coaxial cable that attaches the ablation probe to the microwave generator output cable. The flexible coaxial cable ends into a 24-cm long handle, followed by a 15-cm section of stainless steel hypotube, followed by a highly flexible expanded polytetrafluoroethylene (ePTFE or Teflon^TM) sheath, which contains the moveable microwave energy antenna. The end of the sheath is attached to a polyether block amide elastomer-guide-lead (Pebax®) to aid in the proper placement of the sheath.

Moving the sliding ring on the handle moves the antenna according to numbered locations in the sheath. The emitted microwave energy from the antenna is directed towards the target tissue from the active surface opposite the corresponding numbered segment on the sheath, which creates a continuous lesion approximately, each 26 mm long. The black markers indicate the shielded side of each numbered segment. The ablations are created by independent activation of the microwave ablation antenna at one of the corresponding numbered segments, which are selected by moving the sliding ring on the handle. The position of the antenna within the sheath is also visible for the user by the position indicator of the sliding ring on the handle. When the device is active, the sheath section where the antenna is positioned is pressed against the tissue to be ablated, directing the microwave energy into the target tissue and preventing it from being applied to neighboring tissue.

The microwave generator's output (2450 MHz) is conducted through the output cable to the cabling of the ablation probe and finally out of the antenna at the distal section of the ablation probe. Energy is emitted in a radial pattern to the orientation of the ablation tip. Shielding of the ablating tip inhibits microwave energy emission to nontargeted tissue. Microwave ablation is possible because the target tissue contains polar molecules (most notably water), which vibrate in response to the induced electromagnetic microwave field. This vibration creates heat through friction, resulting in an increased tissue temperature. After reaching a certain temperature, the tissue becomes necrotic and consequently ablated.

History of microwave ablation therapy

After animal research the first open-heart microwave ablation was performed in December 1998 in Dresden, Germany [11]. Initially, the LYNX probe (renamed in FLEX 2) of AFx (Freemont, CA, USA) was used until September 2001. The LYNX probe consisted of a 2-cm long microwave emitting antenna within a rigid distal portion. Opposite of the antenna there is a protective shield preventing emission to adjacent structures. The shaft of the probe was flexible to allow bending in any desired position in the endocardial setting. The LYNX-probe underwent several changes in its design since January 2000. This new probe was then named FLEX 2. In October 2001, we started to use the FLEX 4 probe. The flexibility of the FLEX 4 ablating tip enabled us to change our endocardial-lesion concept [12].

The first epicardial microwave ablation was performed in Dresden in 2000. Mazzitelli *et al.* reported their first FLEX 4 epicardial ablation in the fall of 2001 [13]. Since then, 100 epicardial ablations have been performed in Dresden exclusively on patients with permanent AF who did not require opening of the left atrium (aortic valve replacement [AVR] and/or coronary artery bypass grafting [CABG]). The first true endoscopic, off-pump, microwave ablation was performed in 2002 by Saltman using the FLEX 10 [14, 15]. The stand-alone therapy for AF is only justifiable when it can be done in a minimal invasive setting.

In the following three sections, we present our experiences with microwave ablation at the Dresden Heart Center.

Endocardial microwave ablation

As mentioned before, we started to use microwave for ablation in 1998 and first conducted a prospective registry study. Patients with permanent AF who underwent mitral valve replacement/repair, AVR, and coronary bypass grafting were included. Patients with paroxysmal AF and patients younger than 18 years were excluded. Additional exclusion criteria were emergency operations or foreseeable increased surgical risk, such as (1) stroke or acute myocardial infarction during the last 6 weeks before surgery, (2) acute myocarditis, (3) acute congestive heart failure (NYHA IV), (4) pregnancy and nursing, (5) known drug addiction, and (6) incompetence and/or other conditions which do not allow the patient to understand the nature, significance, and scope of the registry.

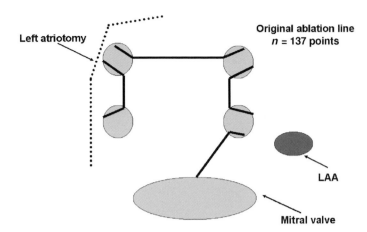

Left atriotomy

Original ablation line
n = 137 points

LAA

Mitral valve

Figure 14.1 Lesion line concept I
(according to Allessie's group [16]).

On the day of admission to the hospital all antiar-rhythmic drugs were stopped, except the remaining cardiovascular medication, which was continued. The benefits and risks of ablation were explained to all patients and an informed consent was obtained prior to surgery, which included the anonymous inclusion of their data in a registry for scientific evaluation.

After the operation, all patients got sotalol to sta-bilize their rhythm and were anticoagulated with Phenprocoumon with a target INR of 2.0–3.0 for CABG patients or 3.0–4.0 for patients with a me-chanical mitral or aortic valve. For all patients who showed stable sinus rhythm at the 3 months follow-up and who had not received a mechanical valve, the anticoagulation and sotalol therapy was stopped.

The first 137 patients underwent ablation accord-ing to the lesion line concept of Allessie, first de-scribed in 1996 [16]. The procedure started under direct view at the posterior part of the mitral valve annulus including all pulmonary veins. The lines connecting the pulmonary veins ended 1 cm inside the veins. The next lesion line started at the same depth but on the contra-lateral side. A sketch of the geometry of the lesion lines is shown in Figure 14.1. We analyzed the data from the first 100 patients with this concept with a minimum follow-up of 6 months. We recognized that not to resect or close the right and left atrial appendage was a criterion for failure. If we did not close the lesion line around the atrial appendages, we saw lower rate of sinus rhythm. This was statistically significant and led us

to change our lesion line concept, where we included both atrial appendages to the ablation lines.

In the next 112 patients, the modified lesion lines were used. The left atrial appendage was always included, while the right atrial appendage was only ablated when the right atrium was opened and an ablation of the isthmus was carried out. Now the pulmonary veins were isolated in a different manner [12]. Figure 14.2 shows a sketch of this new lesion line concept. Two box-lesions are made, one around the left pulmonary veins and one around the right pulmonary veins where the lesion is completed by the left atriotomy. Further, a lesion is made from the left atrial appendage tip towards the posterior leaflet of the mitral valve and finally connected to the left-sided box. A connecting line between the left and right box is made at the backwall of the left atrium. This lesion concept was used in all patients not af-fected by the surgical procedure or patient char-acteristics. Only for patients with an atrial septal defect, tricuspid insufficiency necessitating surgery and partly reoperations, a transseptal approach was chosen. In these patients the box lesion around the right pulmonary veins were exclusively made by ab-lation with an additional lesion to the transseptal incision. In addition, a tricuspid isthmus lesion was done, creating a connection between the transsep-tal incision and the right atriotomy. Left atrial size reduction or additional incisions were not part of our concept.

By now 249 patients, who had endocardial mi-crowave ablation were included in a registry. Follow-up was complete for all patients. Table 14.1 shows

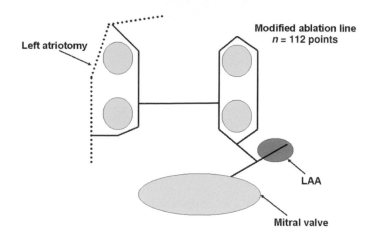

Left atriotomy

Modified ablation line
n = 112 points

LAA

Mitral valve

Figure 14.2 Lesion line concept II.

patient demographics and clinical data. The preoperative demographics and clinical data were comparable for both patient groups. The duration of the intraoperative ablation procedure was 13 ± 5 minutes for both left atrial lesion concepts. Additional lesion lines in the right atrium prolonged the ablation procedure about 3 minutes.

Table 14.1 Demographic and clinical data of both patient groups.

	Lesion line concept I (group A)	Lesion line concept II (group B)	p
Number of patients	137	112	
Female/male	71/66	57/55	ns
Age (yr)	68.4 ± 7.8	68.1 ± 8.0	ns
EF (%)	56.1 ± 11.9	56.9 ± 11.9	ns
Range (%)	32–80	20–83	
LA (mm)	52.6 ± 9.6	53.1 ± 8.7	ns
Range (mm)	30–102	38–76	ns
LA $\geq$ 60 mm	18.2%	17.4%	ns
Duration of AF (yr)	6.5 ± 9.2	6.8 ± 7.0	ns
Range (yr)	0.5–57.2	0.1–42.2	ns
Duration > 7 yr	24.8%	37.0%	ns
Mitral valve surgery (number)	87	72	
Coronary artery by pass grafting (number)	59	33	
Aortic valve replacement (number)	17	36	

EF, ejection fraction; LA, left atrial diameter; AF, atrial fibrillation.

Complications related to the procedure, such as hemorrhage, perforation of the esophagus, or later stenosis of the pulmonary veins never occurred. The 30-day survival rate in group A (line concept I) was 97.8 and 96.4% in group B (line concept II) and did not differ between the lesion line concepts ($p > 0.05$). Seven patients died perioperatively; the causes of death were low cardiac output syndrome, multiorgan failure, and right ventricular failure. Sixty-five percent of patients in group A showed stable sinus rhythm after 6 months, while this was 80% of group B ($p = 0.1573$).

At the 6-month follow-up in group A, 62% of patients with MVS, 68% with CABG, and 78% of patients with AVR were in stable sinus rhythm. In group B, 88% of patients with MVS, 78% with CABG, and 85% of patients with AVR were in stable sinus rhythm ($p = 0.1991$).

All patients with stable sinus rhythm demonstrated good biatrial transport function in echocardiography [12]. Twenty-six percent of all patients had a pacemaker after 6 months. Of these 249 patients, five had a pacemaker before the operation (2 single chambers, 3 double chambers). From this registry, an additional analysis was made to determine if patients, in whom sinus rhythm was restored, had higher survival rates in comparison to patients who remained in AF. In a prospective registry study, all consecutive patients who received endocardial microwave ablation ($n = 111$) added to their primary surgical indication were included as a "treatment group" while patients ($n = 104$) who required comparable surgery without ablation were defined as a "control group."

Table 14.2 Patient characteristics at baseline.

	Microwave ablation	Control	p
Number of patients	111	99	
Female/male	51/60	53/46	ns
Age (yr)	68.5 ± 7.5	72.3 ± 9.3	ns
Range (yr)	45.1–83.5	36.6–86.9	—
pAF before surgery	111 (100%)	99 (100%)	
pAF since (yr)	6.5 ± 8.4	4.2 ± 6.9	ns
Range (yr)	0.1–50.8	0.1–38.5	—
Ejection fraction	56.1 ± 12.1	52.4 ± 2.1	ns
Range (%)	32–80	30–78	—
Echocardiographic left atrial diameter (mm)	52.6 ± 9.9	51.9 ± 9.4	ns
Range (mm)	30–102	24–90	—

pAF, permanent atrial fibrillation.

Exclusively patients with documented permanent AF were included [17] where on the basis of clinical, hemodynamic, or prognostic factors an indication for cardiac surgery was given. Only an ejection fraction of <30% was an exclusion criterion. Death was the endpoint of the study. A complete 2 years follow-up from both groups was obtained. Based on the exclusion criterion (EF < 30%), five patients from the control group were excluded, leaving a total of 99 patients [18] (see Table 14.2).

Preoperatively, the groups did not differ from each other regarding demographical, anatomical, and hemodynamic data. Also, the preoperative duration of AF was comparable. In the ablation group, 68 patients were operated as a single procedure while 43 patients got a combined operation. In the control group, there were 68 single operations and 31combined procedures. Also, the frequency and complexity of the operations in both groups were comparable. The average operation time in the ablation group was 3.17 ± 0.59 hours and in the control group 3.04 ± 0.57 hours. Thirty-day mortality in the ablation group was 1.0% (1 patient), after 1 year 6.3% (7 patients), and after 2 years 8.1% (9 patients). There were no procedure-related deaths. In the control group, the results were as follows: 30-day mortality 5.1% (5 patients), after 1 year 12.1% (12 patients), and 22.2% after 2 years (22 patients). In conclusion, mortality after 2 years

was significantly higher in the control group than in the ablation group [Log–Rank (Mantel–Cox) test: $p = 0.0051$].

The causes of death are shown in Table 14.3. Sinus rhythm restoration rate in the ablation group was seen in 68%, 58%, and 54%, after 6 months, 1 year, and 2 years, respectively. In the control group, this was only 8%, 10%, and 11% in the same time frame. In summary, we were able to demonstrate that endocardial microwave ablation is an effective therapy for the treatment of patients with permanent AF [11, 19–23]. Sinus rhythm was restored between 50 and 80% after 1 year. These are reasonable results compared to the 90% sinus rhythm after the conventional Cox-maze procedure reported by Cox himself [3].

Table 14.3 Causes of death for both groups during the 2 years follow-up period.

Ablation group (n = 111)	Number of death	Control group (n = 99)
Heart failure	1	Bilateral pulmonary embolism
Heart failure	2	Mesenteric ischemia
Sept. multiorgan failure	3	Heart failure
Sept. multiorgan failure	4	Mesenteric ischemia
Cardiogenic shock	5	Malignant cardiac arrhythmia
Heart failure	6	Sept. multiorgan failure
Cranial hemorrhage	7	Stroke
Corpus uteri carcinoma	8	Sept. multiorgan failure
Bronchial carcinoma	9	Acute subdural hematoma
	10	Heart failure
	11	Pulmonary embolism
	12	Sept. multiorgan failure
	13	Stroke
	14	Heart failure
	15	Colon carcinoma
	16	Stroke
	17	Mesenteric hemorrhage
	18	Heart failure
	19	Heart failure
	20	Stroke
	21	Pneumonia
	22	Heart failure

It has to be emphasized that we were able to demonstrate that successful endocardial microwave ablation is able to significantly reduce mortality in patients with permanent AF [18]. This fact was mostly due to a remarkable reduction in complications associated with AF, like thromboembolic events or bleeding under anticoagulation therapy (Table 14.3).

Epicardial microwave ablation as concomitant procedure

The usual endocardial ablation in cardiac surgery, commonly in combination with MVS, necessitates the opening of the left atrium or both atria (depending on lesion concept and access to mitral valve). For patients, who require bypass and/or aortic valve surgery there is a different situation. Opening of the left atrium is normally not required, which leads to a new operative technique in concomitant antiarrhythmic surgery. Ablation can also be performed epicardially, creating a complete box-lesion, isolating the pulmonary vein with a connection line at posterior part of the left atrium. The lesion concept has found a wide acceptance worldwide because it is easy to reproduce and can be done without extracorporeal circulation [9].

The separation of the pulmonary veins plus the opening of the transverse sinus are important steps. The pericardial reflections (venae cavae and pulmonary veins) need to be dissected. This strategy has been evaluated in a randomized study.

Till today, the lesion concept is limited by the fact that an epicardial lesion to the mitral valve annulus is not possible on the beating heart because the risk to injure the circumflex artery and/or coronary sinus is too high. We performed the procedure with a FLEX 4 microwave probe with 65 W and 90 seconds per ablation on the beating heart without extracorporeal circulation. The Dresden lesion line concept for epicardial microwave ablation is depicted in Figure 14.3.

The first experiences with this epicardial lesion line concept provided good results and can facilitate the ablation procedure especially in patients who require coronary bypass grafting and/or AVR. Preliminary results from our prospective study in Dresden ($n = 46$ patients) are demonstrated in Table 14.4.

No procedure-related complications (thromboembolic events, bleeding, pulmonary stenosis or

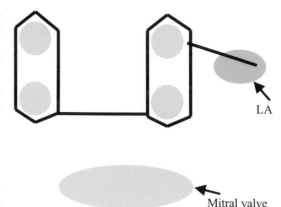

Figure 14.3 Dresden lesion line concept for epicardial ablation.

esophageal perforation) were observed. One patient died during his stay in the rehabilitation clinic. One patient required a pacemaker implant due to a higher grade of AV-block.

Inspired by the experiences from interventional studies by Pappone [24], we also decided to connect the boxes around the pulmonary veins by placing a lesion line on the roof of the left atrium. Pappone did the same from inside the atrium with the idea to additionally modulate the ganglia embedded in the pericardial fat pads.

The epicardial concept has advantages due to its less invasive approach compared to the maze operation or endocardial techniques. This leads to:
—decreased bleeding risk;
—decreased operation time of the antiarrhythmic surgery;
—decreased cross-clamp time;
—possibly decreased morbidity and mortality.

Table 14.4 Results of 46 epicardial microwave ablation patients with permanent atrial fibrillation.

Patients (numbers)	Time (days)	Stable sinus rhythm (%)
46	10	50
42	30	61
34	90	65
27	180	63
17	360	65

This may have a positive impact on the patient in the following topics.

• Total operation time in contrast to the classical maze procedure is significantly reduced, the ablation is carried out on the beating heart, no need for aortic clamping and no additional incisions are required.

• Significant hemodynamic improvement, increasing physical abilities, and quality of life.

• No palpitations and arrhythmic episodes.

• Protection from AF-induced heart insufficiency.

• Reduction of thromboembolic events and its complications.

• Anticoagulation therapy can be stopped in case of stable sinus rhythm. Nevertheless, this has to be outweighed with the potential risks of epi- and endocardial ablation therapy.

• Antiarrhythmic surgery increases total operation time.

• Protected perforation of the atrium with consequential bleeding.

• Development of pulmonary vein stenosis after weeks to months.

• Increased episodes of AF or atrial flutter due to inhomogeneous lesions or gaps in the lesion lines.

• Development of esophageal–atrial fistula (only reported with unipolar radiofrequency ablation [25, 26].

• Injury of coronary arteries due to misplacement of the epicardial probe [23].

These complications may be caused by the lack of experience with the device. Careful review of the instructions for user (IFU) and assistance of an experienced surgeon during the first procedures should prevent unnecessary complications [12].

Based on the until now published results of all actually marketed ablation techniques, independent of which energy source is used, a reduction of morbidity and mortality for treated patients was shown [12, 18]. The positive results of ablation are not only reflected by the restoration of sinus rhythm, but also in its safe application and its easy use. In addition, the economic standpoint has to be emphasized. In times of given budget constraints in several healthcare systems, it could be worthwhile to have a strategy which is able to reduce AF-related complications like thromboembolic events and cerebrovascular bleedings, which cause enormous costs and may be prevented by ablation therapy.

Randomized studies are ongoing now and to evaluate the clinical and scientific evidence of these matters. Also, in our center we conducted a randomized study to evaluate epicardial microwave ablation as a concomitant procedure with CABG and/or AVR in patients with permanent AF. (Epicardial microwave ablation for highly symptomatic permanent atrial fibrillation: prospective, open, controlled, randomized, mono center study.) We expect the first results in the beginning of 2008.

Endoscopic epicardial microwave ablation as "stand-alone" procedure

Cardiac ablation normally is performed through a median sternotomy as a concomitant procedure with other cardiac operations. A minimal invasive approach without sternotomy or thoracotomy using microwave technology on the beating heart without extracorporeal circulation was recently implemented [9, 15, 27]. Improved monitoring techniques for endoscopic applications allow a more extensive use of this technique [28].

There are several milestones in the history and implementation of endoscopic epicardial microwave ablation:

• First microwave ablation on the left atrium through a small right anterior mini-thoracotomy on a patient undergoing a mitral valve reconstruction (March 2002, Argenziano) [29].

• The first robotic microwave application (October 2002, Loulmet, Hill Hospital, New York) [30].

• First closed chest, totally endoscopic microwave ablation as a stand-alone procedure (November 2002, Saltman) [14, 15].

• First combined operation doing microwave ablation and mitral valve reconstruction with the robot (January 2003, Bisleri, Chitwood) [31].

Since then the number of video-supported and totally endoscopic microwave ablation applications has increased. Until August 2005, approximately 700 of these procedures were carried out in 75 centers worldwide.

In Table 14.5, the European centers currently performing endoscopic microwave ablation are listed. A hybrid approach as described by Bisleri *et al.* [32] where surgeon and electrophysiologist work together to offer the patient an optimal treatment for AF may reform the global strategy for the stand-alone ablation treatment. Some clinical relevant

Table 14.5 Actual experiences with endoscopic microwave application (till September 2005).

Center	Place	Application	Number of patients
Univ. Turku	Turku	endoscopic	20
Univ. Helsinki	Helsinki	endoscopic	5
Univ. Tampere	Tampere	endoscopic	10
CHU Erasm	Brussel	robotic	15
OLV Aalst	Aalst	robotic	10
CHU Louvain	Mt Godinne	endoscopic	15
Cleveland	Middlesbrough	endoscopic	35
St Mary	London	endoscopic	2
		robotic	1
Osp. Civile	Brescia	endoscopic	15
Univ. Padova	Padua	robotic	1
Univ. Maastricht	Maastricht	endoscopic	12
		robotic	3
HZ Osnabrück	Bad Rothenfelde	endoscopic	2
Nottingham City H	Nottingham	endoscopic	5
USA in total	several	endoscopic/robotic	ca. 550

issues like the management of the left atrial appendage and the mitral valve lesion still need to be evaluated.

Approximately 60% of these procedures are done through a bilateral endoscopic approach, 40% can be done monolateral approach (including robotic surgery). The pure monolateral endoscopic approach becomes more and more. In the hand of an experienced surgeon, it can be carried out in less than 2 hours.

The table shows that this therapy is still in its experimental phase. Similar to other centers, the Heart Center of Dresden is starting a study of the endoscopic epicardial microwave ablation in highly symptomatic patients with permanent AF. This will be a prospective, open controlled, single center study for the evaluation and applicability of this therapy. The first results will be available at the beginning of 2008. Despite promising perspectives for this technique, one has to emphasize that this approach is still not evidence-based and obviously far from clinical routine.

References

1 Cox JL, Schuessler RB, D'Agostino HJ *et al.* The surgical treatment of atrial fibrillation: III. Development of a definitive surgical procedure. *J Thorac Cardiovasc Surg* 1991; **101**: 569–583.

2 Cox JL, Boineau JP, Schuessler RB *et al.* Five-year experience with the Maze procedure for atrial fibrillation. *Ann Thorac Surg* 1993; **56**: 814–824.

3 Cox JL, Boineau JB, Schuessler RB *et al.* Modification of the maze procedure for atrial flutter and atrial fibrillation: I. Rationale and surgical results. *J Thorac Cardiovasc Surg* 1995; **110**: 473–484.

4 Raine D, Dark J, Bourlee JP. Effect of mitral valve repair/replacement surgery on atrial arrhythmia behavior. *J Heart Valve Dis* 2004; **13**: 615–621.

5 Quader MA, McCarthy PM, Gillinov AM *et al.* Does preoperative atrial fibrillation reduce survival after coronary bypass grafting? *Ann Thorac Surg* 2004; **77**: 1514–1524.

6 Wolf PA, Mitchel JB, Baker CS, Kannel WB, D'Ágostino RB. Impact of atrial fibrillation on mortality, stroke, and medical costs. *Arch Intern Med* 1998; **158**: 229–234.

7 Damiano RJ. Alternative energy sources for atrial ablation: judging new technology. *Ann Thorac Surg* 2003; **75**: 329–330.

8 Borgrefe M, Budde T, Podczeck A *et al.* High frequency alternating current ablation of an accessory pathway in humans. *J Am Coll Cardiol* 1987; **10**: 576–582.

9 Maessen JG, Nijs JF, Smeets JL, Vainer J, Mochtar B. Beating-heart surgical treatment of atrial fibrillation with microwave ablation. *Ann Thorac Surg* 2002; **74**(4): 1307–1311.

10 Viola N, Williams MR, Oz MC, Ad N. The technology in use for the surgical ablation of atrial fibrillation. *Semin Thorac Cardiovasc Surg* 2002; **14**: 198–205.

11 Knaut M, Spitzer SG, Karolyi L *et al.* Intraoperative microwave ablation for curative treatment of atrial fibrillation in open heart surgery—the MICRO-STAF and

MICRO-PASS pilot trial. *Thorac Cardiovasc Surg* 1999; **47**(suppl 3): 379–384.

12 Knaut M, Tugtekin SM, Jung F, Matschke K. Microwave ablation for the surgical treatment of permanent atrial fibrillation—a single center experience. *Eur J Cardiothorac Surg* 2004; **26**: 742–746.

13 Mazzitelli D, Park CH, Park KY, Benetti FJ, Lange R. Epicardial ablation of atrial fibrillation on the beating heart without cardiopulmonary bypass. *Ann Thorac Surg* January 2002; **73**(1): 320–321.

14 Saltman A. A totally endoscopic technique for off-pump epicardial ablation of atrial fibrillation on beating-heart. *Heart Surg Forum* 2003; **6**(2): 119–120.

15 Saltman AE, Rosenthal LS, Francalancia NA, Lahey SJ. A completely endoscopic approach to microwave ablation for atrial fibrillation. *Heart Surg Forum* 2003; **6**(3): E38–E41.

16 Zarse M, Deharo JC, Allessie MA. Radiofrequency ablation of anatomical atrial circuits in a rabbit model of atrial fibrillation. *Circulation* 1996; **94**: 164–171.

17 Fuster V, Ryden LE, Asinger RW *et al.* American College of Cardiology/American Heart Association/European Society of Cardiology Board. ACC/AHA/ESC guidelines for the management of patients with atrial fibrillation: executive summary. *J Am Coll Cardiol* 2001; **38**: 1231–1266.

18 Knaut M, Tugtekin SM, Spitzer SG, Jung F, Matschke K. Mortality after cardiac surgery with or without microwave ablation in patients with permanent atrial fibrillation. *J Heart Valve Dis* 2005; 14: 531–537.

19 Spitzer SG, Knaut M. Intraoperative Mikrowellenablation zur chirurgischen Behandlung von Vorhofflimmern. *Herzschr Elektrophys* 2002; **13**: 225–232.

20 Spitzer SG, Richter P, Knaut M, Schüler S. Treatment of atrial fibrillation in open heart surgery. The potential role of microwave energy. *Thorac Cardiovasc Surg* 1999; **47**(suppl 3): 374–378.

21 Deneke T, Khargi K, Grewe PH *et al.* Efficacy of an additional MAZE procedure using cooled-tip radiofrequency ablation in patients with chronic atrial fibrillation and mitral valve disease. *Eur Heart J* 2002; **23**: 558–566.

22 Schuetz A, Schulze CJ, Sarvanakis KK *et al.* Surgical treatment of permanent atrial fibrillation using microwave energy ablation: a prospective randomized clinical trial. *Eur J Cardiothorac Surg* 2003; **24**: 475–480.

23 Manasse E, Medici D, Ghiselli S, Ornaghi D, Gallotti R. Left main coronary artery lesion after microwave epicardial ablation. *Ann Thorac Surg* 2003; **76**: 276–277.

24 Pappone C, Rosanio S. Evolution of non-pharmacological curative therapy for atrial fibrillation. Where do we stand today? *Int J Cardiol* 2003; **88**: 135–142.

25 Gillinov M, Petterson G, Rice TW. Esophageal injury during radiofrequency ablation of atrial fibrillation. *J Thorac Cardiovasc Surg* 2001; **122**: 1239–1240.

26 Mohr WF, Fabricius AM, Falk V *et al.* Curative treatment of atrial fibrillation with intraoperative radiofrequency ablation: short-term and midterm results. *J Thorac Cardiovasc Surg* 2002; **123**: 919–927.

27 Saltman A. Microwave ablation. The endocardial and epicardial experience. In: *Fourth Annual Conference on the Surgical Treatment of Atrial Fibrillation.* Promedica International, London, 2004.

28 Kypson AP, Nifong LW, Chitwood WR, Jr. Robotic mitral valve surgery. *Semin Thorac Cardiovasc Surg* 2003; **15**(2): 121–129.

29 Garrido MJ, Williams M, Argenziano M. Minimally invasive surgery for atrial fibrillation: toward a totally endoscopic, beating heart approach. *J Card Surg* 2004; **19**(3): 216–220.

30 Loulmet DF, Patel NC, Patel NU *et al.* First robotic endoscopic epicardial isolation of the pulmonary veins with microwave energy in a patient in chronic atrial fibrillation. *Ann Thorac Surg* 2004; **78**(2): E24–E25.

31 Masroor S, Kypson AP, Nifong LW, Chitwood WR, Jr. *Minimally Invasive Microwave Atrial Ablation for Atrial Fibrillation: Short-term Follow-up in 31 Patients.* ISMICS, London, UK, HSF Supplement, 2004: 29.

32 Bisleri GL, Manzato A, Argenziano M, Vigilance D, Munaretto C. The need of a hybrid approach for the treatment of atrial fibrillation. *Heart Surg Forum* 2005; **8**(5): 1125.

CHAPTER 15

Epicardial ablation in the treatment of atrial fibrillation

Stefano Benussi & Ottavio Alfieri

Introduction

In the early nineties, surgery for atrial fibrillation (AF) was reaching its plateau phase, early after being born. At that time the advantages of sinus rhythm restoration were becoming progressively clearer. Although the efficacy of the maze operation turned out to be impressively high, some issues limiting its adoption as the routine cure of AF soon became apparent. Being characterized by an extensive use of right and left atrial incisions, the maze procedure, in fact, required a considerable prolongation of cardiopulmonary bypass and of aortic cross-clamp time, especially when performed in combination with other standard open-heart procedures [1]. Additionally, such operation increased bleeding, blood products requirement, and intubation time [1]. Finally, after concurrent maze operation, postoperative sinus node dysfunction required implantation of a permanent pacemaker in 20–25% of the patients [2].

In 1996, Harada *et al.* reported the constant finding of regular repetitive activation of the left atrium in patients with AF undergoing mitral valve surgery [3]. In the same year, Sueda *et al.* documented in a similar series of patients shorter refractory periods leading to a shorter mean AF cycle length in the left atrium [4]. Both studies indicated that the left atrium as the driving chamber for AF, at least in patients with mitral valve disease. Such findings stimulated the search for simplified techniques lim-

ited to the left atrium to treat AF during mitral valve surgery.

Sueda called "simple left atrial procedure" a surgical encircling of the four pulmonary veins, connected to the mitral valve annulus by two cryoablation lines [4, 5]. The procedure was feasible in less than 30 minutes and SR was restored in 86% of the patients. Nevertheless, the overall rate of recovery of left atrial contraction was 61% probably due to the isolation of the posterior third of the left atrium.

The introduction in AF surgery of radiofrequency (RF) ablation allowed to further simplify left atrial procedures. Melo *et al.* reported a 60% cure of AF in a series of patients undergoing mitral valve surgery and concomitant ablation consisting of two separate endocardial encirclings around the orifices of the left and the right pulmonary veins with a RF linear catheter [6].

The epicardial radiofrequency approach

Therefore, in the mid-nineties the available evidence was starting to focus on the efficacy of a set of linear scars only involving the left atrium during open-heart surgery and on the possibility of performing it with linear catheters.

In 1998, Ruchat and colleagues proved RF to be effective in the animal model even when ablations are performed from the epicardial surface, on the beating heart [7].

In February 1998, we started the first clinical experience with epicardial ablation of AF in patients undergoing concomitant mitral valve surgery [8, 9]. The ablation procedure was carried out using a temperature-controlled multipolar RF linear

Manual of Surgical Treatment of Atrial Fibrillation.
Edited by Hauw T. Sie *et al.* © 2008 Blackwell Publishing,
ISBN: 978-1-4051-4032-4.

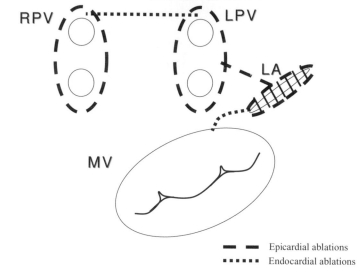

Figure 15.1 Complete left atrial ablation scheme. LPVs, left pulmonary veins; RPVs, right pulmonary veins; LA, sutured left appendage; MV, mitral valve.

catheter. Two encircling lesions around the ostia of the right and of the left pulmonary veins were carried out epicardially together with a short ablation from the left encircling to the base of the left appendage, usually before cardiopulmonary bypass, invariably before aortic cross-clamping, on the beating heart. Through a conventional left atriotomy, the ablation scheme was then completed with two endocardial lesions, one connecting the two encirclings and the other connecting the left appendage to the mitral annulus. After completion of the mitral valve procedure, the left appendage was sutured from within the left atrium (Figure 15.1).

A number of favorable features of epicardial ablation were evident from the very beginning. First of all, epicardial ablation around the PVs allowed to perform most of the lesions before aortic cross-clamping. Such a chance of reducing cardiopulmonary bypass and aortic occlusion time was probably one of the most appealing aspects in the era of the cut-and-sew maze operation.

Additionally, the epicardial approach could actually increase safety of the ablation procedure. In fact, being the heat source on the epicardial surface, the risk of ablation-related thromboembolism was virtually abolished. In addition to that, as it would become painfully evident in the following years [10], the propagation of heat toward the flowing blood, and not in the direction of the structures surrounding the heart could prevent collateral damage.

Finally, the possibility of a complete AF ablation from the epicardium could open the way toward beating heart AF surgery and further on to minimally invasive surgical approaches.

Therefore, by ablating epicardially, AF could be treated during mitral valve surgery with minimal addition to the magnitude of the operation and without increased risk of mortality or morbidity.

Indeed, the ablation pattern was such that all the conceptual criteria of an effective treatment of AF were fulfilled. Encircling of the pulmonary veins resulted in isolation of automatic foci located within the venous ostia, which had been claimed to be responsible for initiation of AF [3, 4]. In addition, the lesions connecting the two encirclings and extending to the mitral annulus created a block for the macroreentrant circuits perpetuating the arrhythmia.

Finally, due to the limited atrial muscle trauma related to RF use and to the electrical exclusion (and relative loss of contraction) of a negligible amount of atrial wall, around the orifices of the pulmonary veins, a complete recovery of the left atrial contractile function could be expected.

Results

When performed in the context of a complete left atrial lesion set (PV isolation and connecting lines) as described above, the epicardial approach could lead to satisfyingly high AF cure rates. In an early series of 132 patients [11] with AF (92% permanent) undergoing open-heart surgery, mainly for mitral disease (98%), such epicardial RF approach yielded a 3-year freedom from recurrence of 77%. As anticipated, the epicardial approach allowed a significant reduction of both the aortic cross-clamp time and the time spent for endocardial ablations. Performing a standard epicardial approach with modern unipolar RF catheters abated the ablation-related open-heart time to about 5 minutes. No procedure-related complication was recorded. Bleeding, intensive care unit, and hospital stay, as well as mortality did not appear to be modified by the addition of the ablation procedure. All patients in stable SR showed an effective contraction (A-wave >10 cm/s) of both the left and the right atrium [11].

After the first clinical reports [8, 9], epicardial ablation became an increasingly popular adjunct in the treatment of AF. Diverse unipolar ablating systems were used for epicardial ablation on the beating heart, with success rates between 77 and 90% [11–13]. Many groups chose to adopt epicardial ablation to cure AF in the context of concomitant ablation [8–13].

Melo *et al.* reported using the above-mentioned unipolar RF device in a small series of patients operated on through sternotomy for the treatment of lone AF [14].

After the description of the first case by Mazzitelli and colleagues in 2002 [15], Maessen described a preliminary surgical experience with microwave ablation on the beating heart. He used a 4-cm-long linear antenna epicardially to carry out a posteriorly connected bilateral pulmonary vein encircling ablation while trying to validate electrical isolation by means of pulmonary vein pacing [12]. AF was successfully cured in 87% of the patients at early control. Interestingly, in some of the patients the acute isolation of the pulmonary veins was not attainable despite multiple parallel or overlapping ablations.

Such open chest clinical experiences led the way to the development of minimally invasive surgical approaches to treat lone AF. Saltman *et al.* recently reported the feasibility of an epicardial ablation approach using a linear microwave probe through a small right thoracotomy or through thoracoscopy [16].

Actually, recently published experimental evidence seem to support that epicardial microwave ablation can allow acute electrical isolation (bidirectional block), but is usually associated with incomplete (not full-thickness) scars [17, 18].

The same phenomenon was also observed independently by Santiago and colleagues [19] and by Thomas *et al.* [20] with unipolar RF. Epicardial ablation with such devices on patients seems to yield transmural lesions at best in 15–20% of the cases. Failure to penetrate has been elated to the composition and to the thickness of the atrial wall [19].

The major obstacle to the progression of the lesion through the subendocardial layer is the convective cooling exerted by blood flowing through the atrial chamber.

Bipolar devices, first introduced in the clinical practice in 2002 [21], seem a promising way to obviate such problems. The clamping mechanism of bipolar ablators, in fact, eliminates convective endocardial cooling and compresses the atrial walls thus reducing tissue thickness and improving contact. Prasad *et al.* demonstrated bipolar RF atrial ablations to be transmural both acutely and after 3 months in pigs [22]. Despite such clear-cut results, in the clinical setting, more than one ablation line may be necessary to achieve isolation [21, 23, 24]. In a recent clinical study with a different bipolar RF device we found a complete conduction block in 92% of the pulmonary vein couples after a single ablation and in 100% after one repeat ablation [25].

In summary, a single bipolar RF ablation can be insufficient to provide acute conduction block. But different authors using different devices all come to the same conclusion: by deploying repeat ablations as necessary, bipolar RF allows a 100% acute efficacy in pulmonary veins isolation [21, 23, 25]. This is no small thing. In fact, while it is true that incomplete lesions can have some efficacy in the cure of AF, there is growing evidence indicating a direct cause–effect relationship between incomplete ablation lines and clinical failure. In addition, incomplete isolation of the pulmonary veins has been related to automatic left atrial arrhythmias (left atrial tachycardia/flutter) that are generally worse than AF itself since they are typically high rate, they are refractory to medical treatment and difficult to ablate [26].

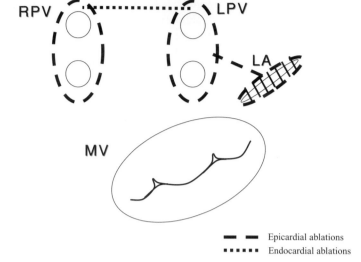

RPV   LPV

LA

MV

Figure 15.2 Simplified left atrial ablation scheme. RPV, right pulmonary veins; LPV, left pulmonary veins; LA, sutured left appendage; MV, mitral valve.

━ ━ Epicardial ablations
▪▪▪▪▪▪ Endocardial ablations

Another important aspect of bipolar ablation is the safety profile. Injury to the esophagus or to the bronchial tree has been found to occur in as much as 1% of patients ablated with unipolar RF [27]. On the contrary, collateral damage of the structures surrounding the heart has not been reported with bipolar ablation so far. In fact, during bipolar ablation, only the outer, inactive part of the clamp is in contact with the parietal pericardium so that only the tissue that is held between the jaws is consistently heated.

One-year follow-up demonstrates left atrial ablation with a bipolar device to allow SR recovery in 72–89% [25, 28] in patients undergoing concomitant ablation. No ablation-related complications are reported. The time required for the ablation procedure is further reduced to a few minutes.

The increased swiftness and safety of the ablation procedure stimulates an expansion of the indications in patients with a poor ventricular function and in those requiring complex and/or multiple open-heart procedures.

The major limitations of bipolar technology are:
—Feasibility in the case of extensive pericardial adhesions (e.g., redo operations). In such cases a fully endocardial approach may be preferable in order to avoid an extensive dissection of the adhesions around the PVs.

—Connecting lines can be more difficult to perform epicardially, on the beating heart with a bipolar device. Actually, the mitral connecting line has been initially omitted by some groups [25, 28] for fear of injuring a major coronary branch in the AV groove (Figure 15.2). But this led to an excess rate of postoperative left atrial flutter and to lower success rates at late follow-up.

Some possible options to carry out the mitral connecting ablation are available:

a Perform the ablation with bipolar RF or with a unipolar ablator after surgical dissection of the AV junction to isolate the coronary artery.

b Completing the mitral line with a different unipolar device (e.g., a reusable cryoprobe when this is available), in the coronary-free segment of the AV groove [29] (Figure 15.3).

c Actually, provided a coronary-free segment is present at all [29] and clearly identifiable on the posterior left AV groove, such connecting line is probably feasible with the same bipolar device, by clamping from the atriotomy up to the mitral anulus. As a practical adjunct, once such coronary-free site is identified by epicardial inspection, a marking can be drawn (e.g., with methylene blue) or a hypodermic needle can be placed in the corresponding atrial point, to make the open-heart identification of the exact portion of the mitral anulus to be targeted more easily and precisely.

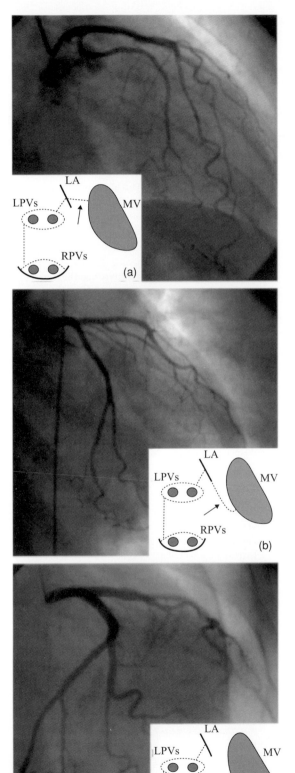

Figure 15.3 Tailoring of the ablation set based on coronary anatomy. Three representative types of coronary anatomy (left angiogram) are shown together with the corresponding suggested routes of the mitral line (arrow): (a) From the appendage to the lateral half of the posterior anulus in patients with a strongly dominant right coronary artery. (b) From the appendage to the medial portion of the posterior anulus, crossing the AV groove perpendicularly, in patients with a mildly dominant right coronary artery. (c) From the right encircling to the medial commissure, close to the interatrial septum in patients with a left-dominant coronary circulation. Dotted line, ablations; solid line, surgical incision; arrow, mitral line. (LA, sutured left appendage; LPVs, left pulmonary veins; MV, mitral valve; RPVs, right pulmonary veins.) (Reprinted from Reference [29]. Copyright 2003, with permission from the Society of Thoracic Surgeons)

Presently, no reliable means of performing a mitral connecting line epicardially, on the beating heart, has been reported.

On the other hand, the epicardial connection between the two PV encirclings seems within reach. In the search of a completely epicardial approach, we have recently described a technique to perform a left atrial connection between the two encirclings epicardially, off-pump by simply clamping tangentially the posterior left atrium with a standard bipolar RF device [30].

An extremely appealing application of bipolar ablation is in the minimally invasive treatment of lone AF. Video-assisted bilateral PV isolation and resection of the left appendage has been recently proposed by Wolf and colleagues for the treatment of lone AF (mainly persistent and paroxysmal) [31]. The procedure requires access to both pleural cavities through non-rib-spreading minithoracotomy and PV separate encircling on the beating heart off cardiopulmonary bypass. Preliminary results on a small series of patients are very promising, with more than 90% of the patients in SR off drugs at 6 months after surgery.

Summary

In the early nineties, surgery opened the way toward nonpharmacologic treatment of AF. Since then, the maze procedure has remained the gold standard for surgical ablation of AF. With the advent of modern physical means, diverse approaches assayed the efficacy of ablating instead of cutting and suturing. Epicardial ablation has emerged as a possible way to treat AF on the beating heart. Nevertheless, a scarce penetration of epicardial ablation scars, mainly related to convective endocardial cooling has been mentioned as a possible cause of failure of unipolar catheters. With the advent of modern bipolar devices, acute transmurality is predictably achievable in every treated patients. A transmural ablation is now feasible as a concomitant procedure within a few minutes, mainly before cross-clamping. Thanks to such new devices, a definite role of beating heart minimally invasive ablation for the treatment of lone AF, appears today within reach.

References

1 Kawaguchi AT, Kosakai Y, Sasako Y, Eishi K, Kiyoharu N, Kawashima Y. Risks and benefits of combined maze procedure for atrial fibrillation associated with organic heart disease. *J Am Coll Cardiol* 1996; **28**: 985–990.

2 Cox JL, Schuessler RB, Lappas DG, Boineau JP. A 8$^1/_2$-year clinical experience with surgery for atrial fibrillation. *Ann Surg* 1996; **224**: 267–273.

3 Harada A, Sasaki K, Fukushima T *et al*. Atrial activation during chronic atrial fibrillation in patients with isolated mitral valve disease. *Ann Thorac Surg* 1996; **61**: 104–112.

4 Sueda T, Nagata H, Shikata H *et al*. Simple left atrial procedure for chronic atrial fibrillation associated with mitral valve disease. *Ann Thorac Surg* 1996; **62**: 1796–1800.

5 Sueda T, Nagata H, Orihashi K *et al*. Efficacy of a simple left atrial procedure for chronic atrial fibrillation in mitral valve operations. *Ann Thorac Surg* 1997; **63**: 1070–1075.

6 Melo JQ, Neves J, Ribeiras R *et al*. When and how to report results of surgery on atrial fibrillation. *Eur J Cardiothorac Surg* 1997; **12**: 739–745.

7 Ruchat P, Schlapfleer J, Fromer M, Garadz JP, Genton CW, von Segesser LK. Atrial fibrillation inhibition by subepicardial radiofrequency ablation in a sheep model [Abstract]. In: *Abstract Book of the 12th Annual Meeting of the EACTS*, 1998: 434.

8 Benussi S, Pappone C, Nascimbene S *et al*. Epicardial radiofrequency ablation of chronic atrial fibrillation during mitral valve surgery: early success rate and atrial function recovery. *Circulation* 1999; **100**: I-854.

9 Benussi S, Pappone C, Nascimbene S *et al*. A simple way to treat atrial fibrillation during mitral valve surgery: the epicardial radiofrequency approach. *Eur J Cardiothorac Surg* 2000; **17**: 524–529.

10 Kottkamp H, Hindricks G, Autschbach R *et al*. Specific linear left atrial lesions in atrial fibrillation: intraoperative radiofrequency ablation using minimally invasive surgical techniques. *J Am Coll Cardiol* 2002; **40**: 475–480.

11 Benussi S, Nascimbene S, Agricola E *et al*. Surgical ablation of atrial fibrillation using the epicardial radiofrequency approach: mid-term results and risk analysis. *Ann Thorac Surg* 2002; **74**: 1050–1056.

12 Maessen JG, Nijs JF, Smeets JL, Vainer J, Mochtar B. Beating-heart surgical treatment of atrial fibrillation with microwave ablation. *Ann Thorac Surg* 2002; **74**: 1307–1311.

13 Raman JS, Seevanayagam S, Storer M, Power JM. Combined endocardial and epicardial radiofrequency ablation of right and left atria in the treatment of atrial fibrillation. *Ann Thorac Surg* 2001; **72**: 1096–1099.

14 Melo J, Adragao P, Neves J *et al*. Endocardial and epicardial radiofrequency ablation in the treatment of atrial

fibrillation with a new intra-operative device. *Eur J Cardiothorac Surg* 2000; **18**: 182–186.

15 Mazzitelli D, Park CH, Park KY, Benetti FJ, Lange R. Epicardial ablation of atrial fibrillation on the beating heart without cardiopulmonary bypass. *Ann Thorac Surg* 2002; 73: 320–321.

16 Saltman AE, Rosenthal LS, Francalancia NA, Lahey SJ. A completely endoscopic approach to microwave ablation for atrial fibrillation. *Heart Surg Forum* 2003; **6**(3): E38–E41.

17 van Brakel TJ, Bolotin G, Salleng KJ *et al.* Evaluation of epicardial microwave ablation lesions: histology versus electrophysiology. *Ann Thorac Surg* 2004; **78**: 1397–1402.

18 Accord RE, van Suylen RJ, van Brakel TJ, Maessen JG. Post-mortem histologic evaluation of microwave lesions after epicardial pulmonary vein isolation for atrial fibrillation. *Ann Thorac Surg* 2005; **80**: 881–887.

19 Santiago T, Melo J, Gouveia RH *et al.* Epicardial radiofrequency applications: in vitro and in vivo studies on human atrial myocardium. *Eur J Cardiothorac Surg* 2003; **24**: 481–486.

20 Thomas SP, Guy DJR, Boyd AC, Eipper VE, Ross DL, Chard RB. Comparison of epicardial and endocardial ablation using handheld probes. *Ann Thorac Surg* 2003; **75**: 543–548.

21 Gillinov AM, McCarthy PM. Atricure bipolar radiofrequency clamp for intraoperative ablation of atrial fibrillation. *Ann Thorac Surg* 2002; **74**: 2165–2168.

22 Prasad SM, Maniar HS, Diodato MD, Schuessler RB, Damiano RJ, Jr. Physiological consequences of bipolar radiofrequency energy on the atria and pulmonary veins: a chronic animal study. *Ann Thorac Surg* 2003; **76**: 836–841.

23 Gaynor SL, Diodato MD, Prasad SM *et al.* A prospective, single-center clinical trial of a modified Cox maze procedure with bipolar radiofrequency ablation. *J Thorac Cardiovasc Surg* 2004; **128**: 535–541.

24 Bugge E, Nicholson IA, Thomas SP. Comparison of bipolar and unipolar radiofrequency ablation in an in vivo experimental model. *Eur J Cardiothorac Surg* 2005; **28**: 76–80.

25 Benussi S, Nascimbene S, Calori G *et al.* Surgical ablation of atrial fibrillation with a novel bipolar radiofrequency device. *J Thorac Cardiovasc Surg* 2005; **130**: 491–497.

26 Ouyang F, Antz M, Ernst S *et al.* Recovered pulmonary vein conduction as a dominant factor for recurrent atrial tachyarrhythmias after complete circular isolation of the pulmonary veins. Lessons from double lasso technique. *Circulation* 2005; **111**: 127–135.

27 Doll N, Borger MA, Fabricius A *et al.* Esophageal perforation during left atrial radiofrequency ablation: is the risk too high? *J Thorac Cardiovasc Surg* 2003; **125**: 836–842.

28 Gillinov AM, McCarthy PM, Blackstone EH *et al.* Surgical ablation of atrial fibrillation with bipolar radiofrequency as the primary modality. *J Thorac Cardiovasc Surg* 2005; **129**: 1322–1328.

29 Benussi S, Nascimbene S, Calvi S, Alfieri O. A tailored anatomical approach to prevent complications during left atrial ablation. *Ann Thorac Surg* 2003; **75**: 1979–1981.

30 Benussi S, Alfieri O. Off-pump connection of the pulmonary veins with bipolar radiofrequency: towards a complete epicardial ablation. *J Thorac Cardiovasc Surg* (in press).

31 Wolf RK, Shneeberger EW, Osterday R *et al.* Video-assisted bilateral pulmonary vein isolation and left atrial appendage exclusion for atrial fibrillation. *J Thorac Cardiovasc Surg* 2005; **130**: 797–802.

CHAPTER 16

Surgical treatment of atrial fibrillation: the Japanese experience

Yoshio Kosakai

Introduction

In 1991, Cox developed the maze procedure in which the atrium is cut and sutured in a maze-like pattern in order to cure atrial fibrillation (AF) [1–4]. He initially applied the maze procedure to cases with isolated AF. The author of the present chapter treated mainly, since 1992 [5, 6], chronic AF associated with mitral valve disease. The results confirmed that the maze procedure was also an effective treatment for such chronic AF. Combined mitral valve disease and AF have a high incidence in the Japanese population, and, for this reason, Japanese surgeons have had the opportunity to master the maze procedure in a plethora of patients. In this regard, the author has acquired a large experience with this operation and the community of Japanese cardiac surgeons has started numerous researches in the field of surgical treatment for AF.

Development of the surgical treatment of atrial fibrillation and Japanese experience

In 1980, Williams *et al.* reported in a series of experiments on animals that total left atrial isolation is an effective treatment for AF [7]. In 1992, Graffigna *et al.* reported that this procedure was also effective in treating AF in patients suffering from associated mitral valve disease [8]. Both these surgical techniques are very similar to pulmonary vein (PV) isolation. The left atrial isolation and the PV isolation are only

Manual of Surgical Treatment of Atrial Fibrillation.
Edited by Hauw T. Sie *et al.* © 2008 Blackwell Publishing,
ISBN: 978-1-4051-4032-4.

different from each other in size. In retrospect, left atrial isolation was a well-motivated approach. In 1985, Guiraudon *et al.* developed the corridor operation between the sinus node, atrial septum, and AV node; in other words, both right and left atrial isolation [9]. These trials were all effective procedures for stabilizing tachycardia or arrhythmic ventricular rhythm. Nonetheless, AF persisted after the operation in all of the above cases, which suggested that synchronous atrial transport was lacking and there was still a risk of thromboembolism.

In 1991, Cox *et al.* developed the maze procedure in which the atrium is incised and sutured in a maze-like pattern in order to cure AF sustained by macro-reentries [1–4]. The maze procedure is the ideal treatment for AF, since it allows both the atrium and ventricle to maintain sinus rhythm (SR), provides synchronous atrial transport, and prevents systemic thromboembolism. Cox himself has developed two modified versions, namely, maze II and maze III [10, 11]. In 1995, Cox reported that the curative rate of Cox-maze III was 98.8% (342/346). However, in a multicentric questionnaire including over 2500 maze cases performed in Japan [12], the author has reported a curative rate for the Cox-maze III of 55% (6/11) in isolated AF (lone group), 76% (558/757) in AF associated with mitral valve disease (mitral group), 91% (48/53) in AF with congenital heart disease (congenital group), and 73% (22/32) in no cause-and-effect relationship between the basic ailment and AF (other group).

In Japan, many modifications of the Cox-maze procedure have been presented. Since 1994, the same author has modified the maze procedure using extensive cryoablation [5, 6 13]. This modification will be described in detail later in this chapter.

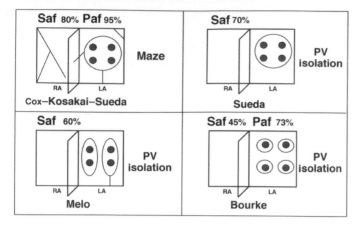

Figure 16.1 Curative rates of maze procedure or PV isolation. Generally, the curative rate of maze procedure is 80% for sustained AF and 95% for paroxysmal AF. Sueda *et al.* reported that the curative rate of the whole four PVs isolation was 70% for sustained AF. Melo *et al.* reported that the curative rate of the each bilateral two PVs isolation was 60% for sustained AF. Bourke *et al.* reported that the curative rate of the each four PVs isolation was 45% for paroxysmal AF and 60% for sustained AF.

In 1994, Lin *et al.* developed an operation for AF associated with mitral valve disease in which the atrium is divided into three compartments: the left atrium, atrial septum, and right atrium [14, 15]. The curative rate of this method, however, is relatively low (64%). Then Lin modified the method to create four compartments instead of three. In 1997, Shyu reported that the curative rate of new compartment operation for AF with mitral valve disease was 86% (14/22) [16]. No further report of the compartment operation is found.

In 1996, Sueda *et al.* considered the hypothesis that AF associated with mitral valve disease occurred only from the left atrium and they conducted research on the left atrial maze in patients undergoing mitral valve surgery [17]. They reported that the curative rate of the left atrium maze procedure (LA maze) was 86% (24/28) [18]. However, in the author's Japanese multicentric questionnaire survey [12] success rate of the LA maze was 50% (1/2) in the lone AF group, 73% (225/310) in the mitral group, and 80% (4/5) in the other group.

In 1999, Nitta *et al.* considered that after the maze procedure the atrium did not contract synchronously. On this basis they developed a radial operation to improve the atrial contribution by means of cutting the left atrium radially [19]. The curative rate of radial operation was 88% (59/67) [20].

In 2001, Isobe *et al.* considered that the atrial appendage may contribute to the contraction of the atrium. The inner diameter of the appendage is smaller than that of the atrium itself and,

therefore, the appendage contributes to the contraction by the Laplace's law. They reported a biatrial preserved (BAP) maze procedure [21]. The curative rate of BAP maze was 96% (48/50). However, the equality among results of each modified maze procedure will be discussed later. The author believes that if the elimination of AF is not complete and the preservation of the left appendage is performed, the patients have a higher risk of thromboembolism.

In 1994, Swartz *et al.* reported a maze procedure with noninvasive catheter ablation [22]. Although numerous complications were observed, this was the first trial of catheter ablation for AF. In 1996, Haissaguerre also reported about right and left atrial radiofrequency catheter ablation for AF [23]. In 1998, Haissaguerre *et al.* reported new catheter ablation, that is, discrete radiofrequency ablation of PVs for focal AF [24]. Consequently, some surgeons tried to isolate only the four PVs without making a maze-like incision pattern. As an after thought, Cox did PV isolation in the maze procedure and maybe this was the main contributor to the success of the maze procedure. Generally speaking, the curative rate of the maze procedure is 80% for sustained AF and 95% for paroxysmal AF. Different patterns of PVs isolation have been proposed with similar success rates. Sueda *et al.* reported curative rate of 70% for sustained AF [25], Melo *et al.* reported success rate of 60% for sustained AF [26], and Bourke *et al.* 45% for paroxysmal AF and 60% for sustained AF [27] (Figure 16.1). Deisenhofer *et al.* reported that foci of AF are not only internal to the PVs but also external to them [28].

Development of devices for surgical ablation of AF and use in Japan

In Cox's original description of the maze procedure, he used mainly a cut and suture technique. This method is time consuming and not hemostatic and the author mainly relies on cryoablation.

The radiofrequent ablation method can achieve blocking lines in the shortest time. However in 2001, Gillinov *et al.* [29] and in 2003, Doll *et al.* [30] reported life-threatening complications such as atrioesophageal fistulas while using unipolar radiofrequent ablation for the maze procedure. Furthermore, invasive cardiologists such as Dr Pappone reported atrioesophageal fistula while using catheter-based radiofrequent ablation [31]. This deadly complication might occur more often than expected and can be completely missed presenting mainly after patient's discharge. In the Japanese experience atrioesophageal fistula postradiofrequency ablation was lethal in four cases. Therefore, the author suggests avoiding unipolar radiofrequent ablation. Since 2004, the bipolar radiofrequent ablator is available in Japan. Although the bipolar radiofrequent ablator seems to be very safe, its widespread application has been limited because the Japanese health insurance system does not cover its use. Other devices e.g., microwave, laser, ultrasound etc. have not yet reached, at the present, the Japanese market.

The equality between results of each modified maze procedure

The author reported findings of a research questionnaire performed on over 2500 maze cases in Japan [12]. This research showed that there were no significant differences in curative rate among different procedures including the Cox-maze, Kosakai-maze, left atrial maze, and so on. The result of the operation was not influenced by the method of the maze procedure, but was influenced by the patient's preoperative condition. This means that the existence of micro-reentry or the acceleration of automaticity influenced the results. The maze procedure can inhibit macro-reentry entirely. However, atrial arrhythmias that are refractory to surgical cure are due to micro-reentry or

acceleration of automaticity. Therefore, such atrial arrhythmias cannot be cured even by means of the maze procedure.

Kosakai modifications to the maze procedure

The author performs the following four modifications of the Cox-maze procedure:

1 The author improves the method further by using freezing as a substitute for incision, and cutting the anterior side of the sinus node without cutting sinus node arteries.

2 To make the maze procedure more effective, atria that have dilated excessively are trimmed to approximately 4 cm in size.

3 Temporarily transecting the SVC is effective for reducing operation time, as it vastly improves mitral valve exposure.

4 The author preserves all of the right atrial appendage and part of the left atrial appendage. See more details in Reference [13].

Patients and method

Between February 1992 and September 2005, 384 cases were treated using the maze procedure or two PV isolations during my tenancy as a staff of The Japanese National Cardiovascular Center and Takarazuka Municipal Hospital. Of these, 196 cases were males, and 188 were females. The average age of patients was 57.8 ± 9.4 years. The average documented duration of AF was 11.1 ± 21.8 years. There were 344 cases of sustained AF, 33 paroxysmal AF, 2 sustained atrial flutter (AFL), and 5 paroxysmal AFL.

The author has applied the maze procedure to 22 cases of isolated AF (lone group), 312 cases of AF associated mainly with mitral valve disease with or without other valve disease (mitral group), 37 cases of AF associated with congenital heart disease, e.g., atrial septal defect, ventricular septal defect, endocardial cushion defect, tricuspid atresia, and so on (congenital group) and 11 cases of no cause-and-effect relationship between the basic ailment and AF, e.g., isolated aortic valve disease, coronary artery disease, and hypertrophic obstructive cardiomyopathy (HOCM) (other group).

Results of lone group (22 cases)

There was no inhospital mortality. In 22 cases, the treatment was completely successful soon after operation. Finally, 21 cases (95%) reverted to SR. In one case that suffered from sustained AF before surgery, paroxysmal atrial tachycardia was documented and controlled by means of an antiarrhythmic drug. A second case developed atrial tachycardia (AT) 12 years after maze procedure. This patient could not be controlled by antiarrhythmic drugs and failed catheter ablation for AT. He eventually underwent ablation of the His bundle to achieve AV block and implantation of a permanent pacemaker.

Results of mitral group (312 cases)

Although four operative deaths (1.3%) and two hospital deaths (0.7%) occurred, the causes of death were not related to the maze procedure. Soon after operation, 93% (286/306) of surviving cases reverted to sinus or junctional rhythm (JR). After few days, 12 cases returned to AF and within 1 year, 31 cases returned to AF. After more than 1 year, 243 cases remained in SR and eight cases were in JR, namely, 82% cases were free from AF. Furthermore, 28 cases returned to sustained AF, one case changed to sustained AFL, and 26 cases changed to sustained AT. Over 1 year after maze procedure, five cases returned to AF and five cases returned to AT. Seventeen cases were implanted with permanent pacemaker. There were four cases of late death, in which the causes of death were liver cancer, cerebral bleeding, ventricular arrhythmia, and sudden death.

Between January 1988 and December 1992, we performed mitral valve surgery without the maze procedure and only 15% (26/176) of the patients returned to SR. On the contrary, in patients where maze procedure and mitral valve surgery was performed, conversion to SR was 80% (243/302).

Results of congenital group (37 cases)

There was no inhospital mortality. Soon after the operation, 100% (37/37) of the cases converted to sinus or JR. After few days, one case returned to AF, and one case became JR. Within 1 year, 97% (36/37) was free from AF. The JR case and another case returned to AT again more than 1 year after

maze procedure. Finally, 92% (34/37) remained in SR.

Results of other group (11 cases)

One case that suffered from HOCM died due to ventricular tachycardia or fibrillation 3 months after operation. Soon after operation 91% (10/11) cases were free from AF. Finally, there were nine cases of SR and one case of AF.

Result of the pulmonary vein isolation

We have done only two PV isolations for AF associated with mitral valve disease. Their AF was sustained but occurred recently. All of them have reverted to SR soon after operation and remain in SR at the present.

Thromboembolism after maze procedure

Throughout the observations over the course of up to 123 months (average 54 mo), among the 115 cases in which a mitral valve prosthesis was not implanted and SR was recovered, there were no confirmed cases of thromboembolism. In case of mitral valve replacement, the incidence of embolism for patients who recovered to SR was 2.4% (4/163) and 8.7% (4/46) for those that did not recover to SR.

In 2002, Bando *et al.* reported the benefit of the maze procedure with concomitant mitral valve replacement (MVR) or mitral valve repair (MVP) [32]. They compared the outcomes between 258 MVR or MVP with maze procedures and 61 control patients without maze procedure during the same interval. Freedom from AF at 5 years was significantly higher in MVR (78%) and MVP (81%) with maze procedure than in MVR (6%) without maze procedure. Freedom from stroke at 5 years was 97% for MVR with maze procedure, 97% for MVP with maze procedure, and only 79% for MVR without maze procedure. They concluded that the addition of the maze procedure to MVR and MVP was safe and effective for selected patients. Elimination of AF significantly decreased the incidence of late stroke.

The maze procedure prevents risks of embolism. Bando *et al.* [33] reported that persistent AF was the most significant risk factor for late stroke after mechanical MVR. Restoration of SR with a maze procedure nearly eliminated the risk of late stroke, whereas neither closure of the left atrial appendage nor therapeutic anticoagulation prevented this complication.

Distinction between atrial flutter and atrial tachycardia

The curative rate of the maze procedure for the isolated AF (lone group) was almost 100%. However, the curative rate of the maze procedure for AF associated with mitral valve disease (mitral group) was 82%. The left atria in the mitral group were larger than in the lone group. Furthermore, atrial muscles in mitral group were extended and degenerated more than those in the lone group. Of unsuccessful cases, half of them changed to AT after the operation. According to conventional differential diagnosis, the occurrence of AFL and AT is determined only by the heart rate. The atrial rate of AFL is 250–350/min and the atrial rate of AT is 140–220/min. However, we observed postoperative regular tachyarrhythmias with a rate of 220–300/min and with isoelectric lines. Postoperatively, three cases that had such arrhythmias underwent electrophysiological studies. The studies showed that these arrhythmias were induced and terminated by pacing, and mappings showed that the electrical excitation radiated in all directions from one point. We believe that these arrhythmias are attributable to micro-reentries, or sometimes to the acceleration of automaticities. Half of the postoperative residual supraventricular arrhythmias associated with mitral valve disease are AT, which has isoelectric lines due to micro-reentry or the acceleration of automaticity.

Indications for the surgical treatment of AF

The isolated atrial fibrillation

The author would like to mention about indications for the maze procedure from his own experience. The isolated AF is not a fatal arrhythmia, and in almost every case, symptoms and complications arising from AF can be controlled by pharmacological therapy. Therefore, surgical indication for lone AF should be considered very carefully. Important

conditions that affect the surgical indications are (1) AF refractoriness to drug therapy, (2) severity of AF symptoms, or systemic embolism, and (3) patient request for a radical operation without pharmacological therapy. Because of recent developments in the catheter-based ablation for AF, the first choice of nonpharmacological treatment for lone AF may be the catheter ablation. However, the maze procedure could be indicated for AF in unsuccessful cases of catheter ablation. Whenever the maze procedure is indicated for isolated AF, a complete maze procedure should be recommended. Presently, simple PV isolation should not be indicated for isolated AF. In addition, if the ECG shows micro-reentry or abnormal automaticity, the maze procedure is, in the author's opinion, contraindicated.

The atrial fibrillation associated with other required cardiac surgery

The concomitant surgical treatment for AF can be indicated generally in patients suffering from other types of heart disease who may require surgery. Some surgeons prefer the simplified maze procedure, namely, LA maze or PV isolation. When LADs exceed 70 mm and CTR (cardio-thoracic ratio) exceeds 80%, the curative rate falls below 60%. In addition, if the patient's cardiac function is unpromising and the operative risk is high, or if the patient has undergone a previous operation and dissection of adhesions is difficult, the simplified maze procedure, for example, PV isolation could be the only procedure indicated. When LADs exceed 87 mm, the curative rate falls to 0%, and it might be a contraindication to perform any AF surgery in such patients.

Summary

The recent successful development of catheter-based ablation for AF has made it the first choice of nonpharmacological treatment for lone AF. However, the maze procedure prevents risks of embolism and increases cardiac output and exercise tolerance. Therefore, the maze procedure could be indicated for lone AF of unsuccessful cases of catheter ablation. The concomitant surgical treatment for AF, namely, the maze procedure and some other heart surgeries, can be indicated generally.

References

1 Cox JL, Schuessler RB, Boineau JP. The surgical treatment of atrial fibrillation. I. Summary of the current concepts of the mechanisms of atrial flutter and atrial fibrillation. *J Thorac Cardiovasc Surg* 1991; **101**: 402–405.

2 Cox JL, Canavan TE, Schuessler RB *et al.* The surgical treatment of atrial fibrillation. II. Intra-operative electrophysiologic mapping and description of the electrophysiologic basis of atrial flutter and atrial fibrillation. *J Thorac Cardiovasc Surg* 1991; **101**: 406–426.

3 Cox JL, Schuessler RB, D'Agostino HJ *et al.* The surgical treatment of atrial fibrillation. III. Development of a definitive surgical procedure. *J Thorac Cardiovasc Surg* 1991; **101**: 569–583.

4 Cox JL. The surgical treatment of atrial fibrillation. IV. Surgical technique. *J Thorac Cardiovasc Surg* 1991; **101**: 584–592.

5 Kosakai Y, Kawaguchi AT, Isobe F *et al.* Cox-maze procedure for chronic atrial fibrillation associated with mitral valve disease. *J Thorac Cardiovasc Surg* 1994; **108**: 1049–1055.

6 Kosakai Y, Kawaguchi AT, Isobe F *et al.* Modified maze procedure for patients with atrial fibrillation undergoing simultaneous open heart surgery. *Circulation* 1995; **92**(suppl 2): 359–364.

7 Williams JM, Ungerleider RM, Lofland GK, Cox JL, Durahum, Sabiston DC. Left atrial isolation, new technique for the treatment of supra-ventricular arrhythmias. *J Thorac Cardiovasc Surg* 1980; **80**: 373–380.

8 Graffigna A, Pagani F, Minzioni G, Salerno J, Vigano M. Left atrial isolation associated with mitral valve operation. *Ann Thorac Surg* 1992; **54**: 1093–1098.

9 Guiraudon GM, Campbell CS, Jones DL, McLellan DG, MacDonald JL. Combined sino-atrial node atrioventricular isolation: a surgical alternative to His bundle ablation in patients with atrial fibrillation. *Circulation* 1985; **72**(suppl 3): 72.

10 Cox JL, Boineau JP, Schuessler RB, Jaquiss RDB, Lappas DG. Modification of the maze procedure for atrial flutter and atrial fibrillation. I. Rationale and surgical results. *J Thorac Cardiovasc Surg* 1995; **110**: 473–484.

11 Cox JL, Jaquiss RDB, Schuessler RB, Boineau JP. Modification of the maze procedure for atrial flutter and atrial fibrillation. II. Surgical technique of the maze III procedure. *J Thorac Cardiovasc Surg* 1995; **110**: 485–495.

12 Kosakai Y. Treatment of atrial fibrillation using the Maze procedure: the Japanese experience. *Semin Thorac Cardiovasc Surg* 2000; **12**: 44–52.

13 Kosakai Y. How I perform the maze procedure. *Oper Tech Thorac Cardiovasc Surg* 2000; **5**: 23–45.

14 Shyu KG, Cheng JJ, Chen JJ *et al.* Recovery of atrial function after atrial compartment operation for chronic atrial fibrillation in mitral valve disease. *J Am Coll Cardiol* 1994; **24**: 399–405.

15 Lin FY, Huang JH, Lin JL Chen WJ, Lo HM, Chu SH. Atrial compartment surgery for chronic atrial fibrillation associated with congenital heart defects. *J Thorac Cardiovasc Surg* 1996; **111**: 231–237.

16 Lin JM, Lin FY, Lin JL, Shyu KG, Hwang JJ, Tseng YZ. Influence of additional partition on the recovery of atrial function after atrial compartment operation for atrial fibrillation. *Am J Cardiol* 1997; **79**: 497–499.

17 Sueda T, Shikata H, Orihashi K, Mitsui N, Nahata H, Matsuura Y. A modified maze procedure performed only on the left atrium for chronic atrial fibrillation associated with mitral valve disease: report of a case. *Surg Today Jpn J Surg* 1996; **26**: 135–137.

18 Sueda T, Nagata H, Orihashi K. Efficacy of a simple left atrial procedure for chronic atrial fibrillation in mitral valve operations. *Ann Thorac Surg* 1997; **63**: 1070–1075.

19 Nitta T, Lee R, Schuessler RB, Boineau JP, Cox JL. Radial approach: a new concept in surgical treatment for atrial fibrillation. I. Concept, anatomic and physiologic bases and development of a procedure. *Ann Thorac Surg* 1999; **67**: 27–35.

20 Nitta T, Lee R, Watandbe H *et al.* Radial approach: a new concept in surgical treatment for atrial fibrillation. II. Electrophysiologic effects and atrial contribution to ventricular filling. *Ann Thorac Surg* 1999; **67**: 36–50.

21 Isobe F, Kumano H, Ishikawa T *et al.* A new procedure for chronic atrial fibrillation: bilateral appendage-preserving maze procedure. *Ann Thorac Surg* 2001; **72**: 1473–1478.

22 Swartz JF, Pellersels G, Silvers J, Patten L, Cervantez D. A catheter-based curative approach to atrial fibrillation in humans. *Circulation* 1994; **90**: I-335.

23 Haissaguerre M, Jais P, Shah DC *et al.* Right and left atrial radiofrequency catheter therapy of paroxysmal atrial fibrillation. *J Cardiovasc Electrophysiol* 1996; **7**: 1132–1144.

24 Haissaguerre M, Jais P, Shah DC *et al.* Spontaneous initiation of atrial fibrillation by ectopic beats originating in the pulmonary veins. *N Engl J Med* 1998; **339**: 659–666.

25 Sueda T, Imai K, Orihashi K, Watari M, Okada K. Pulmonary vein orifice isolation for elimination of chronic atrial fibrillation. *Ann Thorac Surg* 2000; **71**: 708–710.

26 Melo J, Adragao PR, Neves J *et al.* Electrosurgical treatment of atrial fibrillation with a new intraoperative radiofrequency ablation catheter. *Thorac Cardiovasc Surg* 1999; **47**(suppl 3): 370–372.

27 Bourke JP, Dunuwille A, O'Donnell D, Jamieson S, Furniss SS. Pulmonary vein ablation for idiopathic atrial fibrillation: six month outcome of first procedure in 100 consecutive patients. *Heart* 2005; **91**: 51–57.

28 Deisenhofer I, Schneider MA, Bohlen-Knauf M *et al.* Circumferential mapping and electric isolation of pulmonary veins in patients with atrial fibrillation. *Am J Cardiol* 2003; **91**: 159–163.

29 Gillinov AM, Pettersson G, Rice TW. Esophageal injury during radiofrequency ablation for atrial fibrillation. *J Thorac Cardiovasc Surg* 2001; **122**: 1239–1240.

30 Doll N, Borger MA, Fabricius A *et al.* Esophageal perforation during left atrial radiofrequency ablation: is the risk too high? *J Thorac Cardiovasc Surg* 2003; **125**: 836–842.

31 Pappone C, Oral H, Santinelli V *et al.* Atrio-esophageal fistula as a complication of percutaneous transcatheter ablation of atrial fibrillation. *Circulation* 2004; **109**: 2724–2726.

32 Bando K, Kobayashi J, Kosakai Y *et al.* Impact of Cox maze procedure on outcome in patients with atrial fibrillation and mitral valve disease. *J Thorac Cardiovasc Surg* 2002; **124**: 575–583.

33 Bando K, Kobayashi J, Hirata M *et al.* Early and late stroke after mitral valve replacement with a mechanical prosthesis: risk factor analysis of a 24-year experience. *J Thorac Cardiovasc Surg* August 2003; **126**(2): 358–364.

CHAPTER 17

Minimally invasive surgical approach to treat atrial fibrillation

Mustafa Güden, Belhhan Akpınar, & Osman Bayındır

Introduction

Atrial fibrillation (AF) is an insidious disease which is associated with a 1.5- to 2.0-fold increase of mortality and 2- to 5-fold increase for stroke in patients with cardiovascular disease. AF was previously considered as a benign arrhythmia; however, the clinical importance of AF and the necessity to treat AF has gained widespread recognition. The efficacy of pharmacological therapy to convert AF is low with considerable side effects. Overall success at maintaining sinus rhythm with nonsurgical therapies varies but is usually no greater than 60%, with multiple failures due to drug intolerance [1–3]. Thus, nonmedical therapy modalities have emerged with advances in experience and technology, it became evident that catheter-based electrical isolation of pulmonary veins provided better result than medical therapy alone [4–6]. However, this technique remains operator dependent and technically demanding. It can also account for significant complications, such as pulmonary vein stenosis and atypical left atrial flutter [7], not to mention long operation times and being exposed to high levels of radiation [8].

From the surgical aspect, the Cox-maze procedure after several modifications has become the gold standard for the treatment of AF with excellent success rates [9]. However, this was a complex and technically demanding procedure, which could never be universally accepted as a standard practice for the surgical treatment of AF. Most surgeons were reluctant to expose their patients to the risk of the surgical maze because of significantly increased aortic cross-clamping time and the morbidity risks. As a consequence, alternative energy sources have emerged to treat AF surgically; with the aim of replacing some of the incisions of the cut-and-sew technique and creating a conduction block without causing any tissue dehiscence and simplifying the procedure. Various energy sources have been used for this purpose. These energy sources can either be hyperthermic [radiofrequency (RF), microwave, laser, ultrasound] or hypothermic (cryothermy). On the other hand, the efficacy of various energy sources is debated because the creation of continuous linear transmural lesions, which act as an electrophysiological conduction block, is considered to be uncertain and inconsistent. However, most of these energy sources have proven to be safe and efficient in the surgical treatment of AF with good success rates.

The clinical application of these energy sources can be accepted as the first step toward a less invasive approach for the surgical treatment of AF. Indeed these energy sources have reduced the ischemic and cardiopulmonary bypass (CPB) times significantly, thus allowing more surgeons to adopt the technique and offer the treatment chance to their patients.

Another step to reduce the invasiveness of the Cox-maze procedure was to limit it to the left atrium. Various centers reported different ablation lines within the left atrium. This concept came through after the pioneering work of Haissaguerre, who showed that over 90% of the foci that triggered AF was located in the orifices of pulmonary veins [10], although more recent studies suggest a

Manual of Surgical Treatment of Atrial Fibrillation.
Edited by Hauw T. Sie *et al.* © 2008 Blackwell Publishing,
ISBN: 978-1-4051-4032-4.

considerably less percentage [11]. The mini-maze concept was born, which limited the incisions or ablation lines to the left atrium. Success rates of sinus rhythm restoration for long-term ranged between 75 and 82% [12–14], and this procedure found a wide application especially during minimally invasive approaches.

What is minimally invasive?

In cardiac surgery, the term minimally invasive refers to a procedure that either avoids median sternotomy or CPB, or preferably both.

Today, the main candidates for surgical ablation are patients with chronic AF who are undergoing open-heart procedures for various cardiac pathologies. However, these patients constitute the minority of the population who is affected by AF, when compared with lone AF patients.

With the developing coapting technology, such as visualization systems, stabilizers, alternate methods of vascular cannulation, and robotic surgical systems, surgeons have been able to broaden their capabilities to perform minimally invasive procedures. The minimally invasive surgical procedures for the treatment of AF without CPB or median sternotomy would broaden the applicability of this effective procedure, especially for patients with lone AF.

Minimally invasive surgical approaches for treatment of AF

The right minithoracotomy approach on the arrested heart (port-access ablation)

Surgical technique

After standard induction of anesthesia, patients undergo double-lumen intubation for single lung ventilation. Following the administration of 2 mg/kg of heparin, a 17 F arterial cannula (DLP, Inc, Grand Rapids, MI) is introduced through the right internal jugular vein percutaneously to assist venous drainage during CPB. Patients were positioned supine with the right shoulder elevated and external defibrillation pads are placed. A right lateral minithoracotomy (4–6 cm) in the fourth intercostal space is performed. A soft tissue retractor (Heartport Inc, Redwood City, USA) is used for the exposure of the surgical field, avoiding the division

or traction of any rib. A 5-mm camera port (Storz, Karl Storz GmbH and Co, Tuttingen-Ger) is introduced through the fourth intercostal space front axillary line. A second port is introduced through the sixth intercostal space mid-axillary line for left atrial venting and carbon dioxide insufflation, which began immediately after collapsing the right lung. Simultaneously, the right femoral artery and vein are prepared by means of a 2-cm oblique incision in the groin. CPB is established by femoro–femoral cannulation. An 18–20 F arterial cannula (DLP, Inc, Grand Rapids, MI) is used for arterial cannulation. Venous drainage is obtained by a 24–29 F femoral cannula (DLP, Inc, Grand Rapids, MI) and the 17–19 F arterial cannula, previously inserted in the right internal jugular vein, thus allowing adequate venous drainage. The pericardium is opened 2 cm above and parallel to the phrenic nerve. Exposure is optimized with several pericardial stay sutures. Patients are cooled down to 28°C. Both vena cavae are encircled with tapes for a dryer operative field. A transthoracic clamp (Chitwood, Scanlan, Saint Paul, MN, USA) is introduced from the second intercostal space, front axillary line percutaneously. After cross-clamping of the aorta, blood cardioplegia is administered through a custom-made (DLP) antegrade cardioplegia cannula inserted in the ascending aorta. Also, endoaortic balloon can be used to arrest the heart. The left atrium is opened parallel to the interatrial groove. The heart port atrial retractor system (Heart Port Inc, Redwood City, CA) is used for the exposure of the atrium. The ablation is performed through the incision with the aid of endoscopic visualization (Figure 17.1). The ostium of left atrial appendage is closed from inside the left atrium.

Several authors reported their series of patients who underwent a concomitant mitral valve repair or replacement and ablation procedure through a right minithoracotomy [15–18]. The success rate of establishing sinus rhythm was similar in these reports.

Mohr and associates surgically treated AF in 234 patients using a 10-mm T-shaped RF ablation probe (Osypka GmbH, Grenzach-Wyhlen, Germany) targeting a temperature of 60°C for 20 seconds. A minimal invasive approach through a right lateral minithoracotomy was performed in 133 out of 234 patients. Success rate of sinus restoration was

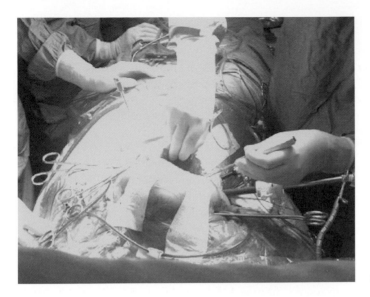

Figure 17.1 The operative field.

81.1 and 72.5% at 6 and 12 months, respectively [15]. Kottkamp and associates operated 70 patients through a right lateral minithoracotomy with the same ablation probe and the incidences of freedom from AF were 93 and 95% at 6 and 12 months, respectively. Kottkamp reported a fistula between the esophagus and the left atrium and another fistula involving the left bronchus system with subsequent left-sided pneumectomy. Also, a significant stenosis of the circumflex artery due to ablation was reported [16].

Ad and Cox used cryoprobe for biatrial ablation through right minithoracotomy. The long-term recurrence of AF was 2.4%. In the series of these authors patients with lone AF were also operated [19]. Doll and colleagues reported their series of 28 patients underwent left atrial cryoablation with the Surgifrost CryoCath (Irvine, CA) in which 20 patients were operated through a right lateral minithoracotomy using video-assistance. The rate of sinus rhythm was 96% postoperatively, 82% at discharge, and 74% at 6 months follow-up [20].

We reported our experience using the irrigated RF ablation probe (Cardioblate, Medtronic Inc., MN) with a similar surgical approach [18]. The Cardioblate RF ablation system consists of a power generator and a pen. The pen-shaped probe allowed sufficient endothoracic movement and enabled the surgeon to perform precise ablation lines through a limited incision. The videoscopic vision allowed

excellent view for the left atrium during the maze procedure.

One of the drawbacks of the right minithoracotomy approach was the difficulty of reaching the left atrial appendage in patients with a deep chest wall. This problem was greatly solved by the introduction of Cardioblate XL pen which has a longer shaft that enables tissue contact in patients with a deep chest.

Our total experience using this approach has reached 80 patients. Conversion to sinus rhythm was 88% at 1 year and 79% at 2 years. Because of saline irrigated RF ablation we did not observe any collateral damage either to the esophagus or coronary arteries in this series. We believe that this method is a valuable approach to patients who have AF and concomitant cardiac pathologies that can be dealt with through a right thoracotomy. A mitral valve can be repaired or replaced, an ASD closure, a tricuspid repair, or myxoma resection can be performed [15–21]. Either a left or a biatrial ablation procedure can be performed, although usually a left atrial ablation was performed.

Ablation through right minithoracotomy approach on the arrested heart is contraindicated in patients with recent amiodarone use. The patients are at a high risk for developing contralateral lung toxicity in the left lung because the right lung is collapsed during this procedure. Therefore, a high FIO_2 is required for the left lung to sustain adequate oxygenation, resulting in parenchymal damage in over 10% of these patients [22, 23].

The validity of this technique has to be redefined in cases with lone AF. Although it is a less invasive approach than a sternotomy, CPB and cardioplegic arrest are still needed for an endocardial ablation. The risks and benefits of such an approach should be redefined and the authors do not use this method for lone AF.

The off-pump median sternotomy approach

Surgical ablation to treat AF has predominantly been combined with mitral valve disease and the success of different energy sources in this aspect has been shown [24–26]. Although the presence of AF in patients undergoing CABG is less than their mitral valve counterparts this percentage is known to increase with older age, male gender, and depressed left ventricle function [27]. This fact, together with the reality that coronary artery surgery still constitutes the main bulk of the cardiac surgical workload in most centers, has created a greater interest toward concomitant CABG and AF treatment.

The surgical treatment of AF has entered a new era with the development of various energy sources and advanced tools. The clinical introduction of bipolar ablation devices and flexible long microwave probes which could be applied epicardially has been one of the advances in this field. The notion of performing ablation in a CABG patient without having to open the left atrium and/or not using CPB seemed to be a valid option [28]. On the other hand, it soon became clear that this would mean making sacrifices from the maze pattern and suffice with pulmonary vein isolation alone [28, 29].

Surgical technique

After the induction of the anesthesia, patients undergo a routine TEE examination, especially to exclude thrombus in the left atrium which will make them ineligible for the procedure.

After median sternotomy and opening of the pericardium, the heparin is administered. The ACT was monitored and maintained above 300 seconds during the procedure. Coronary revascularization is performed prior to ablation for two reasons:

1 Relieving ischemia first further facilitates manipulating the heart, especially if the patient has critical coronary lesions.

2 Manipulating the heart for revascularization after ablation may provoke arrhythmias and sometimes even AF recurrence.

The ablation is performed using a bipolar ablation device.

Right pulmonary vein isolation

After revascularization is completed, the right-sided pulmonary vein isolation is performed first. The right side of the pericardium is suspended with stay sutures. Opening of the right pleural space may be necessary in some cases for exposure. A suction device (heart positioner) is applied on the right ventricle, near the atrioventricular junction and the heart is slightly tilted to the left. This will facilitate the exposure of the right pulmonary veins. This is followed by a blunt dissection around the inferior vena cava (IVC) and the right inferior pulmonary vein, so that the surgeon's index finger can encircle the IVC. Then a plane is developed between the right superior pulmonary vein and the right pulmonary artery. An atraumatic clamp is introduced through this plane (jaws closed) and gently introduced toward the inferior pulmonary vein until the edge of the clamp is seen. A rubber tube (16 Fr, Nelaton) is fed between the two jaws and the clamp is withdrawn and both right pulmonary veins are encircled. The rubber tube will serve as a guide while introducing the lower jaw of the bipolar clamp. The rubber tube is then fed into the lower jaw of the bipolar pen and the lower jaw is then introduced between this plane by pulling the rubber tube until the jaw is visible behind the lower pulmonary vein. Then the jaws are closed, locked, and RF energy applied. The same procedure is applied from the inferior side; that is the inferior jaw is introduced between the plane created between the IVC and the right inferior pulmonary vein and slightly introduced toward the right superior pulmonary vein. The jaws are closed, locked, and ablation repeated. Since the aim is to create a complete conduction block, the right pulmonary veins are paced with two atrial pacemaker wires at a rate of 90 beats/min after each application and the ablation process is repeated until a complete electrical block

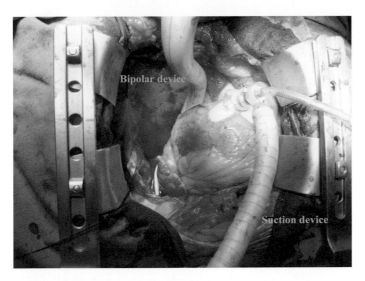

Figure 17.2 Left pulmonary vein ablation is shown. The apex of the heart is tilted toward the patient's right shoulder with suction device.

is achieved. This may occasionally require several applications.

Left pulmonary vein and appendage isolation

The apex of the heart is tilted toward the right shoulder of the patient with the aid of the apical suction device. The pericardium around the pulmonary veins is gently peeled off away from the heart and toward the left pleural cavity. A surgical dissection is performed to create a plane between the left superior pulmonary vein and the left pulmonary artery. The clamp is gently introduced through this plane until its edge is seen coming out behind the left inferior pulmonary vein. Again, both pulmonary veins are isolated with a rubber tube, which is fed into the lower jaw of the bipolar ablation pen. The rubber tube is gently pulled until the lower jaw of the ablation pen is retrieved behind the left inferior pulmonary vein. Both jaws are closed, locked, and ablation is performed (Figure 17.2). After the ablation, the left pulmonary veins are paced with two atrial pacing wires and the conduction block is checked. The ablation procedure is repeated until it is not possible to pace the atria via the pulmonary veins. This may mean several applications of the ablation with the bipolar pen. Usually both pulmonary veins with left atrial tissue can be encircled with this approach. If there is an anomalous location of the pulmonary veins or they are too far from

each other, preferably they are ablated individually. In other words, after the ablation around the left superior pulmonary vein area, the bipolar device is then introduced from the side of the left inferior pulmonary vein and this area is ablated separately. Ablation lines may overlap; however, this detail is negligible.

As the final step of the left atrial appendage is taken in between the jaws of the bipolar ablation device approximately 2 cm above its base. After ablation the appendage is cut 1.5–2 cm above the ablation line while the bipolar device is still clamped. This maneuver facilitates the closure of the appendage. The appendage is closed using 5-0 Prolene continuous and double-layer sutures.

Technical details

To avoid possible pulmonary vein stenosis, the curve of the jaw has to be located toward the left atrium and not the pulmonary veins. The ventilation can be stopped for brief periods to facilitate the dissection around the pulmonary veins and during the ablation. Care should be taken during the left pulmonary vein ablation not to stretch the left internal thoracic artery anastomoses.

One of the difficulties is the inability to perform a complete isolation in one attempt in some patients. Despite the transmurality feedback, one cannot be sure of a conduction block unless pacing of the pulmonary veins is performed. The authors believe that this is an essential step during off-pump ablation.

The introduction of bipolar RF pens had two major impacts on AF surgery. First was the ability to create a transmural lesion and second was the possibility of epicardial application during CABG cases which would eliminate opening of the left atrium [30, 31]. Although bipolar pens were major advancements, their limitations—especially during OPCAB procedures—were soon seen, because it was difficult—if not impossible—to create the interatrial connecting lesions of the maze III procedure. Despite a recent study showing the feasibility of creating maze lesions with bipolar devices on animal models without using CPB, application of these ablation lines in humans so far could not be performed routinely due to anatomical differences and safety reasons [32]. Theoretically, however, creating some of the interatrial connecting lesions should be possible through the left atrial appendage. One of the risks with this method would be air embolism; however, this can be prevented with the use of CO_2 gas. Nevertheless, for the reasons mentioned above, we and most other groups have limited the ablation procedure to pulmonary vein isolation and left atrial appendage ligation during off-pump revascularization.

We operated on 33 patients—21 patients with permanent AF and 12 with paroxysmal AF, with this technique and could restore sinus rhythm in 71 and 73% of cases at 6 and 12 months in this series. Sinus rhythm restoration was 82% for patients with paroxysmal AF versus 59% for patients with permanent AF in 12 months. The difference did not reach statistical significance simply due to the low number of cases; however, there seemed to be a more favorable trend toward the paroxysmal group. During follow-up, maintaining sinus rhythm was more difficult in the permanent AF group; in other words, more patients returned to AF during follow-up in comparison to the paroxysmal group ($p = 0.016$). Female gender, chronic obstructive lung disease, hypertension, and depressed left ventricle function seemed be the risk factors for AF recurrence after the ablation procedure. Pulmonary vein isolation and left atrial appendage ligation could safely be performed without complicating the operation. It seems to be a valid option for cases with paroxysmal

AF who undergo off-pump coronary revascularization.

Maessen and colleagues reported 24 patients undergoing beating-heart epicardial ablation with microwave energy through median sternotomy. The left and right pulmonary veins isolated and connected to each other followed by amputation of the left atrial appendage. Twenty-four of 24 patients were in sinus rhythm in 24 hours, 14 patients at discharge, and 20 patients at 6.4-month follow-up [33].

Totally endoscopic approach for lone AF

The above-mentioned surgical approaches require either median sternotomy or CPB, and the patients operated with these techniques have concomitant cardiac disorders to be cured. Patients who are in AF with concomitant cardiac disorders represent only a minority of patients in general population affected by AF. The ideal operation, especially for the patients with lone AF, should be performed without median sternotomy and CPB, on the beating heart, and epicardially. The successful results with epicardially based pulmonary vein isolation and the development of visualization systems and energy sources with new devices has opened a new era for the minimally invasive surgical treatment of AF. Although the original Cox-maze procedure may have superior results, epicardially based pulmonary vein isolation is a noninvasive method that can be offered to patients with lone AF.

Surgical technique

After double-lumen general endotracheal anesthesia, intraoperative TEE is used to confirm that there is no thrombus in the left atrium. The patient is positioned supine with arms abducted 90°. After deflation of the right lung, three ports (5 mm at the third intercostal space, midaxillary line, 5 mm at the fourth or fifth intercostals space, midaxillary line, and 10 mm at the fifth intercostal space, anterior axillary line) are introduced in the right pleural space. Carbon dioxide insufflation is used to have a better vision.

After opening the pericardium from the superior vena cava (SVC) to IVC approximately 2 cm anterior to the phrenic nerve, blunt dissection is performed underneath the SVC and IVC to establish access to the transverse and oblique sinuses.

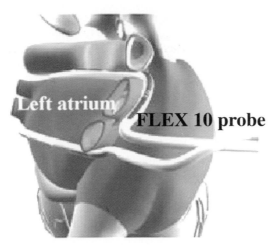

Figure 17.3 The position of the FLEX 10 probe around the pulmonary veins.

Two 14-F red rubber catheters are guided through the sinuses with the aid of stylets. The red rubber catheters are exited through the inferior right chest port and the right lung is reinflated. The left lung is deflated and the same ports are positioned on the left side. The pericardium is opened sharply, 2 cm anterior to the phrenic nerve, just long enough to expose the left atrial appendage. The two red rubber catheters are retrieved and taken out of the chest through the inferiormost port. The catheters are sutured together tip to tip, placed back in the chest, and drawn around the pulmonary veins with gentle traction from the right side. Once the position is confirmed posterior to the left atrial appendage the tip of the FLEX 10 microwave energy probe (AFx, Fremont, CA, USA) is sutured to the end of the transverse sinus catheter and the entire assembly is guided around the pulmonary veins with gentle traction on the inferior catheter. Position of the probe is confirmed and observed from the right side (Figure 17.3).

Ablation around the pulmonary veins (Box lesion) is performed at 90 seconds per lesion and 65 W per application. Mostly, 8–10 lesions are enough to encircle the pulmonary veins. An additional lesion is then placed to connect the pulmonary vein box lesion to the left atrial appendage. For permanent and persistent AF patients, right-sided lesions, which are laterally from the SVC to the IVC along the sulcus terminalis, toward the coro-

nary sinus over the IVC and finally to the tip of the right atrial appendage can be performed, and FLEX 10 probe is withdrawn. After the deflation of the left lung, left atrial appendage is removed with a 45-mm endoscopic stapler (Endo-GIA; Ethicon, New Brunswick, NJ, USA) through 10-mm midclavicular port on the left side.

This technique was reported by Saltman and colleagues. The patient was operated for paroxysmal AF which is resistant to drug therapy. After the operation, during 1 month follow-up the patient remained in sinus rhythm [34].

Salenger and colleagues operated 14 patients with this technique. Their success rate of sinus rhythm is 71% at discharge, 100% at 6 months follow-up, and 67% at 12 months follow-up [35].

Balkhy and colleagues operated a patient, with failed electrical cardioversions and failed percutaneous pulmonary vein isolation, through thoracoscopic approach. The patient was in rate-controlled AF when he was discharged. He was electrically converted to sinus rhythm and at latest follow-up he was in sinus rhythm [36].

Two port thoracoscopic approach

The sole right-sided approach for thoracoscopic ablation depends on the surgeon's ability to perform pericardioscopy. A standard endoscope with a conal covering enables surgeons to perform endoscopy around the entire heart. This protected scope allows the surgeon to dissect out the pericardial reflection around the transverse sinus, oblique sinus, and to scope along the entire back wall of the cardiac surface. In the meantime the surgeon is able to view proper placement of the ablation probe to the back of the heart along its entire extent and also to confirm an appropriate lesion around the pulmonary veins.

The patient is placed under anesthesia with double-lumen endotracheal intubation in supine position. TEE is performed to confirm that there is no thrombus in the left atrium. After deflation of the right lung two 12-mm ports over the right thorax at the 2nd–3rd and 4th–5th intercostal spaces are positioned in the mid-axillary line. The pericardium is opened and the dissection of the pericardial reflection under the SVC and above the right pulmonary artery, right superior pulmonary vein is performed. The protected conus dissecting scope is used to pass between the SVC and just superior to the right superior pulmonary vein into the transverse sinus along the dome of the left atrium until the left atrial appendage is fully visualized. Afterward, the scope is retracted into the right hemithorax and is then used to pass through the pericardial reflection underneath the IVC just inferior to the right inferior pulmonary vein. The scope is introduced through the oblique sinus until the left atrial appendage is seen.

A soft silastic nasogastric tube is passed through the transverse sinus and is directed by the left pericardial surface along the left atrial appendage. With the visualization of the protected endoscope introduced through the oblique sinus the nasogastric tube is grasped and pulled through the oblique sinus. The probe of the energy source is tied onto the distal end of the nasogastric tube. The nasogastric tube is used as a guide to encircle the pulmonary veins. Confirmation of the positioning and laying of the probe is performed by passing the protected scope around the heart. Ablation is initiated to perform pulmonary vein isolation. With this technique described by Li Poa, the early success rate in restoring sinus rhythm is reported to be 86% [37].

Totally endoscopic approach with the aid of robotic surgical system

With the development of robotic surgical systems, surgeons could perform totally endoscopic procedures such as CABG, ASD closure, and mitral valve repair [38–40]. The superior 3D visualization and dexterity offered by the new surgical robotic devices, combined with the flexibility of the ablation probes, have led surgeons to operate patients for ablative therapy using minimally invasive approaches.

Surgical technique
After the induction of anesthesia the patient is intubated with a double-lumen endotracheal tube to allow single lung ventilation. TEE is used to confirm that there is no thrombus in the left atrium. The patient is placed in supine position and three ports are created on the chest at the 2nd, 3rd, and 5th intercostal spaces posterior to the right anterior axillary line. The port's location is selected especially

to have a better access to SVC and transverse sinus. After right lung exclusion and CO_2 inflation, the pericardium is incised 1 cm above the right phrenic nerve. The SVC and IVC are dissected circumferentially to have free access to the transverse and oblique sinuses. The fat pad on the roof of the left atrium is dissected carefully through an additional port on the medium axillary line (third intercostal space). A 16-F Foley catheter containing a guidewire is introduced beneath the SVC. The aorta and the pulmonary artery are lifted up (lifting maneuver), while the guidewire, extracted for the Foley, is advanced across the transverse sinus. The guidewire is pushed along the lateral wall of the pericardial cavity, reaching the diaphragmatic surface of the heart. It is progressed across the oblique sinus, beneath the IVC, and finally surfaced outside the thoracic wall through the same port. Outside the chest, the tail of the guidewire is tied to the microwave probe FLEX 10 (Afx, Fremont, CA, USA). The guidewire is pulled out carrying the probe inside the chest. The probe is advanced up to encircle the orifices of both right and left pulmonary veins. Lifting maneuver and the introduction of the robotic camera into the transverse sinus enables the surgeon to visualize directly the proper orientation of the probe beneath the left atrial appendage, while guarding the circumflex artery. The detachable markers on the probe's back help optimize the placement of the probe, avoiding any inappropriate twisting. A continuous circular lesion, encircling the pulmonary veins (box lesion) is produced (65 W for 90 s for each 2 cm). It is important to keep the probe away from the sinus node, the left main and the circumflex coronary arteries.

First robotic endoscopic epicardial isolation of the pulmonary veins was performed by Loulmet and colleagues on October 23, 2002. The patient was in sinus rhythm after the operation; however, he was diagnosed with intermittent atrial flutter 8 months after the surgery. After transcatheter ablation of the tricuspid isthmus he was in stable sinus rhythm [41].

Jansens and colleagues operated seven patients with this technique. In one patient, the operation was converted to small right thoracotomy due to the trauma to the right pulmonary artery. After a follow-up period ranging 6–11 months, four of the

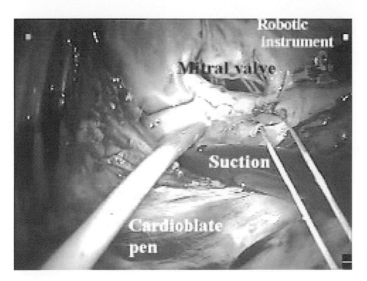

Figure 17.4 Interatrial view ablation process through the robotic endoscope.

five patients were in sinus rhythm. In the fourth postoperative month, one of the patients had atrial atypical flutter, which was cured with a percutaneous ablation. The last two patients continued to have AF, but the symptoms were much less severe than before the ablation procedure [42].

Bolotin and colleagues operated a patient for left AF ablation and mitral valve repair through a right minithoracotomy with the aid of the da Vinci robotic surgical system. The patient underwent off-pump, beating heart epicardial peripulmonary vein microwave ablation using the FLEX 10 catheter, followed by supplemental on-pump endocardial lesions. At the third month follow-up, the patient was in sinus rhythm [43].

The authors' experience on robotically enhanced AF treatment is based on patients with concomitant cardiac pathologies. We used the Cardioblate XL pen (Medtronic Inc, MN, USA) for ablation in three patients undergoing mitral valve repair with the aid the da Vinci robotic surgical system. All three patients underwent a totally closed procedure and the RF ablation was performed through a 2-cm service port (Figure 17.4). The longer shaft of the Cardioblate XL pen enabled us to maneuver the pen easily looking at the 2D view on the monitor. All three patients came out of the operating room in sinus rhythm and remained in sinus rhythm 3 months after the operation. The authors believe that this is a feasible option for patients undergoing a combined procedure and the left atrium has to be opened anyway.

Conclusion

The ideal minimally invasive procedure should be reproducible, and be applicable to all patients with AF, and be performed with minimal access. On the other hand, a higher incidence of complications, compared to conventional methods, cannot be acceptable for the sake of minimally invasiveness.

With the help of new energy sources and probes, visualization techniques and robotic surgical system, the development of the minimally invasive procedures will offer surgeons the potential to treat AF in a large number of patients, especially with lone AF.

Today, merely simple pulmonary vein isolation and sometimes LAA exclusion can be performed with the minimally invasive approaches for the treatment of AF, avoiding CBP and median sternotomy. With simple pulmonary vein isolation better success rates are observed for paroxysmal AF, while considerably lower success rates are reported for permanent AF.

In the light of the studies so far, the maze III lesion pattern seems to be the only alternative for the treatment of permanent AF (Figure 17.5).

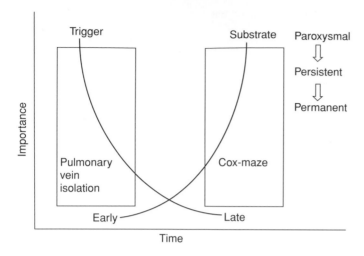

Figure 17.5 This figure shows the complex relation between time and atrial fibrillation and suggests the lesion set to be chosen according to the patient.

The improvement of techniques and new devices, which will enable the performance of maze III lesion patterns without CBP and median sternotomy, will eventually lead to an increase in the success rates of the minimally invasive approaches, especially for the patients with permanent AF.

References

1 Roy D, Talajic M, Dorian P *et al.* Amiodarone to prevent recurrence of atrial fibrillation. Canadian trial of atrial fibrillation investigators. *N Engl J Med* March 30, 2000; **342**(13): 913–920.

2 Singh S, Zoble RG, Yellen L *et al.* Efficacy and safety of oral dofetilide in converting to and maintaining sinus rhythm in patients with chronic atrial fibrillation or atrial flutter: the symptomatic atrial fibrillation investigative research on dofetilide (SAFIRE-D) study. *Circulation* November 7, 2000; **102**(19): 2385–2390.

3 Wyse DG, Waldo AL, DiMarco JP *et al.* Atrial Fibrillation Follow-up Investigation of Rhythm Management (AFFIRM) Investigators. A comparison of rate control and rhythm control in patients with atrial fibrillation. *N Engl J Med* December 5, 2002; **347**(23): 1825–1833.

4 Pappone C, Rosanio S, Oreto G *et al.* Circumferential radiofrequency ablation of pulmonary vein ostia: a new anatomic approach for curing atrial fibrillation. *Circulation* November 21, 2000; **102**(21): 2619–2628.

5 Pappone C, Oreto G, Rosanio S *et al.* Atrial electroanatomic remodeling after circumferential radiofrequency pulmonary vein ablation: efficacy of an anatomic approach in a large cohort of patients with atrial fibrillation. *Circulation* November 20, 2001; **104**(21): 2539–2544.

6 Oral H, Scharf C, Chugh A *et al.* Catheter ablation for paroxysmal atrial fibrillation: segmental pulmonary vein ostial ablation versus left atrial ablation. *Circulation* November 11, 2003; **108**(19): 2355–2360.

7 Saad EB, Rossillo A, Saad CP *et al.* Pulmonary vein stenosis after radiofrequency ablation of atrial fibrillation: functional characterization, evolution, and influence of the ablation strategy. *Circulation* December 23, 2003; **108**(25): 3102–3107.

8 O'Callaghan PA, Meara M, Kongsgaard E *et al.* Symptomatic improvement after radiofrequency catheter ablation for typical atrial flutter. *Heart* August 2001; **86**(2): 167–171.

9 Cox JL, Jaquiss RD, Schuessler RB, Boineau JP. Modification of the maze procedure for atrial flutter and atrial fibrillation. II. Surgical technique of the maze III procedure. *J Thorac Cardiovasc Surg* August 1995; **110**(2): 485–495.

10 Haissaguerre M, Jais P, Shah DC *et al.* Spontaneous initiation of atrial fibrillation by ectopic beats originating in the pulmonary veins. *N Engl J Med* September 3, 1998; **339**(10): 659–666.

11 Schmitt C, Ndrepepa G, Weber S *et al.* Biatrial multisite mapping of atrial premature complexes triggering onset of atrial fibrillation. *Am J Cardiol* June 15, 2002; **89**(12): 1381–1387.

12 Guden M, Akpinar B, Caynak B *et al.* Left versus bi-atrial intraoperative saline-irrigated radiofrequency modified maze procedure for atrial fibrillation. *Card Electrophysiol Rev* September 2003; **7**(3): 252–258.

13 Deneke T, Khargi K, Grewe PH *et al.* Left atrial versus bi-atrial maze operation using intraoperatively cooled-tip radiofrequency ablation in patients undergoing open-heart surgery: safety and efficacy. *J Am Coll Cardiol* May 15, 2002; **39**(10): 1644–1650.

14 Benussi S, Nascimbene S, Agricola E *et al.* Surgical ablation of atrial fibrillation using the epicardial radiofrequency approach: mid-term results and risk analysis. *Ann Thorac Surg* October 2002; **74**(4): 1050–1056.

15 Mohr FW, Fabricius AM, Falk V *et al.* Curative treatment of atrial fibrillation with intraoperative radiofrequency ablation: short-term and midterm results. *J Thorac Cardiovasc Surg* May 2002; **123**(5): 919–927.

16 Kottkamp H, Hindricks G, Autschbach R *et al.* Specific linear left atrial lesions in atrial fibrillation: intraoperative radiofrequency ablation using minimally invasive surgical techniques. *J Am Coll Cardiol* August 7, 2002; **40**(3): 475–480.

17 Wellens F, Casselman F, Geelen P *et al.* Combined atrial fibrillation and mitral valve surgery using radiofrequency technology. *Semin Thorac Cardiovasc Surg* July 2002; **14**(3): 219–225.

18 Guden M, Akpinar B, Sagbas E, Sanisoglu I, Ergenoglu MU, Ozbek U. A radiofrequency modified maze and valve procedure through a port-access approach. *Heart Surg Forum* 2003; **6**(5): 292–296.

19 Ad N, Cox JL. The Maze procedure for the treatment of atrial fibrillation: a minimally invasive approach. *J Card Surg* May–June 2004; **19**(3): 196–200.

20 Doll N, Kiaii BB, Fabricius AM *et al.* Intraoperative left atrial ablation (for atrial fibrillation) using a new argon cryocatheter: early clinical experience. *Ann Thorac Surg* November 2003; **76**(5): 1711–1715.

21 Guden M, Akpinar B, Ergenoglu MU, Sagbas E, Sanisoglu I, Ozbek U. Combined radiofrequency ablation and myxoma resection through a port access approach. *Ann Thorac Surg* October 2004; **78**(4): 1470–1472.

22 Van Dyck M, Baele P, Rennotte MT, Matta A, Dion R, Kestens-Servaye Y. Should amiodarone be discontinued before cardiac surgery? [Review]. *Acta Anaesthesiol Belg* 1988; **39**(1): 3–10.

23 Dimopoulou I, Marathias K, Daganou M *et al.* Low-dose amiodarone-related complications after cardiac operations. *J Thorac Cardiovasc Surg* July 1997; **114**(1): 31–37.

24 Benussi S, Pappone C, Nascimbene S *et al.* A simple way to treat chronic atrial fibrillation during mitral valve surgery: the epicardial radiofrequency approach. *Eur J Cardiothorac Surg* 2000; **17**: 524–529.

25 Guden M, Akpinar B, Sanisoglu I, Sagbas E, Bayındır O. Intraoperative saline irrigated radiofrequency modified maze procedure for atrial fibrillation. *Ann Thorac Surg* 2002; **74**: S1301–S1306.

26 Akpinar B, Guden M, Sagbas E *et al.* Combined radiofrequency modified maze and mitral valve procedure through a port access approach: early and mid-term results. *Eur J Cardiothorac Surg* 2003; **24**: 223–230.

27 Khargi K, Lemke B, Deneke T. Concomitant anti-arrhythmic procedures to treat permanent atrial fibrillation in CABG and AVR patients are as effective as in mitral valve patients. *Eur J Cardiothorac Surg* 2005; **27**: 841–846.

28 Prasad SM, Maniar HS, Diodato MD, Schuessler RB, Damiano RJ, Jr. Physiological consequences of bipolar radiofrequency energy on the atria and pulmonary veins: a chronic animal study. *Ann Thorac Surg* 2003; **76**: 836–842.

29 Khargi K, Hutten B, Lemke B, Deneke T. Surgical treatment of atrial fibrillation: a systematic review. *Eur J Cardiothorac Surg* 2005; **27**: 258–265.

30 Damiano RJ, Jr. Alternative energy sources for atrial ablation: judging the new technology. *Ann Thorac Surg* 2003; **75**: 329–330.

31 Prasad SM, Maniar HS, Moustakidis P, Schuessler RB, Damiano RJ, Jr. Epicardial ablation on the beating heart: progress towards an off-pump maze procedure. *Heart Surg Forum* 2001; **5**: 100–104.

32 Gaynor SL, Ishii Y, Diodato D *et al.* Successful performance of Cox-maze procedure on beating heart using bipolar radiofrequency ablation: a feasibility study in animals. *Ann Thorac Surg* 2004; **78**: 1671–1677.

33 Maessen JG, Nijs JF, Smeets JL, Vainer J, Mochtar B. Beating-heart surgical treatment of atrial fibrillation with microwave ablation. *Ann Thorac Surg* October 2002; **74**(4): S1307–S1311.

34 Saltman AE, Rosenthal LS, Francalancia NA, Lahey SJ. A completely endoscopic approach to microwave ablation for atrial fibrillation. *Heart Surg Forum* 2003; **6**(3): E38–E41.

35 Salenger R, Lahey SJ, Saltman AE. The completely endoscopic treatment of atrial fibrillation: report on the first 14 patients with early results. *Heart Surg Forum* 2004; **7**(6): E555–E558.

36 Balkhy HH, Chapman PD, Arnsdorf SE. Minimally invasive atrial fibrillation ablation combined with a new technique for thoracoscopic stapling of the left atrial appendage: case report. *Heart Surg Forum* 2004; **7**(6): 353–355.

37 Li Poa. Two port thoracoscopic approach for pulmonary vein isolation. In: *Postgraduate Course: 5th Annual Surgical Treatment for Atrial Fibrillation.* ISMICS Meeting, New York, 2005.

38 Wimmer-Greinecker G, Deschka H, Aybek T, Mierdl S, Moritz A, Dogan S. Current status of robotically assisted coronary revascularization. *Am J Surg* October 2004; **188**(suppl 4A): 76S–82S.

39 Chitwood WR, Jr, Nifong LW, Elbeery JE *et al.* Robotic mitral valve repair: trapezoidal resection and prosthetic annuloplasty with the da Vinci surgical system. *J Thorac Cardiovasc Surg* December 2000; **120**(6): 1171–1172.

40 Torracca L, Ismeno G, Alfieri O. Totally endoscopic computer-enhanced atrial septal defect closure in six patients. *Ann Thorac Surg* October 2001; **72**(4): 1354–1357.

41 Loulmet DF, Patel NC, Patel NU *et al.* First robotic endoscopic epicardial isolation of the pulmonary veins with microwave energy in a patient in chronic atrial fibrillation. *Ann Thorac Surg* August 2004; **78**(2): e24–e25.

42 Jansens JL, Ducart A, Preumont N *et al.* Pulmonary vein isolation by robotic-enhanced thoracoscopy for symptomatic paroxysmal atrial fibrillation. *Heart Surg Forum* 2004; **7**(6): E595–E598.

43 Bolotin G, Kypson AP, Nifong LW, Chitwood WR, Jr. Robotically-assisted left atrial fibrillation ablation and mitral valve repair through a right mini-thoracotomy. *Ann Thorac Surg* October 2004; **78**(4): e63–e64.

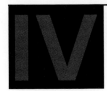

PART IV
The invasive cardiologist approach

Percutaneous treatment of atrial fibrillation

Carlo Pappone & Vincenzo Santinelli

Introduction

Atrial fibrillation (AF) is the most common arrhythmia because of the rising average age of the population that has a substantial effect on the mortality and health-care costs. In the United States, it currently affects about 2.4 million Americans, and by the year 2050, the number will be about 5.6 million. As a consequence, in industrialized countries, the number of affected individuals is projected to more than double in the next 50 years. Two principal clinical problems are associated with AF. One is that if ventricular response rate is not adequately controlled, patients may develop a tachycardia-mediated cardiomyopathy. The other problem is the risk of stroke and death. Indeed, AF is associated with an increased number of hospitalization, and sometimes frequent electrical cardioversions are required despite the use of antiarrhythmic drugs. These observations indicate how imperative it is to promote coordinated efforts on behalf of cardiologists, electrophysiologists, neurologists, and primary-care providers in order to meet the increasing challenge of stroke prevention and rhythm management in the growing AF population. The classification scheme has four categories for AF unrelated to an immediate, reversible cause: (1) first detected episode (uncertainty about duration); (2) paroxysmal (recurrent, but can terminate spontaneously in <7 days, and commonly <48 h); (3) persistent (recurrent, lasting >7 days, and typically requires cardioversion to terminate); and (4) permanent (fails to terminate after cardiover-

sion or relapses <24 h after termination or no cardioversion attempted) [1, 2]. The rate of progression from paroxysmal to permanent AF has been estimated to be 8% at 1 year [3], with nearly 20% entering permanent AF by 3–4 years [4, 5]. It appears clear that for patients with persistent AF, progression rates to permanent AF are higher, reaching 40% by the end of 1 year in a Finnish cohort [6]. Despite important advances in its treatment, AF remains an independent predictor of morbidity and mortality. It seems that the optimum pharmacological approach is a therapy tailored to the individual patient, and, even with optimum therapy, drug treatment is rarely curative while successful treatment is usually defined as a reduction in frequency, duration, and severity of AF episodes. Actually, selection of antiarrhythmic drugs to maintain the sinus rhythm is essentially based on safety rather than efficacy. To date, inability of drugs to control AF recurrences, or to relieve patients of limiting symptoms has provided an incentive for development of nonpharmacological therapies such as percutaneous catheter ablation that can now be considered the primary alternative to drug therapy offering the possibility of a lasting cure. The objectives in the treatment of AF are to reduce symptoms and to minimize the risk of stroke. Catheter ablation is an evolving field and an increasingly used approach, which is highly successful when performed by experienced operators. We have made a lot of progress and complications may occur only in a small minority of patients. Percutaneous catheter ablation has now evolved as an established approach for the treatment of paroxysmal, persistent, and permanent AF and can be performed on a daily basis in electrophysiology laboratories. The first decade of catheter

Manual of Surgical Treatment of Atrial Fibrillation.
Edited by Hauw T. Sie *et al.* © 2008 Blackwell Publishing,
ISBN: 978-1-4051-4032-4.

AF ablation has been characterized by new observations and concepts, and improvement in technology. At present, most techniques aim at ablation around the pulmonary veins with or without additional lesions, which is associated with low complication rates and high success rates [5–16]. In the late 1990s, a group in Bordeaux demonstrated that muscle sleeves surrounding pulmonary veins may be arrhythmogenic frequently supplying triggers that set off AF. This opened up a new therapeutic avenue which is based on the electrical disconnection of the PV from the atrial substrate. This approach is founded on the fact that PV ectopy is the main trigger for AF initiation. PV mapping is performed by the circular ring catheter, which is positioned inside the ostia of the veins. Subsequently, it became clear that only 60% of patients with paroxysmal AF were cured, and for permanent AF, PV isolation has a success rate of only about 20–25%. About 6 years ago, we reported that electrical isolation of the PV may not be required as demonstrated by higher success rates after circumferential PV ablation (CPVA) which is based on a >80% reduction in the bipolar voltage amplitude in and within the ablation lines.

AF ablation approaches

Currently, multiple approaches are used to increase the success rate for catheter ablation of AF. These involve, either singly or in combination, extending the PV encircling lesions posteriorly to include much of the PV antrum (antrum isolation), adding linear left atrial lesions, ablation within or around coronary sinus, and/or ablating sites in the right and left atria exhibiting fractionated atrial potentials during AF recorded by manual or even automated detection. Recent studies, however, have emphasized limitations of automated complex fractionated atrial electrograms detection for AF ablation because the software has inherent weakness in detecting noise and precisely recognizing beginning and ending of the complex affecting measurement of atrial cycle length. Finally, as demonstrated by our group for the first time, recent experimental studies in canine models suggest that activation of the intrinsic cardiac autonomic nervous system plays a role in the generation of AF. Despite several and different AF approaches, in the last few years

two have emerged as dominant approaches in current clinical practice: the segmental ostial ablation to electrically isolate the PVs from the left atrium and our approach, in which we encircle the PVs 1 or 2 cm away from their ostia, with additional ablation lines in the posterior left atrium and adjacent to the mitral isthmus. Although endpoints of the two strategies are different, there are other methodological differences. PV isolation requires identification of PV potentials, which may be difficult to separate from atrial electrograms, while CPVA is a purely anatomic approach. Also, segmental ostial ablation requires insertion of two catheters into the left atrium, while CPVA requires only a single catheter in the left atrium. The 3D mapping system, which is used during CPVA, has the advantage of limiting radiation exposure to patients and operators. Whether one of the two ablation strategies is superior, segmental ostial ablation was compared to the circumferential left atrial ablation strategy in a randomized study of 80 patients with paroxysmal AF [12]. The endpoint of the study was freedom from symptomatic AF after a *single* ablation procedure. In this study, CPVA was more effective than PV isolation, with success rate at 6 months being 87 and 67%, respectively. No differences between the two ablation strategies in the complication rates were reported. At 6 months, 67% of patients randomized to segmental ablation were in sinus rhythm without any repeat procedure, as 88% of those randomized to CPVA. In patients with AF recurrence after PV disconnection subsequently treated with CPVA, no AF recurrence was observed. The authors suggested that by encircling the PVs, ablation lines may eliminate: (1) the triggers, (2) the anchor points for rotors or mother waves that drive AF, (3) the vein of Marshall, which has a left atrial insertion in close proximity to the left superior PV; (4) may exclude up to 30% of the posterior left atrial wall limiting the area available for circulating wavelets that may be needed to perpetuate AF. These findings suggest that CPVA is preferable to PV isolation alone as the first approach. In the last few years, the two initial different strategies have reported similar success rates and are going toward a unified strategy, that is the circumferential approach as isolation alone is insufficient. A wider ablation design which includes additional lines appears to be indeed crucial to cure patients with both paroxysmal and permanent AF.

Indeed, the vast majority of centers performing AF ablation are empirically isolating all four PVs. It was quickly recognized that any of the PVs can serve as a trigger and that ablating only a single "culprit" could unmask triggers in another PV. Ablating all four PVs was also found to be more effective than ablating only three. Furthermore, some groups are ablating "outside" the tubular portion of the PV to avoid the risk of PV stenosis and to improve the efficacy of the procedure. Therefore, to encompass as much of the PV structure as possible, ablation needs to be performed at least 10–20 mm outside PV ostia, when possible. Although different groups may refer to ablation in this region by different names such as pulmonary vein antrum isolation, left atrial catheter ablation, circumferential PV antrum ablation, or extraostial isolation, the lesion sets produced by the procedures are all very similar.

AF ablation as first-line therapy

When AF ablation was first described, this approach was considered as a "last-line" treatment and reserved only for highly symptomatic patients with refractory AF. However, over the past 5 years, high success rates with few complication rates have been reported by many centers worldwide suggesting that this procedure could be appropriate to expand its indications. To date, we have performed CPVA in >8000 patients. We include patients with structural heart disease, and many of the patients had either idiopathic AF or hypertension. At 5 years, our success rate was about 90% for paroxysmal AF and about 80% for persistent/permanent AF. Our results demonstrate that CPVA is safe and effective in patients with paroxysmal, persistent, and permanent AF and/or with associated heart diseases. In our opinion, AF ablation can be now offered as first-line therapy in experienced centers particularly in patients with permanent AF to maintaining long-term sinus rhythm.

The importance of maintaining sinus rhythm

Recently, the importance of maintaining sinus rhythm in patients with AF has been questioned [17, 18]. Unfortunately, drugs or devise-based therapies for maintaining sinus rhythm have poor efficacy and significant drawbacks. We believe that failure of AFFIRM, RACE, or STAF studies in demonstrating

any difference between rate and rhythm control is not a positive finding for the rate control strategy but rather evidence of ineffectiveness of methods used for rhythm control. We compared the outcomes of 589 patients undergoing catheter ablation of AF with those of 582 patients treated with drug therapy in a nonrandomized trial [9]. The results of this study suggested that restoration of sinus rhythm by circumferential pulmonary vein ablation was associated with a subsequent survival rate equivalent to age-matched patients in the general population with AF. Conversely, patients treated with antiarrhythmic drugs had a lower survival rate than the same age-matched population. These results for the first time strongly emphasize the need to maintain the sinus rhythm without the use of antiarrhythmic drugs in patients with AF [9].

AF mechanisms

The mechanisms of AF are complex and not yet well defined. Improvements in catheter ablation techniques will essentially depend on better understanding of the mechanisms of this arrhythmia [19]. Permanent AF is a highly heterogeneous and complex disease, and there are different mechanisms in different patients. However, it has became increasingly evident that PV ectopy, as firstly demonstrated by Haissaguerre *et al.*, is only the tip of the iceberg. AF is a disease of the posterior wall of the LA which also includes autonomic innervation. We have recently localized vagal fibers and/or ganglia around PV ostia at the venoatrial junction by eliciting vagal reflexes [10]. Their ablation results in heart rate variability attenuation during follow-up and no AF recurrences in almost all patients in whom it is possible to elicit and ablate such vagal reflexes (overall, 30% of patients in our series). The usual sites of left atrial lesions needed to ablate AF coincide with regions of vagal innervation [10]. Therefore, CPVA is able to eliminate both triggers and the substrate, which include local vagal denervation.

Circumferential pulmonary vein ablation technique

Patient population

Over the last years more than 8000 patients with paroxysmal, persistent, and permanent AF, many

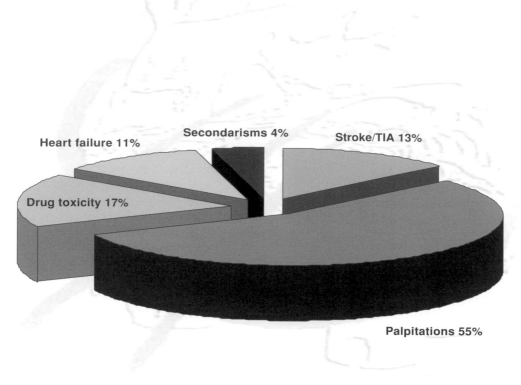

Heart failure 11%

Secondarisms 4%

Stroke/TIA 13%

Drug toxicity 17%

Palpitations 55%

Figure 18.1 Main indications to circumferential pulmonary vein ablation.

of whom with associated structural heart disease, were referred to our Department of Arrhythmology in Milan for CPVA (Figure 18.1). In our series the presence of heart failure, coronary artery disease, and mechanical prosthetic valves did not affect the outcome. The main indication for ablation was the presence of severe symptoms (Figure 18.2).

Mapping and ablation

Three catheters are usually used: a standard bi- or quadripolar catheter in the RV apex to provide backup pacing; a quadripolar catheter in the coronary sinus to allow pacing of the left atrium; and a deflectable ablation catheter is advanced through the transseptal sheath. A pigtail catheter is temporarily positioned above the aortic valve to act as a landmark at the time of transseptal puncture. A reference patch is also placed on the back of the patient. A 3D reconstruction of the LA is created with an electroanatomical mapping system. Tubular models of

the PVs and the outline of mitral valve annulus are also depicted as anatomical landmarks for the navigation system and we create the map by entering each PV in turn. Three locations are recorded along the mitral annulus to tag the valve orifice. To acquire PVs we use three criteria based on (1) fluoroscopy, (2) impedance, and (3) electrical activity. Entry into the vein is clearly identified as the catheter leaves the cardiac shadow on fluoroscopy, the impedance usually rises above 140–150 Ω, and the electrical activity disappears. To better differentiate between PVs and LA, we use voltage criteria (fractionation of local bipolar electrogram) and impedance (a rise of >4 Ω above mean left atrial impedance) to define PV ostium. Clearly, the anatomical appearance acts as added confirmation of catheter entry into the PV ostium, and an 8-mm tip-deflectable catheter or a 4-mm tip-irrigated catheter is used for mapping and ablation. The mapping and ablation procedures are performed by using the coronary

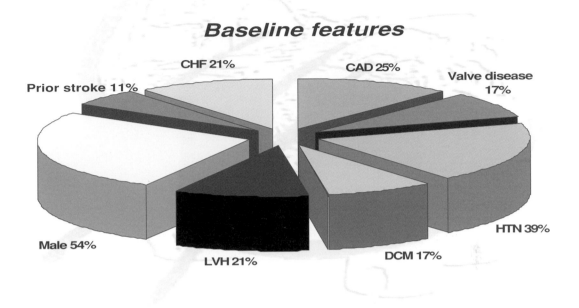

Figure 18.2 Cumulative Milan experience (*n* = 8682 points) from January 1998 to December 2005.

sinus (CS) atrial signal if the patient is in SR or the right ventricular signal if the patient is in AF, as the synchronization trigger for the CARTO system. Each endocardial location is recorded while a stable catheter position is maintained, as assessed by both end-diastolic stability (a distance, 2 mm between two successive locations) and LAT stability. Atrial volumes are calculated at the end of diastole independently of the underlying rhythm (AF or SR). The mapping catheter is introduced into the left atrium under fluoroscopic guidance, and its location is recorded relative to the location of the fixed reference. Usually, 100 points are required to create adequate maps of LA and PVs and up to 200 points for accurate mapping of left AT. The anatomic reconstruction of the LA obtained with the CARTO system or Endocardial Solutions system is reliable as compared with magnetic resonance imaging. By moving the catheter inside the heart, the mapping system continuously analyzes its location and

orientation and presents it to the user on the monitor of a graphic workstation, thereby allowing navigation without the use of fluoroscopy. The mapping procedure is performed by moving the catheter to numerous and sequential points within the LA and PVs and acquiring the location in 3D space together with the local unipolar and bipolar voltages and the local activation time (LAT) relative to the chosen reference interval. The acquired information is then color coded and displayed. As each new site is acquired, the reconstruction is updated in real time to progressively create a 3D chamber geometry color encoded with activation time. Additionally, the collected data can be displayed as voltage maps depicting the magnitude of the local peak voltage in a 3D model. The chamber geometry is reconstructed in real time by interpolation of the acquired points. Local activation times can be used to create activation maps, which are of importance when mapping and ablating focal or macro-reentrant atrial tachycardia

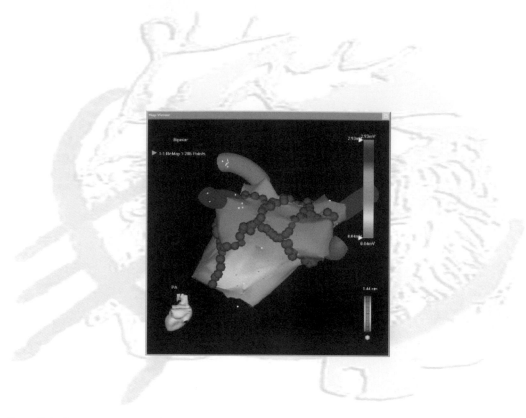

Figure 18.3 Electroanatomic map after circumferential pulmonary vein ablation.

(AT), but are not used during ablation of patients in AF.

Ablation procedure

Our initial ablation strategy was to encircle the four PVs by creating circumferential lesions around each PV (Figure 18.3). These lines consisted of contiguous focal lesions initially deployed at >5 mm from the PV ostia. However, from 2001 lesions are deployed 1–2 cm from the ostia, when possible, to include much more substrate. Additional ablation lines on the posterior wall connecting both the superior and inferior PVs and the mitral annulus to the left inferior PV (mitral isthmus line) are performed (Figure 18.3) in order to prevent postablation left atrial flutters [14, 15]. Radiofrequency (RF) current is usually applied with a target temperature of 55–65 °C and a maximum power of 100 W. However, RF energy is applied in the posterior wall with a maximum power of 50 W and a temperature target of

55 °C to minimize the risk of injury. RF energy is applied continuously on the circumferential planned ablation lines, as the catheter is gradually dragged along the line. Continuous catheter movement, often in a to and fro fashion over a point helps keep catheter tip temperature down due to passive cooling. The end point of ablation is voltage abatement of the local atrial electrogram by 90% or to less than 0.05 mV. In some patients, if necessary, additional ablation lines are created along the left atrial roof, septum/anterior wall, or along the posterior mitral annulus. On average, a total of 10–15 seconds of RF is required. Circumferential ablation lines are usually performed starting at the lateral mitral annulus and withdrawing posteriorly then anterior to the left-sided PVs, passing between the left superior PV (LSPV) and the LAA before completing the circumferential line on the posterior wall of the LA. The "ridge" between the LSPV and LAA can be identified by fragmented electrograms due to collision of

activity from the LAA and LSPV/LA. We observe termination of AF during the procedure in around a third of patients. If AF does not terminate during RF, then transthoracic cardioversion is performed at the end of the procedure. If there are immediate recurrences of AF after the cardioversion, then the completeness of the lines are reassessed. Ablation is performed in the cavotricuspid isthmus in patients with a history of typical atrial flutter, and in patients in cavotricuspid isthmus-dependent atrial flutter is induced by atrial pacing.

Pulmonary vein denervation

Potential vagal target sites are identified during the procedure in at least one third of patients [10]. Vagal reflexes are considered sinus bradycardia (<40 bpm), asystole, AV block, or hypotension that occurs within a few seconds of the onset of RF application. If a reflex is elicited, RF energy is delivered until such reflexes are abolished, or for up to 30 seconds. The end point for ablation at these sites is termination of the reflex, followed by sinus tachycardia or AF. Failure to reproduce the reflexes with repeat RF is considered confirmation of denervation. Complete local vagal denervation is defined by the abolition of all vagal reflexes. The most common sites are tagged on electroanatomical maps [10]. Vagal denervation is associated with reduced heart rate variability consistent with vagal withdrawal up to 6 months after the procedure.

Among patients in SR, postablation remap is performed utilizing the preablation map for the acquisition of new points to permit accurate comparison of pre- and post-RF bipolar voltage maps. Among patients in AF, after restoration of SR, postablation remap is done with the anatomic map acquired during AF to have the same landmarks and lesion tags for accurate lesion validation. Gaps are defined as breakthroughs in an ablated area, and identified by sites with single potentials and by early local activation. The completeness of the mitral isthmus line is usually demonstrated during coronary sinus pacing by endocardial and coronary sinus mapping looking for widely spaced double potentials across the line of block. In our experience, usually the double potential interval at the mitral isthmus during coronary sinus pacing after block is achieved is approximately 150 milliseconds, depending on the atrial dimensions and the extent of scarring

Table 18.1 Safety (*n* = 8682).

Death	0 (0%)
Pericardial effusion	6 (0.07%)
Stroke	1 (0.012%)
TIA	4 (0.05%)
Tamponade	5 (0.05%)
Atrial–esophageal fistula	1 (0.012%)
PV stenosis	0 (0%)
Incisional LA tachycardia	479 (6%)

and lesion creation [14]. If incomplete block is revealed by impulse propagation across the line, further RF applications are given to complete the line of block.

In patients who are in AF at the beginning of the procedure, RF ablation is performed without an initial attempt at cardioversion. If AF does not terminate during ablation, cardioversion is performed at the end of the procedure.

Safety and efficacy

Complications of circumferential left atrial ablation are reported in Table 18.1. Postablation left atrial flutters are relatively common but usually they do not require a redo procedure as most of them resolve spontaneously within 5 months after the index procedure. Atrioesophageal fistula is very rare but its occurrence is dramatic and devastating [11]. Lower RF energy application is recommended when ablating on the LA posterior wall and now we make the line on the posterior wall near to the roof of the LA, where the LA is not in direct contact with the esophagus. Success rates are 90% among patients with paroxysmal AF and 80% among those with persistent/permanent AF. In patients with paroxysmal AF in whom vagal reflexes are elicited and abolished by RF applications long-term success rate is about 100% [10]. A recent randomized study from our laboratory demonstrated that early recurrence of AF or iatrogenic left AT may occur within the first few months after the procedure particularly in patients without additional ablation lines but usually they do not require a repeat procedure as they resolve spontaneously during long-term follow-up [14]. Another recent randomized study from our laboratory demonstrated that CPVA is superior to amiodarone in maintaining long-term sinus rhythm in patients with chronic AF.

Anatomic, electrical, and functional remodeling following CPVA

Restoration of SR after ablation (usually at 5-mo follow-up) results in "reverse" electrical and mechanical atrial remodeling and improved atrial function transport. Enlarged atria may become smaller and this is associated with electrical and mechanical changes. In patients with mitral regurgitation, anatomic remodeling is much more pronounced and, interestingly, is associated with reduced mitral regurgitation and improved left ventricular function as compared with patients in whom SR is maintained by drugs alone. In our experience, anatomic, electrical, and functional remodeling after ablation is associated with good long-term outcome in patients with paroxysmal, persistent, and permanent AF.

Fully remote-controlled catheter ablation of atrial fibrillation

A potentially exciting technical advance in the procedure of catheter ablation for AF is remote magnetic navigation as the current strategy of manual catheter manipulation is highly operator dependent, with a long and variable learning curve and a great potential for both inefficacy and complications in inexperienced hands [20–21]. Fully remote-controlled catheter ablation of AF with a magnetically guided catheter system may increase the ability of inexperienced operators to perform this procedure easily and safely. This navigation system is integrated with a newly developed electroanatomical CARTO-RMT mapping system, which allows to obtain many mapping points much more easily than with manual catheter manipulation. A magnetic 4-mm tip catheter, the NaviStar-RMT catheter, has been developed to function with both magnetic navigation and CARTO system. The CARTO-RMT system sends real-time catheter tip location and orientation data to the magnetic navigation system. Magnetic field orientations of specific points can be stored on the navigation system, and reapplied if desired to previously visited locations on the map. We have now developed a protocol for remote CPVA procedure. The learning curve with this system is not too long and no complications have been observed. Based on our preliminary experience with fully remote-controlled ablation under magnetic guidance of different substrates such as PV, slow pathways, and/or accessory pathways, a new era in interventional electrophysiology is beginning as magnetic catheters can be navigated in the left atrium more precisely and safely than manually without risk of major complications even in less experienced centers.

Conclusions

The circumferential pulmonary vein approach as performed in Milan can be safely performed in the majority of patients with paroxysmal, persistent, and permanent AF, with high success rates, which are maintained long term. With practice and new technology development, the CPVA procedure can become shorter and safely performed even in less experienced centers, making it well tolerated and exposing the patient to less risk of complications.

References

1 Fuster V, Ryden LE, Asinger RW *et al.* ACC/AHA/ESC guidelines for the management of patients with atrial fibrillation: executive summary. *Circulation* 2001; **104**: 2118–2150.

2 Levy S, Camm AJ, Saksena S *et al.* International consensus on nomenclature and classification of atrial fibrillation: a collaborative project of the Working Group on Arrhythmias and the Working Group of Cardiac Pacing of the European Society of Cardiology and the North American Society of Pacing and Electrophysiology. *J Cardiovasc Electrophysiol* 2003; **14**: 443–445.

3 Levy S, Maarek M, Coumel P *et al.* Characterization of different subsets of atrial fibrillation in general practice in France: the ALFA study. *Circulation* 1999; **99**: 3028–3035.

4 Al-Khatib SM, Wilkinson WE, Sanders LL *et al.* Observations on the transition from intermittent to permanent atrial fibrillation. *Am Heart J* 2000; **140**: 142–145.

5 Humphries KH, Kerr CR, Connolly SJ *et al.* New-onset atrial fibrillation: sex differences in presentation, treatment, and outcome. *Circulation* 2001; **103**: 2365–2370.

6 Lehto M, Kala R. Persistent atrial fibrillation: a population based study of patients with their first cardioversion. *Int J Cardiol* 2003; **92**: 145–150.

7 Pappone C, Rosanio S, Oreto G *et al.* Circumferential radiofrequency ablation of PV ostia. *Circulation* 2000; **102**: 2619–2628.

8 Pappone C, Oreto G, Rosanio S *et al.* Atrial electroanatomic remodeling after circumferential radiofrequency PV ablation. Efficacy of an anatomic approach in a large cohort of patients with AF. *Circulation* 2001; **103**: 2539–2544.

9 Pappone C, Rosanio S, Augello G *et al.* Mortality, morbidity, and quality of life after circumferential PV ablation for AF: outcomes from a controlled nonrandomized long-term study. *J Am Coll Cardiol* 2003; **42**: 185–197.

10 Pappone C, Santinelli V, Manguso F *et al.* Pulmonary vein denervation enhances long-term benefit after circumferential ablation for paroxysmal AF. *Circulation* 2004; **109**: 327–334.

11 Pappone C, Oral H, Santinelli V *et al.* Atrio-esophageal fistula as a complication of percutaneous transcatheter ablation of AF. *Circulation* 2004; **109**: 2724–2726.

12 Oral H, Scharf C, Chugh A *et al.* Catheter ablation for paroxysmal AF: segmental PV ostial ablation vs. left atrial ablation. *Circulation* 2003; **108**: 2355–2360.

13 Oral H, Knight BP, Tada H *et al.* PV isolation for paroxysmal and persistent AF. *Circulation* 2002; **105**: 1077–1081.

14 Pappone C, Manguso F, Vicedomini G *et al.* Prevention of iatrogenic atrial tachycardia after ablation of atrial fibrillation: a prospective randomized study comparing circumferential pulmonary vein ablation with a modified approach. *Circulation* 2004; **110**: 3036–3042.

15 Pappone C, Santinelli V. The who, what, why, and how-to guide for circumferential pulmonary vein ablation. *J Cardiovasc Electrophysiol* 2004; **15**: 1226–1230.

16 Haissaguerre M, Jais P, Shah DC *et al.* Spontaneous initiation of atrial fibrillation by ectopic beats originating in the pulmonary veins. *N Engl J Med* 1998; **339**: 659–666.

17 Wyse DG, Waldo AL, DiMarco JP *et al.* AF Follow-up Investigation of Rhythm Management (AFFIRM) Investigators. A comparison of rate control and rhythm control in patients with AF. *N Engl J Med* 2002; **347**: 1825–1833.

18 Van Gelder IC, Hagens VE, Bosker HA *et al.* Rate Control versus Electrical Cardioversion for Persistent AF Study Group. A comparison of rate control and rhythm control in patients with recurrent persistent AF. *N Engl J Med* 2002; **347**: 1834–1840.

19 Pappone C, Santinelli V. Towards a unified strategy for atrial fibrillation ablation? *Eur Heart J* 2005; **26**: 1687–1688.

20 Pappone C, Santinelli V. Atrial fibrillation ablation: state of the art. *Am J Cardiol* 2005; **96**: 59L–64L.

21 Pappone C, Santinelli V. Atrial fibrillation ablation: a realistic alternative to pharmacologic therapy? *Nat CV Med* 2005; **2**: 608–609.

22 Pappone C, Vicedomini G, Manguso F *et al.* Robotic magnetic navigation for atrial fibrillation ablation. *J Am Coll Cardiol* 2006; **47**: 1390–1400.

CHAPTER 19

Surgical ablation of arrhythmias associated with congenital cardiopathies

Nestor Sandoval, Fernando Rosas, & Victor Manuel Velasco

Introduction

The definitive surgical treatment for cardiac arrhythmias began in the late 1960s when Seally performed the first surgery for Wolf–Parkinson–White (WPW) syndrome in 1968 [1]. This endocardial technique was modified and made popular later by Cox [2]. On the basis of the works of cryoinjury by Cooper [3], Guiraudon introduced a different technique for the treatment of WPW syndrome that consists in epicardial dissection and cryoablation [4], with the same results as those obtained when using endocardial approaches.

Experimental intracavitary studies [5] allowed identifying completely the ectopic foci and the accessory pathways, which made easier the application of techniques for the ablation of different arrhythmias as the intranodal reentry tachycardia [6], atrial tachycardia [7], and ventricular tachycardia [8]. These techniques obtained excellent results with a success rate of 95% [9], and with the introduction of percutaneous radiofrequency cardiac interventionism [10], surgical indication decreased until the introduction of the treatment of atrial fibrillation and atrial flutter by the Cox–Maze procedure at the beginning of 1990s [11, 12]. This technique did not become popular, for the complexity and technical difficulty involved, until the introduction and use of other methods of intraoperative ablation such as the radiofrequency, ultrasound, and flexi-

ble cryoablation, which simplified the concept of the Maze procedure. The results using alternative sources of energy can be compared but are not similar to those obtained with the classic Maze III of cutting and suturing in which a complete section exists of the atrial wall, assuring the transmurality [13–15].

The number of patients with previous corrected congenital cardiopathies that arrive to adolescence or to adult age is increasing, thanks to the improvement of surgical results. The frequent occurrence of tachyarrhythmias, their variety, the complexity of cardiac malformations involved, and the poor hemodynamic tolerability has forced us to a distinct understanding, classification, and treatment of those tachyarrhythmias that are not amenable to pharmacologic therapy or to catheter-mediated radiofrequency treatment and therefore require surgical treatment or combination of this with the implantation of a pacemaker or antitachycardia device [16, 17].

Although the main focus of this book is on the surgical treatment of atrial fibrillation, in this chapter we will also focus, for completeness, on surgical treatment of both atrial and ventricular tachycardias in the pediatric population.

The atrial arrhythmias are an important cause of morbidity and mortality in pediatric patients with congenital heart disease even following previous cardiac surgery. The tolerance to ventricular response is equally different in this group of patients. For this reason some important differences must be considered, and atrial arrhythmias must be

Manual of Surgical Treatment of Atrial Fibrillation.
Edited by Hauw T. Sie *et al.* © 2008 Blackwell Publishing, ISBN: 978-1-4051-4032-4.

Table 19.1 Distribution of SVT by age.

Study	Population	AV nodal	Anomalous pathway	Atrial primary
Josephson et al. [22]	Adult	51%	34%	15%
Gillette [23]	Pediatric	24%	33%	42%
Ko et al. [24]	Pediatric	13%	73%	14%
Naheed et al. [20]	Fetal	—	73%	27%

compared with the arrhythmias that appear in the adult. The tachycardias can be well tolerated during several hours by an infant but can produce syncope in a young adult; therefore, not only the frequency rate of the arrhythmias is determinant but also the physiological response according to age [18].

The fetus has poorer tolerance of supraventricular tachycardias (SVT) than the newborn and the infant, thus developing hydrops fetalis (severe cardiac insufficiency) in few hours of high-frequency heart rates, which would be well tolerated for much longer periods by the newborns [19, 20].

The two most common mechanisms of SVT in the fetus are the primary atrial tachycardia (atrial flutter) and the atrioventricular (AV) tachycardia by reentry through an anomalous pathway. These fetal cardiac arrhythmias can be primary in the absence of cardiac structural disease or secondary when associated with congenital or acquired cardiac disease. In the newborn, atrial flutter is common and appears without structural disease and later appears in older children or adolescents with cardiac anomalies [21]. The most frequent SVT in newborns, infants, and in general in the pediatric population is the AV reentry tachycardia secondary to an anomalous pathway (syndrome of WPW).

Table 19.1 shows the incidence of the different types of SVT in the fetal, pediatric, and adult population, according to several studies [20, 22–24].

The *ventricular arrhythmias*, such as ventricular tachycardia, are the second-most common type of tachyarrhythmia in children, although their incidence is much smaller than the SVT.

Patients with ventricular paroxysmal tachycardia constitute a heterogeneous group from the etiologic point of view. These tachyarrhythmias can be secondary to myocarditis of viral etiology or rheumatic myocarditis, heart tumors (hamartoma), and arrhythmogenic right ventricular dysplasia *or* secondary to ventriculotomy scars during surgical repair such as tetralogy of Fallot [25].

Idiopathic ventricular tachycardias are rare in children but can be incessant and can lead to a tachycardiomyopathy. These forms can be cured by radiofrequency catheter ablation in more than 90% of the cases. Some arrhythmias of potentially serious nature in children without cardiopathy, such as the long QT syndrome, bear little relation with congenital cardiopathies but can lead to a syncope and sudden death in 50% of the patients.

Sinus *bradycardia* is present in children with vagotomy or in young asymptomatic sportsmen. Union rhythm and the second-degree, Wenckebach-type AV block do not need medical treatment nor a pacemaker implantation.

Complete congenital AV block is common and in 50% of the cases associated with congenital malformations [26].

The subject of the arrhythmias in pediatric population is vast and interesting, but in this chapter we are going to especially emphasize on tachyarrhythmias associated with congenital cardiopathies and on those generated after surgical repairs.

There are several aspects to be considered such as the genesis, origin, treatment, and relation to the AV node. There are also different types of classification (Table 19.2) and two major types of cardiac arrhythmia based on the arrhythmogenic substrate. Group I includes the younger patients (congenital tachycardias), and group II, the adolescents and the older patients (acquired tachycardias) [16].

Supraventricular tachycardias

Supraventricular tachycardias (SVT) are tachycardias that originate above the bifurcation of the His bundle or in which this region participates in the circuit of the tachycardia. They are classified into two further groups (Table 19.3). In the *first group*, the tachycardia requires the AV node or the ventricular tissue for its initiation and/or maintenance and includes the following:

1 *AV tachycardia by secondary reentrant to an accessory pathway.* This is the most frequent supraventricular paroxysmal tachycardia in the pediatric population.

Table 19.2 Classification of tachyarrhythmia by mechanism, genesis, and origin.

Mechanism
Enhanced focal automaticity
   AET/JET
   VPBs/SVBPs
   Focal VT
Triggered activity
   VPCs/SVBCs
Reentry
   AP (WPW)/Mahaim/PJRT
   AVNRT/A flutt, IART,
   Reentry VT

Genesis
Congenital
   AP/Mahaim/PJRT
   AVNRT
   focal AT/focal VT
Acquired
   A flutt/IART/focal AT/A fib
   Focal VT/reentry VT/V fib

Origin
Focal
   AET/JET/SVPBs/A fib (focal triggered)
   AP (WPW)/Mahaim/PJRT
   VPBs/focal VT
Regional
   A flutt/IIART
   Reentry VT
Global
   Chronic A fib., V fib

AET, automatic ectopic tachycardia; JET, junctional ectopic tachycardia; VPCs, ventricular premature contractions; SVPCs, supraventricular premature contractions; VT, ventricular tachycardia; AP, accessory pathway; WPW, Wolff–Parkinson–White syndrome; PJRT, permanent junctional reentry tachycardia; AVNRT, AV-nodal-reentry-tachycardia; A flutt, atrial flutter; IIART, intra (incisional) atrial reentry tachycardia; A fib, atrial fibrillation; V fib, ventricular fibrillation.

Table 19.3 Classification of SVT by dependence of AV node.

A. Tachycardias dependent on the AV node
  1. AV reentrant tachycardia
    • Orthodromic reciprocant (WPW manifest or concealed)
    • Antidromic reciprocant (WPW manifest)
    • Orthodromic permanent reciprocant (Coumel)
    • Variants of preexcitation (Mahaim)
  2. Nodal reentry AV tachycardia
    • Variety common
    • Variety no common
  3. Union AV ectopic tachycardia
B. Tachycardias nondependent of the AV node (primary atrial tachycardias)
  1. Focal atrial tachycardia
  2. Inappropriate sinus tachycardia
  3. Macroreentry atrial tachycardia
  4. Atrial flutter (horary or antihorary)
    • Atopic atrial flutter
    • Incisional atrial tachycardia
  5. Atrial fibrillation

The second group includes the primary atrial tachycardias that are defined as the supraventricular arrhythmias that do not require AV node or ventricular tissue for their initiation and/or maintenance. The classification of the atrial tachycardias proposed by Lesh [27] is based on the probability of treatment with catheter and is divided into the following categories:

1 *Focal atrial tachycardias.* These tachycardias can be cured with applications of radiofrequency energy at the trigger site. According to their anatomical location they can be subclassified as:

  a Atrial tachycardia originated in the crista terminalis of the right atrium;

  b Atrial tachycardia originated in the pulmonary veins;

  c Septal atrial tachycardias; and

  d Other focal atrial tachycardias.

The mechanism leading to them is almost impossible to identify. More important than to know the underlying mechanism is to obtain an exact location of the trigger point with endocardiac mapping so that ablation is successful.

2 The *syndrome of inappropriate sinus tachycardia* is rare and its leading mechanism is not clear.

3 *Atrial tachycardias by macro-reentrant* are those that use a macro-anatomic circuit (fixed or

2 *AV tachycardia by nodal reentrant,* where the reentry circuit is confined to compact AV node and its extensions are confined in the atrium. This is the most common form of supraventricular paroxysmal tachycardia in the adult population.

3 The *ectopic tachycardia of the AV union,* which is a rare form of tachycardia triggered by an automatic mechanism.

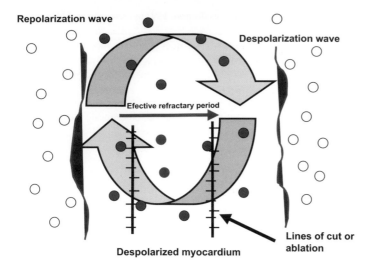

Repolarization wave

Despolarization wave

Efective refractory period

Despolarized myocardium

Lines of cut or ablation

Figure 19.1 Reentry circuit and ablation mechanism. The picture shows the reentry wavelet with the same size of the effective refractory period that may be ablated by any form, cut, or energy.

functional) and/or a surgical barrier. They can be subclassified as:

  a Typical atrial flutter;
  b Atypical atrial flutter; and
  c Incisional atrial tachycardia.

In this category, ablation with radiofrequency energy and surgery are successful when a barrier that interrupts the circuit of the macro atrial reentry is produced and has a high percentage of healing. The most common type of atrial tachycardia by macro reentrant is the typical atrial flutter characterized for the presence of negative F waves in DII, DIII, and AVF and positive in V_1.

The challenge is greater in patients with previous complex atrial procedures, such as Mustard and Senning for transposition of great vessels and Fontan surgery for hearts with functional single ventricle, because in those cases they present atrial arrhythmias by reentry, such as typical atrial flutter and incisional tachycardia, with macro variable circuits by the combination of multiple natural and surgical barriers, where the endocardiac mapping is more difficult and the possibilities of success by catheter ablation is low.

4 *Atrial fibrillation* has many anatomic and pathophysiologic substrates such as the presence of intracavitary shunt and enlargement of the auricles, ventricular hypertrophy secondary to obstruction of the ventricular outlet, valvular defects with incensed intracavitary pressure and thickness of the atrial wall or fibrosis, or scar in the atrium by previous surgery.

The pathophysiologic mechanism is maintained by multiple macro reentries in both atria; nevertheless, different theories exist to explain this and other arrhythmias, as discussed in other chapters of this book. In the case of atrial fibrillation, the mechanism of the arrhythmia involves two processes: (1) a focal trigger of automaticity and (2) multiple wavelets of macro reentries that migrate in the atria. Nevertheless, the definitive mechanism of fibrillation continues being controversial. The first theories of the circular disorganized movements or multiple reentries proposed by Moe [28], which were confirmed later by Allessie [29], continue being effective as the basic mechanism of atrial fibrillation.

Experimental studies in animals with fast atrial pacing stimulation could reproduce the arrhythmia and have demonstrated that the shortening of the refractory period is another cause of atrial fibrillation with rapid response, which auto limits and in some patients could play an important role in the recurrence of the arrhythmia after the electrical cardioversion [30].

The remodeling and enlargement of the atria, which in addition has important anatomic alterations such as loss of myofibrils, alterations of the sarcoplasmic reticulum, and alterations in the effective refractory period (minimum distance between the depolarization and repolarization wave), facilitate the formation of macro reentry wavelets especially in large atria. This concept generated the idea of being able to section these reentries in a surgical way to cure the disease [31] (Figure 19.1).

The theory of "mother rotor" has based its last studies with optical mapping and it challenges the theory of multiple reentry waves. This rotor has been defined as a stable rotational pattern of reaction and diffusion that begins in a fixed point, turns counterclockwise, and consists of an established source of high frequency that initiates and maintains the entire atrial fibrillation episode [32].

Haissaguerre and colleagues [33] demonstrated that up to 90% of the paroxysmal or intermittent episodes of atrial fibrillation originates around the pulmonary veins as a reentry which persists or autolimits itself by the tendency of the atria to remain in sinus rhythm. These findings justified its treatment by isolation of the pulmonary veins. Nevertheless, for other authors [34] the origin of the premature contractions is distributed almost 50% in both atria, suggesting that the presence of an automatic focus, located in a different place than the pulmonary veins, could be the origin of the atrial fibrillation.

When atrial fibrillation becomes *chronic* or *permanent,* the macro reentries, which are the basis of this type of fibrillation, appear, perpetuated by the mechanism that Allessie [35] has denominated the "atria remodeling," and with which the chronic fibrillation predisposes to more fibrillation and its healing will only be obtained with surgery in either atria or Maze III.

SVT involving the AV node

AV reentrant tachycardia by anomalous pathway

This tachycardia uses an anomalous pathway as one of the circuit arms of the reentry and is the form of SVT that is most frequently found in children. According to Gillette, almost 50% of the pediatric patients studied for SVT have anomalous pathways [18]. Most of them are male and in 20% of the cases they have associated structural cardiac disease, mainly Ebstein's anomaly in 10–20%. The WPW syndrome is diagnosed when the anomalous pathway is apparently in sinus rhythm, with delta wave at the beginning of QRS complex and short PR interval due to the ventricular preexcitation through the accessory pathway. Later, with the maturation of the conduction tissue and the development of the adrenergic innervation, the accessory pathways will stop being active with the consequent disappearance of the arrhythmia. The anomalous pathway can have capacity to travel in both ways or only in retrograde manner (concealed). Half of the children with SVT who use an accessory pathway do not have preexcitation during sinus rhythm and the anomalous pathway is concealed. The most frequent age for occurrence of SVT is the first 2 months of age, and by the first year of life, two thirds of these infants no longer have tachycardias. The second top age groups of recurrence or occurrences of SVT are the groups of 5–8 and 10–13 years [21].

AV reentrant tachycardia can be *orthodromic reciprocant* (the most common, 80–90% of the cases). In rare occasions tachycardia is antidromic reciprocant (less than 5% of the cases). The tachycardia has an AV relation of 1:1 and ends in the presence of AV block. The primary atrial tachycardias such as atrial flutter and fibrillation can also lead to the ventricles through an accessory pathway. If the conduction through the anomalous pathway is very fast, these patients can pass from atrial fibrillation to ventricular fibrillation with high risk of sudden death. Atrial fibrillation is rare during childhood; it appears in less than 1% of the infants with WPW. Nevertheless, the risk of atrial or ventricular fibrillation increases in the second decade of life, particularly in adolescents of masculine sex, with permanent preexcitation.

A variety of tachycardias by reentrance is the *orthodromic permanent reciprocant* of the AV union described by Coumel in 1967 [36]. In most of these cases the accessory pathway is in the right posteroseptal region of the heart, with a very slow conduction between the ventricle and the atrium characterized by a tachycardia of narrow QRS complexes, usually incessant which leads to cardiomyopathy if it is not recognized. There is a retrograde P wave with long RP′ interval, usually greater than 150 ms (the interval P′R is smaller than the RP″ interval) and the retrograde P waves are negative in DII, DIII, and AVF.

Age, weight, symptoms, and existence of tachycardiomyopathies or associated congenital cardiopathy of the patient play an important role in the indications for catheter radiofrequency ablation [37] (Table 19.4).

Most of the accessory pathways have a left lateral location (50% of the cases) and posteroseptal

Table 19.4 Catheter radiofrequency energy ablation in pediatric population indications by age groups

	Infant	1–4 yr (<15 kg)	5–13 yr (>15 kg)	>13 yr
Mild symptoms	−	−	±	+
Moderate symptoms	−	±	+	+
Severe symptoms	±	+	+	+
Tachycardiomyopathy	±	+	+	+
Congenital cardiopathy associated	±	+	+	+

+, Usually indicated; ±, indicated in some patients; −, usually not indicated.

pathways (30%). The rarest localizations are the anteroseptal and the right lateral. More accessory pathways can be found in 5–15% of the cases, particularly in patients with Ebstein's anomaly, and this is a reason for recurrence of arrhythmia after ablation [38, 39]. In the initial studies, the early success of catheter radiofrequency ablation of accessory pathways was from 89 to 100%, the recurrence from 3 to 9%, and the long-term success from 85 to 100% [40–42]. Surgery is indicated in symptomatic patients in whom the medical treatment and radiofrequency catheter ablation have not been successful. This can be due to cases of anomalous posterior bundle with epicardiac trajectory, which makes access difficult with radiofrequency [43].

In patients with Ebstein's anomaly that requires surgical repair, some authors recommend the ablation of the bundle before surgery; nevertheless, we as other authors perform surgical correction and resection of the anomalous pathway during the same operation [44, 45].

Nodal AV reentrant tachycardia

In childhood it has an incidence of 2.2%. Between 6 and 10 years of age, 31% of the cases with SVT are due to nodal reentrant. More than 50% of the SVT in adults correspond to this arrhythmia. A double physiologic nodal pathway is documented in 40% of the children and in 80% of the adults.

This tachycardia is a reentry rhythm in the AV node between two functional pathways anatomically different. One fast pathway is localized at the anterior-superior atrial septum of the compact AV node (His bundle), and a slow pathway

localized inferior and posterior to the AV node. The normal conduction during sinus rhythm is made through the fast pathway and the PR interval is normal. When an extrasystole blocks the fast pathway, the conduction is made through the slow pathway and goes back to the atrium in a retrograde way through the fast pathway (slow–fast circuit), and if this mechanism continues, it will initiate the tachycardia.

The most common variety of nodal reentrant is the slow–fast, which is characterized in the ECG for the presence of a pseudo-S in derivations DII, DIII, AVR and a pseudo-R in derivation V_1 due to simultaneous activation at the atrium and the ventricles. The inverse form of nodal reentrant (fast–slow), also known as *noncommon variety*, uses the fast pathway as antegrade and the slow pathway as retrograde, which originates an RP' interval longer than the P'R interval. In these cases the P wave is negative in derivations DII, DIII, AVF, and from V_2 to V_6.

The pharmacotherapeutic options for the AV nodal reentrant tachycardia are similar to those described for the acute and chronic management of the SVT by accessory pathways. In the recurrent or refractory cases to medical treatment, ablation is indicated with radiofrequency energy or surgical treatment. Ablation of the fast pathway conduction is a long-term success in 82–96% of the cases, with a recurrence of 5–14% of the patients and an incidence of AV block of 0–10%. Better results are obtained with ablation of the slow conduction pathway because a long-term success is obtained in 98–100% of the cases, with a recurrence of 0–2% and an incidence of AV block of 0–1.3%. With the use of an appropriate technique, the risk of inducing a complete AV block during ablation of the pathway of slow conduction can be reduced to less than 1% without exposing the success of the procedure. For this reason, ablation of this pathway is preferred in the treatment of nodal reentrant [38, 46, 47].

Union ectopic tachycardia

The union ectopic tachycardia is an infrequent form of supraventricular paroxistic or permanent tachycardia which appears in pediatric patients and is associated with a high morbidity and mortality. It can be of acquired origin in the postoperative period of correction of congenital cardiopathy, particularly in the closure of ventricular septal defect, associated with low magnesium levels. It can be of congenital origin and is observed almost always in patients less than 6 months of age associated with heart failure in 62% of the patients and associated with cardiac malformations in 35% of the patients. The mechanism involved is abnormal automatism [48, 49].

Ablation of the His bundle is indicated when tachycardia cannot be treated with pharmacologic therapy and ventricular function is compromised. Ablation of the ectopic focus without disturbing the AV synchrony would be ideal but it is difficult to obtain. It is almost always necessary to carry out ablation of the AV node and later implant a definitive pacemaker [50, 51].

SVT independent from AV node (primary atrial tachycardias)

Focal atrial tachycardias

Atrial tachycardias are rare in pediatric population and are caused by multiple mechanisms: (1) abnormal automatism of one or more ectopic atrial focuses, (2) triggered activity, or (3) reentry.

The triggering mechanism in many of the cases is difficult to confirm. The atrial reentry tachycardias can be induced by programmed stimulation protocols, are well tolerated, and easy to control with digital and beta blockers, whereas tachycardias by automatic or ectopic focus are almost always incessant, refractory to medicines, and can conduce to a tachycardiomyopathy. For their treatment they need ablation with radiofrequency energy.

Atrial reentry tachycardia is associated with structural cardiac disease, especially in the late postoperative stage of atrial surgeries such as Mustard or Senning in 20–50% [52] and Fontan surgery in 40–50% [53, 54].

Some patients can develop fibrillation or atrial flutter, which is not easily cured with catheter ablation, but sometimes this arrhythmia can be mistakenly diagnosed as atrial flutter although the atrial frequency is less than 250 bpm and the F waves of the flutter are not present [27, 55]. The effectiveness of the treatment with radiofrequency catheter ablation is from 30 to 80%, with a high recurrence up to 50% in short-term especially in patients associated with previous Fontan-type surgery or associated with a

complex congenital cardiopathy [56, 57]. For this reason the option of corrective surgery arose along with the ablation of the arrhythmia that is actually applied [58–62].

On the contrary, automatic or ectopic atrial tachycardia is present in patients with a structurally normal heart. Most of the focuses are located in the right atrium, and 20–30% of the cases have more than one focus. The automatic atrial tachycardia frequently induces tachycardiomyopathy and a subsequent heart failure. It relates with duration of tachycardia (almost always incessant) and with the cardiac frequency rate higher than 140 bpm. Cure with radiofrequency catheter ablation is obtained in more than 80% of the cases [25, 27], and the surgical treatment is another alternative with resection of the tissue responsible for the origin of the arrhythmia [63].

The multifocal atrial tachycardia is characterized electrocardiographically by the presence of three or more different morphologies of P wave. Multifocal atrial tachycardia is associated with a high mortality and disappears if the treatment of the underlying disease is effective. Catheter ablation is not indicated in multifocal atrial tachycardia [27].

Syndrome of unsuitable sinus tachycardia

Patients with unsuitable sinus tachycardia have a cardiac frequency rate at rest higher than 100 beats/min or a heart rate faster than 100 beats/min with minor efforts. It is probably due to an abnormal autonomic influence in the sinus node with excessive sympathetic tone and reduced vagal tone [27].

It is frequent in young women with average age of 30 and who are professionals in health areas. The initial handling is made with beta blockers or verapamil. In the refractory cases, the modification of the sinus node with radiofrequency catheter ablation can be made and is obtained in 75% of the cases; nevertheless, the recurrence is high (30–35%). In the cases of recurrence, a more aggressive ablation must be made that can include total ablation of the sinus node function and implant of definite pacemaker.

Flutter and atrial fibrillation

Unlike the adult population, flutter and atrial fibrillation are rare in pediatric population. Most of the cases of atrial flutter are found in fetal and neonatal periods. In older children, cases of atrial flutter and fibrillation are observed when advanced valvular disease exists, especially of rheumatic origin or myocardiopathies with atrial dilatation. In adult population with atrial septal defect, the incidence of flutter and atrial fibrillation is 14–22% [64–66] and it persists in a high percentage after surgical repair, unlike those who undergo simultaneous Maze procedure [67–69].

The newborns with atrial flutter can pass to sinus rhythm with fast transesophagic stimulation or electrocardioversion, and usually they do not require chronic antiarrhythmic pharmacotherapy. In older children with atrial flutter or fibrillation, the objective is to obtain and maintain the sinus rhythm. Previous to cardioversion, a transesophageal echocardiogram must be practiced to exclude intra-atrial thrombus and anticoagulant therapy, especially in high-risk cases of thromboembolism, as patients with Fontan or Mustard surgery must be maintained. In the postoperative period, atrial fibrillation or flutter can appear as an acute answer to the surgery. In these cases antiarrhythmic therapy must be maintained for 3–6 months. The development of atrial tachycardias in the postoperative period by macro reentry, such as typical atrial flutter, atypical, or incisional atrial tachycardia, can be due to residual defects that must be evaluated particularly after Fontan surgery.

In refractory cases, radiofrequency catheter ablation must be considered just like in the typical atrial flutter where healing is obtained in 80–90% of the cases. In atypical atrial flutter and in incisional atrial tachycardia by reentry, healing with ablation is obtained only in 30–50% of the cases; nevertheless, with electro-anatomic mapping [70] a better success can be obtained.

Ventricular tachycardia

Nonischemic ventricular tachycardia is a nonfrequent entity in pediatric population and is associated more frequently with alterations in the ventricular wall, such as arrhythmogenic dysplasia of the right ventricle, long Q-T syndrome, scars by previous surgeries, or the presence of cardiac tumors.

Nonischemic ventricular tachycardias

Arrhythmogenic right ventricle dysplasia

This is a rare and poorly defined entity. It is characterized by repeated episodes of ventricular tachycardia with a pattern of left branch blockage. The free wall of the right ventricle is replaced by very thin wall, with fat and fibrous tissue. This process can jeopardize the septum and the left ventricle. Ventricular tachycardia can be developed from childhood. The mechanism of arrhythmia is a reentry generated from a slow conduction localized in the infiltration sites of the right ventricle, usually polymorphic and multifocal, which makes the treatment difficult by radiofrequency, [71] and the surgical treatment consists in the isolation of the right ventricle, the section through the arrhythmogenic zone, or the partial ventriculectomy [72]. Final option is the use of implantable automatic cardioverter-defibrillator (IACD), and in extreme cases heart transplantation.

Idiopathic ventricular tachycardia

The site of origin of the arrhythmia can be located in the posterosuperior fascicle of the left ventricle or in the septum, and although the first option of treatment is medical with calcium antagonists, but a surgical possibility exists and is the subendocardiac resection of the place of origin or ablation with radiofrequency catheter [73].

Late postoperative in tetralogy of Fallot

Premature ventricular contractions or nonsustained ventricular arrhythmia on the Holter monitoring of patients after a surgical repair of tetralogy of Fallot are common (up to 60%). Nevertheless, its relation with sudden death is not clear. Ventricular ectopy with more than 30 uniform ventricular extra systoles in 1 hour seems to be associated with risk of sudden death, but recent studies have not shown such a relationship [74].

Sustained monomorphic ventricular tachycardia is not frequent and the mechanism of reentry is the most common cause [75]. The focus is generally located in the outflow tract in the area of the patch or infundibulectomy or in the borders of the closure of the septal defect. Approximately in 20% of the cases the reentry can be multiple, compromising the body of the right ventricle.

The incidence of sustained ventricular tachycardia is among 5 and 8% [74, 76] and the risk of sudden death between 0.5 and 6% over 30 years [77, 78]. The risk factors in the development of ventricular tachycardia are older age at the repair, residual right ventricular hypertension, use of patch in the outflow tract or aneurysm formation, important pulmonary insufficiency, and prolonged QRS greater than 180 milliseconds in ECG at rest in sinus rhythm [74, 79–81]. Approximately 15% of the patients who have been operated for tetralogy of Fallot require reoperation due to residual defects and these patients are in greater risk of developing sustained ventricular tachycardia [82–84]. In this case they must undergo an electrophysiologic study previous to surgery and the repair must include cryoablation in the possible places of origin of the arrhythmia and resection of the right ventricular scar [85]. Also, it is recommended to make this repair before the symptomatology becomes severe and the life of the patient is at risk [86].

Long Q-T syndrome
It has been associated with recurrent attacks of syncope and cardiac arrest. It is believed that it is the congenital result of a dysbalance in the sympathetic innervation that results in a dominance of the neural left side sympathetic activity and generates arrhythmias that are triggered by an increase in the sympathetic activity mediated by the left stellate ganglion. Another theory sustains its etiology in a neuritis triggered by a viral process. Other theory is that this syndrome is the result of a congenital alteration of some channels responsible for the action potential associated with phenotypes that are clinically manifested by prolongation of the QT interval associated with sudden death, episodes of polymorphic ventricular tachycardia, and ventricular fibrillation. The medical treatment is with beta blockers and if it fails, surgical treatment is recommended, consisting in the resection of the left stellate ganglion and high thoracic sympathectomy with adequate results. A last alternative is to place an IACD [87–89].

Ventricular tachycardia of chagasic origin
In our environment the Chagas disease is diagnosed more frequently, especially in rural areas due to poor socioeconomic and housing conditions. Its presentation consists in a cardiomyopathy event with ventricular arrhythmia that can be treated medically or controlled with an IACD or jointly with radiofrequency and surgery [90].

Other causes of ventricular arrhythmia
The surgical treatment has been used for other causes of ventricular arrhythmia like in the cases of sarcoidosis and in patients with heart tumors. Incessant ventricular tachycardia, particularly in infants, is frequently caused by myocardial hamartoma that appears as either microscopic or macroscopic. It is identified by mapping, and the surgical technique consists in tumor resection or cryoablation [91].

Surgical treatment
Supraventricular arrhythmias
Arrhythmia surgery could be a final alternative for a growing number of patients with congenital heart disease who have not been treated properly by the catheter radiofrequency method or require a corrective procedure associated with any arrhythmia substrate. Together with the surgical techniques, a variety of new sources of ablation are now available, such as cryoablation, radiofrequency, laser, and ultrasound.

The complexity of some entities as the heterotaxia that sometimes is associated with the absence of the coronary sinus, anomalous venous return, and tricuspid valve atresia requires the accomplishment of ablation lines different from the conventional right-sided Maze and must be replaced by others like isolation of the cavae ablation of the segment that runs from the inferior vena cava to the ring of the AV valve, connection of the area of the interatrial septum with the atrial appendix orifice, and crossing of the sulcus terminalis to confine and section the possible reentry circuits [92]. In patients with tricuspid valve atresia, some authors suggest an ablation line between the coronary sinus and the rudiment of the tricuspid valve; nevertheless, the proximity of this line to the AV node increases the risk of AV block [93]. Patients with automatic tachycardia are treated with resection of the compromised zone as in the case of origin in the right side. Successful cases have been reported with the removal of the right atrial appendage, and some cases associated with

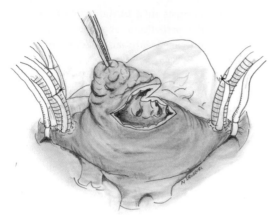

Figure 19.2 Removal of a dysplastic tissue on the right atrial appendage

auricular tumor [94] or isolation of the left atrium [7] (Figure 19.2).

Accessory-pathways-type WPW

This surgery has been one of the greatest successes through the years for the treatment of the accessory pathways and also it is the type of surgery that only a few surgeons actually know as an alternative when radiofrequency fails or some kind of anomaly coexists that must be treated simultaneously. As mentioned at the beginning of the chapter, endocardial and epicardial approaches are both effective. The endocardial approach requires the use of extracorporeal circulation, but it is a safe technique and carries high effectiveness [2, 9].

Intraoperative mapping in the operating room is necessary and we still routinely use epicardial intraoperative mapping in all patients. After placing bipolar electrodes in the right and left atrial appendages and on the right ventricular surface, a programmed stimulation is made to reproduce the arrhythmia and if that is not possible, then with ventricular or auricular stimulation and with another manual bipolar electrode, epicardial mapping is made at the level of the AV sulcus following predetermined map and confirming the shortest site of activation and the place where ablation must be made [95, 96].

In the last cases we have used the octopus starfish arm (Medtronic Inc.) to make easier the rise of the heart and the mapping in the posterior face

without deterioration of the hemodynamics of the patient.

If the accessory pathway is found at the right side, even when anteroseptal, lateral right, or posteroseptal, no aortic clamp is needed, and although we have used cryoablation at −60°C in two patients who have not received radiofrequency previously, we prefer to perform a surgical endocardial cut that assures a complete section of the muscular pathway. In some patients that had previous catheter radiofrequency ablation and require surgical intervention we have also found a zone of endocardial fibrosis with intact inner muscular tissue as if transmurality was not achieved during the catheter ablation.

When the pathway is confined to the left side, a short period of cardiac arrest is required. We approach the left atrium transseptally and through the roof of the left atrium to make the procedure easier, since usually these patients have a normal size left atrium.

Intranodal AV reentry tachycardia

This entity is currently healed by means of percutaneous catheter radiofrequency ablation [97]. Surgical ablation is an option when a concomitant anomaly exists, such as the atrial septal defect. In these cases with the use of extracorporeal circulation, the closing of the septal defect is made initially and later with cryoablator at −60°C and injuries of cryoablation are made around the AV node close to the ostium of the coronary sinus where the slow conduction tissue is located without producing prolongation of the PR interval. When a 2:1 AV block appears, the use of cryoablation must be suspended immediately to wait for the recovery of the conduction. Then the procedure is continued until the final electrophysiologic tests demonstrate the disappearance of the anomalous reentry (Figure 19.3).

Atrial flutter

This arrhythmia is highly susceptible to ablation during surgery of the concomitant congenital entity. Several techniques or variations of the same are actually used with different ablation methods. For the typical flutter, an ablation line can be made at the level of the isthmus between the inferior vena cava, the coronary sinus, and the tricuspid ring, but the addition of right-sided Maze is recommended

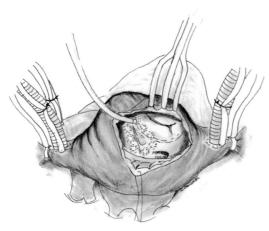

Figure 19.3 Cryoprobe around the AV node–His bundle along the perimeter of the Kock's triangle. The specific position of the probe shown in the figure should be monitored particularly closely for the development of right bundle branch block.

in the cases of coexistence of other reentries [98] (Figure 19.4).

In the cases of atrial flutter and atrial fibrillation, the accomplishment of Maze III, especially if the left atrium is enlarged, is recommended. Atrial reentry tachycardia localized in the edge of the septal defect can be treated with the resection or

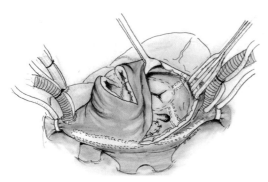

Figure 19.4 Right-sided Maze procedure in patient with a concomitant atrial septal defect. The atrial septal defect is already closed with a patch. Two incisions are made: the superior going through the atrial appendage to the superior tricuspid annulus; the second inferior incision goes from the inferior tricuspid annulus ring to the crista terminalis. Cryoablation lines are made (−60°C for 90 s) connecting the superior and inferior vena cava. A third line of cryoablation is made at the isthmus between inferior vena cava, coronary sinus, and tricuspid annulus.

cryoablation of the place of origin of the arrhythmia. In patients who need a Fontan conversion, only a modified right-sided Maze can be added with ablation lines at the edge of the septal defect or previously placed patch and the right lateral wall and the previous atriopulmonary anastomosis, and ablation line of the cavo-tricuspid isthmus [98–100].

Atrial fibrillation

Maze procedure is being used in patients with atrial fibrillation with or without structural cardiac disease and is highly effective in patients who need a concomitant mitral valve repair or atrial septal defect closure [101–106].

Fontan conversion is indicated in cases of compression of pulmonary veins, deterioration of functional class, increased cyanosis, protein-losing enteropathy syndrome, and untreatable atrial arrhythmia. Before the introduction of the Fontan conversion, a right atrial wall reduction was employed in order to reduce the venous pressure on the atrial wall resulting in arrhythmia ablation. Unfortunately the arrhythmia recurrence was high, leading in antiarrhythmic medical therapy and cardiac transplantation in most severe cases. With the experience gained with the Maze procedure, cryoablation lesions were added to interrupt the areas of slow conduction during the arrhythmia cycle, in particular based on intraoperative epicardial mapping. In general, there are three mayor anatomic sites that are critical to tachycardia circuits: the area between the coronary sinus ostium and the inferior vena cava ostium; the area between the AV valve annulus and the inferior vena cava ostium; and the lateral atriotomy and its relationship to the length of the crista terminalis and the region of the superior limbus, corresponding to the rim of the previous atrial defect patch (Figures 19.5a,b). In the cases of tricuspid atresia, a linear lesion is also made from the border of the cut of the transected inferior vena cava toward the coronary sinus (Figures 19.5b,c). When atrial fibrillation is the major concomitant arrhythmia, normally the left atrium is enlarged and surgery must include a modified right-sided Maze and left-sided Maze (Cox Maze III) (Figure 19.6). This is the best surgical alternative for these patients and can be performed with radiofrequency and cryoablation (Figure 19.7) [107–09]. The right-sided Maze can create a new arrhythmia substrate resulting in

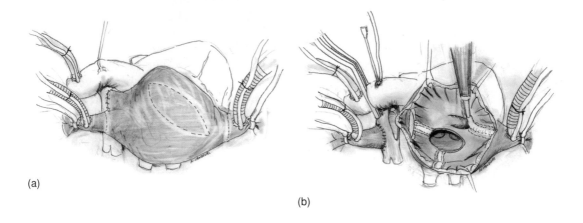

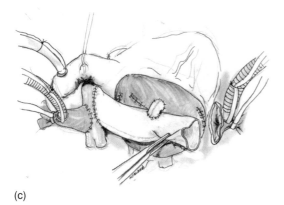

Figure 19.5 (a) Classical Fontan procedure in a patient with tricuspid atresia (right atrium to pulmonary artery anastomosis). The dashed line shows where the superior and inferior vena cava are going to be transected. The elliptic dashed lines in the middle show the area to be resected. (b) In the same patient, after aortic cross clamping and antegrade cardioplegic arrest, division of superior vena cava and take down of the atrio pulmonary anastomosis are made. Right atrium is opened and atrial septal patch is removed. A bidirectional Glenn shunt is performed. Modified right-sided Maze is performed using three lines of cryoablation (−60°C for 90 s): (1) superior from the atrial septal defect (ASD) to the superior border of the atrium in the previous anastomosis defect; (2) from the ASD border to the crista terminalis and the incision edge; (3) the isthmus ablation line from coronary sinus to the inferior vena cava. In cases with existing tricuspid valve, a fourth line is made from the inferior border of the atrium to the tricuspid annulus. (c) The final step of the extracardiac Fontan procedure is performed. A Gore-Tex graft tube is anastomosed from the pulmonary artery to the inferior vena cava and a fenestration is performed with a 6-mm Gore-Tex tube from the graft and the right atrium.

postoperative tachycardia and, consequently, the rationale of a concomitant pacemaker implantation is to have an alternative in the event of arrhythmia surgery failure. This is important since after the operation there is limited venous access to the heart either for percutaneous pacemaker electrodes implantation or for access to the radiofrequency ablation catheter. If an antitachycardia pacemaker is implanted, this can detect and terminate the early atrial arrhythmia that normally occurs during the first 3 months of the postoperative period. Sinus dysfunction is common after the operation and the pacemaker guarantees an adequate heart rate and AV synchrony resulting in improved cardiac output.

In patients with atrial septal defect and concomitant atrial fibrillation, the same standard technique is indicated. The left incisions are performed with aortic clamp, and after closure of the atrial septal defect, with the heart beating, the incisions of the

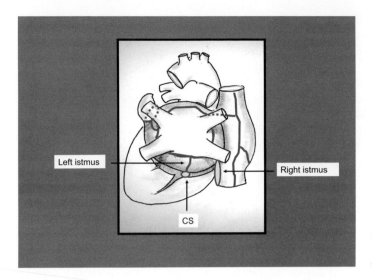

Figure 19.6 Maze III. The cartoon shows a posterior view of the heart and the black lines represent the left and right side incision, including ablation of the right and left isthmus. CS, coronary sinus.

right side are performed. Some authors suggest that the right-sided Maze is not effective in patients with atrial fibrillation associated with atrial septal defect; nevertheless, recent publications have shown effectiveness when right-sided Maze is performed with a right isthmus lesion even in the case of left atrium enlargement [104, 110].

Atrial reentry tachycardia

This arrhythmia is frequent after Fontan operation and, as mentioned at the beginning, it can be

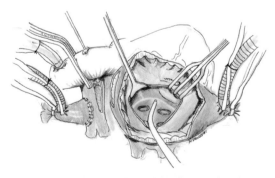

Figure 19.7 In patients with atrial fibrillation, after the right-sided Maze is complete, left atrium is exposed through the atrial septal defect. Using a monopolar irrigated radiofrequency device, pulmonary vein isolation is performed completing the Maze III procedure. This modification saves ischemic time in these patients.

confused with atrial fibrillation. Many surgical techniques have been proposed, such as the blockade of the cavo-tricuspid isthmus and modified right-sided Maze. Comparative studies have shown better results when modified right-sided Maze is used [100]. Catheter radiofrequency ablation has been used intraoperatively, with good results in the treatment of this supraventricular arrhythmia concomitant to congenital cardiac surgery [111].

Ventricular tachycardia

Intraoperative epicardial mapping is necessary to determine more exactly the site of origin of the arrhythmia and to appropriately perform subendocardial resection. In patients with tetralogy of Fallot, as mentioned before, the technique used consists in the resection of the incisional scar, ablation of the transitional zone with cryoprobe, and implant of a valved conduit between the right ventricle and pulmonary artery to prevent the progressive right ventricular dilatation or aneurysmal formation of the transannular patch, resulting from chronic pulmonary insufficiency. Homograft can be used in small children or biological prosthesis in adolescents [81].

Surgical results

Our experience with surgical treatment of arrhythmias associated with congenital cardiopathies at Clinica Shaio and Fundación Cardio Infantil in

Bogota, from 1993 to 2005 Colombia includes a total of 26 patients treated using mainly cryoablation and in some cases intraoperative irrigated monopolar radiofrequency.

Fourteen patients (age 44.8 ± 20.1 yr) with atrial fibrillation and atrial septal defect underwent either Maze III or modified right-sided Maze with cryoablation of the cavo-tricuspid isthmus. Duration of the atrial fibrillation was of 6.9 ±−5.4 years. All patients were followed up for an average of 116 ± 17 months. There was no early or late mortality and all patients are in sinus rhythm at follow-up, although two patients with right-sided Maze required medication to control the arrhythmia.

Seven patients (age 18.6 ± 5 yr) with Ebstein's anomaly associated with WPW syndrome received tricuspid valvuloplasty and endomyocardial resections (five using cut and sew, and two using cryoablation at −60°C). One patient had an episode of recurrent arrhythmia due to second accessory pathway located in a different place, and another patient required reoperation for residual tricuspid regurgitation.

One 11-year-old patient with permanent incessant tachycardia required a perinodal cryoablation, and one patient with right endomyocardial fibrosis and atrial flutter required one and a half ventricular repair and right-sided Maze with ablation of the cavo-tricuspid isthmus.

Three patients with previous Fontan surgery, one classic atriopulmonary anastomosis and two right atrial to right ventricle outflow tract anastomosis (Bjork-type modification) associated with atrial flutter, required extra cardiac Fontan conversion and modified right-sided Maze with isthmus cryoablation lesions. Two were in functional class III and one in functional class IV. Age was 19.6 ± 3.2 years. They had an adequate postoperative course without mortality.

At 20-month (3–14 mo) follow-up, one patient had automatic tachycardia that required pharmacologic treatment and presented sinus node dysfunction requiring pacemaker implantation. The functional class of every patient in this series was improved, especially in those with Fontan conversion [112].

In recent and larger series [113, 114], 133 patients in the pediatric population had arrhythmia surgery, 50% (67/133) associated with Fontan conversion, 22% (38/133) as accomplishment of initial Fontan, and 28% (38/133) for various arrhythmias in 95% of the cases associated with structural heart disease. Mean age was of 20 ± 7.6 years and mortality included three patients in the immediate postoperative and three in the late postoperative period. All of them had congenital complex cardiopathy with high risk of mortality [115]. Recurrence of the arrhythmia appeared in patients undergoing combined right-sided Maze and Maze III with Fontan conversion, but especially in those patients where only the blockade of the cavo-tricuspid isthmus was used initially. The arrhythmia recurrence rate was 13% and of these only 9% required antiarrhythmic medication.

The mortality in the Fontan conversion group was 1.5%, and 6% required heart transplantation as the last alternative.

Other authors have reported improvement in the functional class and suggested medical treatment to manage persistent arrhythmias [116, 117].

Conclusions

The actual catheter radiofrequency ablation techniques are highly effective for the treatment of most of the cardiac supraventricular arrhythmias associated with congenital cardiopathies [118]. In patients with complex cardiopathies and previous cardiac surgery, the anatomic and hemodynamic alterations make percutaneous catheter radiofrequency ablation difficult and cumbersome.

Fontan conversion to total cavo-pulmonary connections in association with arrhythmia surgery is safe and highly effective, improving the functional class and increasing the tolerance to exercise.

In general, patients with severe ventricular dysfunction, cyanosis, and protein-losing enteropathy are not excluded and may actually benefit from this approach.

The best option for these patients is a right-sided Maze procedure with ablation of the right isthmus in the cases of atrial reentry tachycardia, flutter type. Adding a Maze III when atrial fibrillation is the main arrhythmia is recommended, although this procedure requires prolonged ischemic time and additional intraoperative dissection. Atrial and atrioventricular dysfunction is frequent in the postoperative period, affecting directly the improvement of the functional class. Bicameral pacemaker and IACD implantation may be suggested, since during the first three postoperative months there are a variety of atrial arrhythmias and complications, such as protein-losing enteropathy, that could improve with this management [119]. Surgical fenestration and oral medications can also relieve these complications [120–122].

In spite of these measures, some cases progress toward the deterioration of the function and require an evaluation for heart transplantation or conversion in one and a half ventricular repair [123–125].

In general, it is recommended to follow these patients very closely and perform early surgery since the risks are low and the results in terms of postoperative functional class, quality of life, and exercise tolerance are better.

References

1 Cobb FR, Blumenschein SD, Sealy WC, Boineau JP, Wagner GS, Wallace AG. Successful surgical interruption of the bundle of Kent in a patient with Wolff–Parkinson–White syndrome. *Circulation* 1968; **38**:1018–1029.

2 Cox JL, Gallagher JJ, Cain ME. Experience with 118 consecutive patients undergoing operation for the Wolff–Parkinson–White syndrome. *J Thorac Cardiovasc Surg* 1985; **90**:490–501.

3 Cooper, IS. Cryobiology as viewed by the surgeon. *Cryobiology* 1964; **1**: 44–54.

4 Guiraudon GM, Klein GJ, Galamhusein S *et al*. Surgical repair of Wolf—Parkinson–White syndrome: a new closed heart technique. *Ann Thorac Surg* 1984; **37**: 67–71.

5 Sodi Pallares D, Medrano GA, Bisteni A, DeMichelli A. Electrograms of the conductive tissue in the normal dog's heart. *Am J Cardiol* 1959; **4**: 459.

6 Holman Wl, Ikeshita M, Lease JG, Smith PK, Ferguson TB, Jr, Cox JL. Alteration of antegrade atrioventricular conduction by cryoablation of peri-atrioventricular nodal tissue. *J Thorac Cardiovasc Surg* 1984; **88**: 67–75.

7 Williams JM, Ungerleider RM, Lofland GK, Cox JL. Left atrial isolation: new technique for the treatment of supraventricular arrhythmias. *J Thorac Cardiovasc Surg* 1980; **80**: 373–380.

8 Guiraudon G, Fontaine G, Frank R *et al*. Encircling endocardial ventriculotomy: a new surgical treatment for life-threatening ventricular tachycardias resistant to medical treatment following myocardial infarction. *Ann Thorac Surg* 1978; **26**: 438–444.

9 Cox JL, Ferguson TB, Jr. Surgery for the Wolff–Parkinson–White syndrome: the endocardial approach. *Semin Thorac Cardiovasc Surg* 1989; **1**: 34–46.

10 Lesh MD, Van Hare GF, Epstein LM *et al*. Radiofrequency catheter ablation of atrial arrhythmias: results and mechanisms. *Circulation* 1994; **89**: 1074–1089.

11 Cox JL, Schuessler RB, Dagostino HJ *et al*. The surgical treatment of atrial fibrillation. III: Development of a definitive surgical procedure. *J Thorac Cardiovasc Surg* 1991; **101**: 569–583.

12 Cox JL. The surgical treatment of atrial fibrillation. IV: Surgical technique. *J Thorac Cardiovasc Surg* 1991; **101**: 584–592.

13 Sie H, Beukema W, Ramdat AR *et al*. Radiofrequency modified maze in patients with atrial fibrillation undergoing concomitant cardiac surgery. *J Thorac Cardiovasc Surg* 2001; **122**: 249–256.

14 Williams MR, Garrido M, Oz MC, Argenziano M. Alternative energy sources for surgical atrial ablation. *J Card Surg* May–June 2004; **19**(3): 201–206.

15 Sandoval N. Estado actual del tratamiento quirúrgico de la fibrilación auricular. *Rev Col Cardiol* 2005; **12**(1): 1–9.

16 Hebe J. Role of catheter and surgical ablation in congenital heart disease *Cardiol Clin* 2002; **20**: 469–486.

17 Schultz AH, Wernovsky G. Late outcomes in patients with surgically treated congenital heart disease. *Semin Thorac Cardiovasc Surg Pediatr Card Surg Annu* 2005; **8**: 145–156.

18 Gillette PC, Zeigler VL, Case CL. Pediatric arrhythmias: are they different? In: Zipes DP, Jalife J, eds, *Cardiac Electrophysiology: From Cell to Bedside*. WB Saunders, Philadelphia, 1995: 1265–1268.

19 Case CL, Fyfe DA. Fetal dysrrhythmias. In: Gillete PC, Garson A, Jr, eds, *Pediatric Arrhythmias: Electrophysiology and Pacing*. WB Saunders, Philadelphia, 1990: 637–647.

20 Naheed ZJ, Strasburger JF, Deal BJ *et al*. Fetal tachycardia: mechanisms and predictors of hydrops fetalis. *J Am Coll Cardiol* 1996; **27**: 1736–1740.

21 Deal BJ. Supraventricular tachycardia: mechanisms and natural history. In: Deal BJ, Wolff GS, Gelband H, eds, *Current Concepts in Diagnosis and Management of Arrhythmias in Infants and Children*. Futura, New York, 1998: 117–143.

22 Josephson ME, Wellens HJJ. Differential diagnosis of supraventricular tachycardia. *Cardiol Clin* 1990; **8**: 411–442.

23 Gillette PC. The mechanisms of supraventricular tachycardia in children. *Circulation* 1976; **54**: 133–139.

24 Ko JK, Deal BJ, Strasburger JF *et al*. Supraventricular tachycardia mechanisms and their age distribution in pediatric patients. *Am J Cardiol* 1992; **69**: 1028–1032.

25 Iturralde P. Arritmias en Pediatría. In: Iturralde P, ed., *Arritmias Cardíacas*. McGraw-Hill Interamericana, México DF, 1997: 437–459.

26 Schmidt KG, Ulmer HE, Silverman NH, Kleinman CS, Copel JA. Perinatal outcome of fetal complete atrioventricular block: a multicenter. *J Am Coll Cardiol* May 1991; **17**(6): 1360–1366.

27 Lesh MD, Roithinger FX. Atrial tachycardia. In: Camm AJ, ed., *Clinical Approaches to Tachyarrhythmias*, Volume 11. Futura, New York, 2000: 1–97.

28 Moe GKRW, Abildskov JA. A computer model of atrial fibrillation. *Am Heart J* 1964; **67**: 200–220.

29 Allessie M, Lammers WJEP, Bonke FIM *et al.* Experimental evaluation of Moe's multiple wavelet hypothesis of atrial fibrillation. In: Zipes DP, Jalife J, eds, *Cardiac Electrophysiology and Arrhythmias*. Grune and Straton, Orlando, FL, 1985: 265–275.

30 Morillo CA, Klein GJ, Jones DL *et al.* Chronic rapid atrial pacing. Structural, functional, and electrophysiological characteristics of a new model of sustained atrial fibrillation. *Circulation* 1995; **91**: 1588–1595.

31 Mary-Rabine L, Albert A, Pham TD *et al.* The relationship of human atrial cellular electrophysiology to clinical function and ultrastructure. *Circ Res* 1983; **52**: 188–199.

32 Mandapati R, Skanes A, Chen J, Berenfeld O, Jalife J. Stable micro re-entrant sources as a mechanism of atrial fibrillation in the isolated sheep heart. *Circulation* 2000; **101**: 194–199.

33 Haissaguerre M, Jais P, Shah DC *et al.* Spontaneous initiation of atrial fibrillation by ectopic beats originating in the pulmonary veins. *N Engl J Med* 1998; **339**: 659–666.

34 Schmitt C Ndrepepa G, Weber S *et al.* Biatrial multisite mapping of atrial premature complexes triggering onset of atrial fibrillation. *Am J Cardiol* 2002; **89**(12):1381–1387.

35 Allessie MA. Atrial electrophysiology remodeling: another vicious circle? *J Cardiovasc Electrophysiol* 1998; **9**: 1378–1393.

36 Coumel J, Carbol C, Fabiato A *et al.* Tachycardie permanent par rhythm reciproque. Preuves du diagnosis par stimulation auriculaire et ventric. *Arch Mal Coeur* 1967; **60**: 1830.

37 Walsh EP. Ablation therapy. In: Deal BJ, Wolff GS, Gelband H, eds., *Current Concepts in Diagnosis and Management of Arrhythmias in Infants and Children*. Futura, New York, 1998; 329–367.

38 Bockeria L, Golukhova E, Dadasheva M *et al.* Advantages and disadvantages of one-stage and two-stage surgery for arrhythmias and Ebstein's anomaly. *Eur J Cardiothorac Surg* October 2005; **28**(4): 536–540.

39 Reich JD, Auld D, Hulse E, Sullivan K, Campbell R. The Pediatric Radiofrequency Ablation Registry's experience with Ebstein's anomaly. *J Cardiovasc Electrophysiol* 1998; **9**: 1370–1377.

40 Rosas F, Velasco VM, Rodríguez DA, Jumbo LA. Ablación con catéter. Aspectos generales e indicaciones. In:

Velasco VM, Rosas F, eds., *Arrítmias Cardíacas—Temas Selectos*. Sociedad Colombiana de Cardiología, Bogota, Colombia, 2001; 179–191.

41 Lesh MD, Van Hare GF, Schamp DJ *et al.* Curative percutaneous catheter ablation using radiofrequency energy for accessory pathways in all locations: results in 100 consecutive patients. *J Am Coll Cardiol* 1992; **19**: 1303–1309.

42 McDaniel GM, Van Hare GF. Catheter ablation in children and adolescents. *Heart Rhythm* January 2006; **3**(1): 95–101.

43 Langberg JJ, Man KC, Vorperian VR *et al.* Recognition and catheter ablation of subepicardial accessory pathways. *J Am Coll Cardiol* 1993; **22**: 1100–1104.

44 Dubin AM, Van Hare GF. Radiofrequency catheter ablation: indications and complications. *Pediatr Cardiol* 2000; **21**: 551–556.

45 Khositseth A, Danielson GK, Dearani JA, Munger TM, Porter CJ. Supraventricular tachyarrhythmias in Ebstein anomaly: management and outcome. *J Thorac Cardiovasc Surg* December 2004; **128**(6): 826–833.

46 Kay GN, Epstein AE, Dailey SM *et al.* Selective radiofrequency ablation of the slow pathways for the treatment of atrioventricular nodal reentrant tachycardia: evidence for involvement of perinodal myocardium within the reentrant circuit. *Circulation* 1992; **85**: 1675–1688.

47 Jackman WM, Beckman KJ, McClelland JH *et al.* Treatment of supraventricular tachycardia due to atrioventricular nodal reentry by radiofrequency catheter ablation of slow-pathway conduction. *N Engl J Med* 1992; **327**: 313–318.

48 Damiano RL, Tripp HF, Small KF *et al.* The functional consequences of prolonged supraventricular tachycardia. *J Am Coll Cardiol* 1985; **5**: 541.

49 Garson A, Gillette P. Junctional ectopic tachycardia in children: electrocardiography, electrophysiology and pharmacologic response. *Am J Cardiol* 1979; **44**: 298–302.

50 González FJ, Iturralde P, Calderón J *et al.* Taquicardia congénita de la unión A-V. Respuesta favorable a los antiarrítmicos. *Arch Inst Cardiol Mex* 1999; **69**: 55–62.

51 Rosas F, Eslami M, Elias J *et al.* His bundle ablation in incessant automatic junctional tachycardia [abstracts]. *Eur J Card Pacing Electrophysiol* 1994; **4**: 852.

52 Gatzoulis MA, Walters J, McLaughlin PR, Merchant N, Webb GD, Liu P. Late arrhythmias in adults with the Mustard procedure for transposition of great arteries: a surrogate marker for right ventricular dysfunction? *Heart* 2000; **84**: 409–415.

53 Ghai A, Harris L, Harrison DA, Webb GD, Siu SC. Outcomes of late atrial tachyarrhythmias in adults after the Fontan operation. *J Am Coll Cardiol* 2001; **37**: 585–592.

54 Peters NS, Somerville J. Arrhythmias after the Fontan procedure. *Br Heart J* 1992; **68**: 199–204.

55 Jumbo LA, Velasco VM, Rosas F, Rodríguez DA. Taquicardias supraventriculares incesantes y taquicardiomiopatía. In: Velasco VM, Rosas F, eds, *Arritmias Cardíacas—Temas Selectos*. Sociedad Colombiana de Cardiología, Bogota, Colombia, 2001: 101–114.

56 Triedman JK, Bergau DM, Saul JP, Epstein MR, Walsh EP. Efficacy of radiofrequency ablation for control of intraatrial reentrant tachycardia in patients with congenital heart disease. *J Am Coll Cardiol* 1997; **30**: 1032–1038.

57 Kanter RJ, Garson A, Jr. Atrial arrhythmias during chronic follow-up of surgery for complex congenital heart disease. *Pacing Clin Electrophysiol* 1997; **20**: 502–511.

58 Conte S, Gewillig M, Eyskens B, Dumoulin M, Daenen W. Management of late complications after classic Fontan procedure by conversion to total cavopulmonary connection. *Cardiovasc Surg* 1999; **7**: 651–655.

59 Deal BJ, Mavroudis C, Backer CL, Johnsrude CL, Rocchini AP. Impact of arrhythmia circuit cryoablation during Fontan conversión for refractory atrial tachycardia. *Am J Cardiol* 1999; **83**: 563–568.

60 McElhinney DB, Reddy VM, Moore P, Hanley FL. Revision of previous Fontan connections to extracardiac or intraatrial conduit cavopulmonary anastomosis. *Ann Thorac Surg* 1996; **62**: 1276–1282.

61 Mavroudis C, Backer CL, Deal BJ, Johnsrude CL. Fontan conversion to cavopulmonary connection and arrhythmia circuit cryoablation. *J Thorac Cardiovasc Surg* 1998; **115**: 547–556.

62 Mavroudis C, Deal BJ, Backer CL, Johnsrude CL. The favorable impact of arrhythmia surgery on total cavopulmonary artery Fontan conversion. *Semin Thorac Cardiovasc Surg Pediatr Card Surg Annu* 1999; **2**: 143–156.

63 Lowe JE, Hendry PJ, Packer DL, Tang AS. Surgical management of chronic ectopic atrial tachycardia. *Semin Thorac Cardiovasc Surg* 1989; **1** :58–66.

64 Berger F, Vogel M, Kramer A *et al.* Incidence of atrial flutter/fibrillation in adults with atrial septal defect before and after surgery. *Ann Thorac Surg* 1999; **68**: 75–78.

65 Brenburg RO, Jr, Holmes DR, Brandenburg RO, McGoon D. Clinical follow-up study of paroxysmal supraventricular tachyarrhythmia after operative repair of a secundum type atrial septal defect in adults. *Am J Cardiol* 1983; **51**: 273–276.

66 Gatzoulis MA, Freeman MA, Siu SC, Webb GD, Harris L. Atrial arrhythmia after surgical closure of atrial septal defects in adults. *N Engl J Med* 1999; **340**: 839–846.

67 Bonchek LI, Burlingame MW, Worley SJ, Vazales BE, Lundy EF. Cox/maze procedure for atrial septal defect with atrial fibrillation: management strategies. *Ann Thorac Surg* 1993; **55**: 607–610.

68 Kobayashi J, Yamamoto F, Nakano K, Sasako Y, Kitamura S, Kosakai Y. Maze procedure for atrial fibrillation

associated with atrial septal defect. *Circulation* 1998; **98**(19, suppl): II-399–II402.

69 Sandoval N, Velasco V, Orjuela H *et al.* Concomitant mitral valve or atrial septal defect surgery and the modified Cox maze procedure. *Am J Cardiol* 1996; **77**: 591–596.

70 Pappone C, Santinelli V. Atrial fibrillation ablation: state of the art. *Am J Cardiol* December 19, 2005; **96**(12A): 59L–64L.

71 Fontaine G, Rosas F, Frank R *et al.* Displasia arritmogénica del ventrículo derecho. Una nueva entidad clínica. *Scientia Cardiol Shaio* 1994; **14**: 1–4, 20–31.

72 Cox JL, Bardy GH, Damiano RJ *et al.* Right ventricular isolation procedure for nonischemic ventricular tachycardia. *J Thorac Cardiovasc Surg* 1985; **90**: 212.

73 Klein LS, Shih HT, Hackett FK *et al.* Radiofrequency catheter ablation of ventricular tachycardia in patients without structural heart disease. *Circulation* 1992; **85**: 1666.

74 Gatzoulis MA, Balaji S, Webber SA *et al.* Risk factors for arrhythmia and sudden cardiac death late after repair of tetralogy of Fallot: a Multicentre study. *Lancet* September 16, 2000; **356**(9234): 975–981.

75 Marie PY, Marcon F, Brunotte F *et al.* Right ventricular overload and induced sustained ventricular tachycardia in operatively "repaired" tetralogy of Fallot. *Am J Cardiol* March 15, 1992; **69**(8): 785–789.

76 Gatzoulis MA, Till JA, Somerville J, Redington AN. Mechanoelectrical interaction in tetralogy of Fallot. QRS prolongation relates to right ventricular size and predicts malignant ventricular arrhythmias and sudden death. *Circulation* 1995; **92**: 231–237.

77 Jonsson H, Ivert T. Survival and clinical results up to 26 years after repair of tetralogy of Fallot. *Scand J Thorac Cardiovasc Surg* 1995; **29**: 43 51.

78 Nollert G, Fischlein T, Bouterwek S, Bohmer C, Klinner W, Reichart B. Long-term survival in patients with repair of tetralogy of Fallot: 36-year follow-up of 490 survivors of the first year after surgical repair. *J Am Coll Cardiol* 1997; **30**: 1374–1383.

79 Tateno S, Niwa K, Nakazawa M *et al.* Risk factors for arrhythmia and late death in patients with right ventricle to pulmonary artery conduit repair—Japanese multicenter study. *Int J Cardiol* January 26, 2006; **106**(3): 373-381.

80 Owen AR, Gatzoulis MA. Tetralogy of Fallot: late outcome after repair and surgical implications. *Semin Thorac Cardiovasc Surg Pediatr Card Surg Annu* 2000; **3**: 216–226.

81 Therrien J, Marx GR, Gatzoulis MA. Late problems in tetralogy of Fallot recognition, management and prevention. *Cardiol Clin* August 2002; **20**(3): 395–404.

82 Knott-Craig CJ, Elkins RC, Lane MM, Holz J, McCue C, Ward KE. A 26-year experience with surgical management of tetralogy of Fallot: risk analysis for

mortality or late reintervention. *Ann Thorac Surg* 1998; **66**: 506–511.

83 Oechslin EN, Harrison DA, Harris L *et al.* Reoperation in adults with repair of tetralogy of Fallot: indications and outcomes. *J Thorac Cardiovasc Surg* 1999; **118**: 245–251.

84 Zhao HX, Miller DC, Reitz BA, Shumway NE. Surgical repair of tetralogy of Fallot. Long-term follow-up with particular emphasis on late death and reoperation. *J Thorac Cardiovasc Surg* 1985; **89**: 204–220.

85 Harken AH, Horowitz LN, Josephson ME. Surgical correction of recurrent sustained ventricular tachycardia following complete repair of tetralogy of Fallot. *J Thorac Cardiovasc Surg* 1980; **80**: 779.

86 Therrien J, Siu SC, McLaughlin PR, Liu PP, Williams WG, Webb GD. Pulmonary valve replacement in adults late after repair of tetralogy of Fallot: are we operating too late? *J Am Coll Cardiol* November 1, 2000; **36**(5): 1670–1675.

87 Moss AJ, McDonald J. Unilateral cervicothoracic sympathetic ganglionectomy for the treatment of long QT interval syndrome. *N Engl J Med* 1971; **285**: 903.

88 Platia EV, Griffith LSC, Watkins L *et al.* Management of prolonged QT syndrome and recurrent ventricular fibrillation with an implantable automatic cardioverter defibrillator. *Clin Cardiol* 1985; **8**: 490.

89 Lankipalli RS, Zhu T, Guo D, Yan GX. Mechanisms underlying arrhythmogenesis in long QT syndrome. *J Electrocardiol* October 2005; **38**(4, suppl): 69–73.

90 Rosas F, Velasco V, Arboleda F *et al.* Catheter ablation of ventricular tachycardia in Chagasic cardiomyopathy. *Clin Cardiol* February 1997; **20**(2): 169–174.

91 Garson A, Jr, Smith RT, Moak JP *et al.* Incessant ventricular tachycardia in infants: myocardial hamartomas and surgical cure. *J Am Coll Cardiol* 1987; **10**: 619–626.

92 Deal BJ, Mavroudis C, Backer CL, Johnsrude CL. New directions in surgical therapy of arrhythmias. *Int J Cardiol* 2004; **97**: 39–51.

93 Thoele DG, Ursell PC, Ho SY *et al.* Atrial morphologic features in tricuspid atresia. *J Thorac Cardiovasc Surg* 1991; **102**: 606–610.

94 Ross BA, Crawford FA, Jr, Whitman V, Gillette P. Atrial automatic tachycardia due to an atrial tumor. *Am Heart J* 1988; **115**: 606.

95 Guiraudon GM, Klein GJ, Sharma AD, Jones DL, McLellan DG. Surgical ablation of posterior septal accessory pathways in the Wolff—Parkinson–White syndrome by a closed heart technique. *J Thorac Cardiovasc Surg* September 1986; **92**(3, pt 1): 406–413.

96 Velasco VM, Rosas F, Rodríguez D, Sandoval N. Arritmias en Pediatría. In: En Díaz G, Sandoval N, Carrillo G & Vélez JF, eds. *Cardiología Pediátrica*. McGraw Hill, Bogota, Colombia, 2003: 875–892.

97 Cox JL, Holman WL, Cain ME. Cryosurgical treatment of atrioventricular node reentrant tachycardia. *Circulation* 1987; **76**: 1329–1336.

98 Mavroudis C, Deal BJ, Backer CL. Arrhythmia surgery in association with complex congenital heart repairs excluding patients with Fontan conversion. *Semin Thorac Cardiovasc Surg Pediatr Card Surg Annu* 2003; **6**: 33–50.

99 Deal BJ, Mavroudis C, Backer CL. Beyond Fontan conversion: surgical therapy of arrhythmias including patients with associated complex congenital heart disease. *Ann Thorac Surg* 2003; **76**: 542–554.

100 Deal BJ, Mavroudis C, Backer CL, Buck SH, Johnsrude C. Comparison of anatomic isthmic block with modified right atrial maze procedure for late atrial tachycardia in Fontan patients. *Circulation* 2002; **106**: 575–579.

101 Cox JL, Jaquiss RD, Schuessler RB, Boineau JP. Modification of the maze procedure for atrial flutter and atrial fibrillation. II: Surgical technique of the maze III procedure. *J Thorac Cardiovasc Surg* 1995; **110**: 485–495.

102 Cox JL, Boineau JP, Schuessler RB *et al.* Electrophysiologic basis, surgical development, and clinical results of the maze procedure for atrial flutter and atrial fibrillation. *Adv Card Surg* 1995; **6**: 1–67.

103 Cox JL, Boineau JP, Schuessler RB, Jaquiss RD, Lappas DG. Modification of the maze procedure for atrial flutter and atrial fibrillation. I: Rationale and surgical results. *J Thorac Cardiovasc Surg* 1995; **110**: 473–484.

104 Theodoro DA, Danielson KD, Porter CJ *et al.* Right-sided maze procedure for right atrial arrhythmias in congenital heart disease. *Am Thorac Surg* 1998; **65**: 149–154.

105 Sandoval N, Caicedo V, Orjuela H *et al.* Corrección Tipo Uno y Medio Ventrículo y Cirugía de Laberinto en el Tratamiento de Pacientes con Fibrosis Endomiocárdica, Arritmia y Severo Compromiso del Ventrículo Derecho. *Cardiol Día* 2000; **3**: 68–72.

106 Harada A, D'Agostino HJ, Jr, Schuessler RB, Boineau JP, Cox JL. Right atrial isolation: a new surgical treatment for supraventricular tachycardia: surgical technique and electrophysiologic effects. *J Thorac Cardiovasc Surg* 1988; **95**: 643–650.

107 Deal BJ, Mavroudis C, Backer CL, Johnsrude CL. New directions in surgical therapy of arrhythmias. *Pediatr Cardiol* 2000; **21**: 576–583

108 Mavroudis C, Deal BJ, Backer CL. The beneficial effects of total cavopulmonary conversion and arrhythmia surgery for the failed Fontan. *Semin Thorac Cardiovasc Surg Pediatr Card Surg Annu* 2002; **5**: 12–24.

109 Mavroudis C, Backer CL, Deal BJ, Johnsrude C, Strasburger J. Total cavopulmonary conversion and maze procedure for patients with failure of the Fontan operation. *J Thorac Cardiovasc Surg* 2001; **122**: 863–871.

110 Sandoval N, Jaramillo C, Orjuela H *et al.* Cirugía de laberinto (Maze) derecho vs. Maze III para

fibrilación auricular crónica y comunicación interauricular asociada. *Portuguese J Cardiol* 2004; **23**(suppl IV): 16.

111 Kopf GS, Mello DM, Kenney KM, Moltedo J, Rollinson NR, Zinder CS. Intraoperative radiofrequency ablation of the atrium: effectiveness for treatment of supraventricular tachycardia in congenital heart surgery. *Ann Thorac Surg* 2002; **74**: 797–804.

112 Sandoval N, Caicedo V, Orjuela H *et al.* Cirugía de arritmias en pacientes con cardiopatía congénita asociada o post operatorio de Fontan. *Rev Col Cardiol* 2006; **12**(5): 216.

113 Mavroudis C, Deal BJ, Becker CL. Surgery for arrhythmias in children. *Int J Cardiol* 2004; **97**: 39–51.

114 Backer CL, Deal BJ, Mavroudis C, Franklin WH, Stewart RD. Conversion of the failed Fontan circulation. *Cardiol Young* February 2006; **16**(suppl 1): 85–91.

115 Jenkins KJ. Risk adjustment for congenital heart surgery: the RACHS-1 method. *Semin Thorac Cardiovasc Surg Pediatr Card Surg Annu* 2004; **7**: 180–184.

116 Sheikh AM, Tang AT, Roman K *et al.* The failing Fontan circulation: successful conversion of atriopulmonary connections. *J Thorac Cardiovasc Surg* July 2004; **128**(1): 60–66.

117 Mott AR, Feltes TF, McKenzie ED *et al.* Improved early results with the Fontan operation in adults with functional single ventricle. *Ann Thorac Surg* April 2004; **77**(4): 1334–1340.

118 McDaniel GM, Van Hare GF. Catheter ablation in children and adolescents. *Heart Rhythm* January 2006; **3**(1): 95–101.

119 Cohen MI, Rhodes LA, Wernovsky G, Gaynor JW, Spray TL, Rychik J. Atrial pacing: an alternative treatment for protein-losing enteropathy after the Fontan operation. *J Thorac Cardiovasc Surg* 2001; **121**: 582–583.

120 Rychik J, Rome JJ, Jacobs ML. Late surgical fenestration for complications after the Fontan operation. *Circulation* 1997; **96**: 33–36.

121 Therrien J, Webb GD, Gatzoulis MA. Reversal of protein-losing enteropathy with prednisone in adults with modified Fontan operations: long-term palliation or bridge to cardiac transplantation? *Heart* 1999; **82**: 241–243.

122 Donnelly JP, Rosenthal A, Castle VP, Holmes RD. Reversal of protein-losing enteropathy with heparin therapy in three patients with univentricular hearts and Fontan palliation. *J Pediatr* 1997; **130**: 474–478.

123 Gamba A, Merlo M, Fiocchi R *et al.* Heart transplantation in patients with previous Fontan operations. *J Thorac Cardiovasc Surg* February 2004; **127**(2): 555–562.

124 Jayakumar KA, Addonizio LJ, Kichuk-Chrisant MR *et al.* Cardiac transplantation after the Fontan or Glenn procedure. *J Am Coll Cardiol* November 16, 2004; **44**(10): 2065–2072.

125 Chowdhury UK, Airan B, Talwar S *et al.* One and one-half ventricle repair: results and concerns. *Ann Thorac Surg* December 2005; **80**(6): 2293–2300.

PART V

Perioperative complications, reporting results, and statistical analysis

Perioperative complications during surgical treatment of atrial fibrillation: tips and pitfalls

Nicolas Doll, Alexander M. Fabricius,
Virginia Dietel, Piotr Suwalski, Thomas Walther,
Jan F. Gummert, & Friedrich W. Mohr

Overview

Atrial fibrillation is the most frequent sustained ar-rhythmia affecting more than 5% of the population older than 65 years, resulting in a reduced quality of life and life expectancy. Since the introduction of the maze procedure, an increasing number of surgical approaches have been implemented for the treatment of atrial fibrillation. During the past years a variety of devices such as unipolar and bipolar radiofrequency, cryothermal therapy, microwave, laser, and ultrasound systems have been described. All new methods have undergone thorough evalu-ations, in that course technical systems have been redesigned and surgical approaches were modified. Before reaching a widespread clinical application a thorough analysis in terms of therapeutic bene-fits and possible complications is required. Several studies have reported success rates leading to rein-stitution of atrial rhythm in 60–80% of the patients treated. However, there is no overview on possi-ble complications using surgical ablation therapy. In this chapter we have focused on different en-ergy sources, time of occurrence of postoperative arrhythmias, and patients symptoms and related diagnostic processes. Various published reports of surgical ablation therapy were evaluated with regard to complications that have occurred. In addition, our own experience was considered.

Introduction

Atrial fibrillation is the most frequent sustained ar-rhythmia especially affecting the elderly. The preva-lence of 11% in patients older than 70 years even rises up to 17% in persons older than 84 years. Nev-ertheless, the younger population (over 50 yr) is also affected. The incidence of atrial fibrillation in the general population is 0.5% [1–5].

Atrial fibrillation is characterized by irregular contractions of the atrium with frequencies ranging from 300 to 600 beats/min, thus entailing a confuse conduction to the ventricle.

Risk factors for atrial fibrillation, such as hy-pertension, congestive heart failure, and rheumatic heart disease, have already been delineated by the Framingham study [6]. Since then other under-lying causes, such as diabetes mellitus, hypoxia, hyperthyroidism, coronary artery disease, toxic and genetic abnormalities, and nonrheumatic valve heart diseases—especially in association with mitral valve, have been established [5–10].

Clinically, atrial fibrillation can be divided into a paroxysmal, a persistent, and a permanent form. Pathophysiologically, initiating triggers and a sus-taining substrate are responsible for the mainte-nance and perpetuation of atrial fibrillation [11, 12]. The exact pathological mechanisms leading

Manual of Surgical Treatment of Atrial Fibrillation.
Edited by Hauw T. Sie *et al.* © 2008 Blackwell Publishing,
ISBN: 978-1-4051-4032-4.

the transition from a physiological rhythm to pathological fibrillation, especially on the molecular level, are unclear at present and remain to be elucidated by future research. However, modification or elimination of either triggers or maintaining substrates are promising curative approaches for atrial fibrillation. Triggers are considered to be correlated with sympathetic or parasympathetic stimulation, bradycardia, accessory pathways, acute atrial stretch, and especially with ectopic "firing" foci within the pulmonary and caval veins, as pointed out by Haissaguerre *et al.* in 1998 [13]. Once the atrial fibrillation is present, recovery of the pathologically altered substrate to *restitutio ad integrum* is impossible. Even after treatment the patient remains susceptible with a low threshold for repeat occurrence of atrial fibrillation [14].

Morbidity and mortality associated with atrial fibrillation led to the awareness that effective treatment is required. Knowing more about the pathophysiology of atrial fibrillation and about the concept of modifying or eliminating either the trigger or maintaining substrates subsequently stimulated the rapid development of a wide variety of surgical approaches. Of special importance is the 4.8-fold increased risk of stroke and thromboembolism associated with atrial fibrillation requiring long-term anticoagulation therapy with the risk of life-threatening bleedings [15]. A recent review revealed that about one third of patients suffer adverse events in relation to oral anticoagulation therapy [5]. Clinical symptoms and comorbidities result in a loss of patient's quality of life and life expectancy [2].

Today, besides the highly efficient Cox's maze procedure a variety of different surgical ablation techniques using different energy sources as well as different surgical techniques exist [16, 17]. New concepts for the intraoperative use of ablation techniques have been developed by several research groups, among them unipolar and bipolar radiofrequency, cryo- and microwave technologies, and ultrasound and laser systems. Methods have been improved, refined, and completed; nevertheless, they require further studies. Results, and especially the success rates, reported with the restoration of sinus rhythm are varying, with still some potential for further improvement [18].

In summary, all the new surgical ablation techniques are promising. However, there is some concern due to a rare but severe postoperative complications rate. Such complications may appear early postoperatively as well as with a delay up to several months. This chapter will provide an overview on the incidence and severity of complications and will analyze the related clinical symptoms. The diagnosing process, especially emphasizing on rapid early clinical recognition with the use of diagnostic means, will be thoroughly analyzed. All complications are directly related to the application of the ablation energy through the surgical device. The following three major complications reported will be analyzed: esophageal perforations or fistulae, coronary artery stenosis, and pulmonary vein stenosis.

Esophageal perforation and esophagoatrial fistula after unipolar radiofrequency ablation

Till today, five cases of esophageal injuries in patients after treatment with intraoperative unipolar radiofrequency ablation for atrial fibrillation are reported, which turned out to be fatal in two cases. It is assumed that the radiofrequency energy applied to the left atrium causes thermal damage to the adjacent tissue. Histopathological examinations of the esophagus confirmed the thermal injury and the enclosing inflammation in histological staining. Gillinov *et al.* published a case report on one patient in May 2001. One year later a paper concerning four cases was published by our group. Subsequently, we observed another event of esophageal perforation despite a change in the perioperative technique applied. In April 2003, the complete results of the IRAAF study were summarized and complications described by our group [19–21].

Gillinov described a 60-year-old female patient as cachectic and underweight. He explained the esophageal perforation with the lack of tissue between esophagus and left atrium. The patient suffered from rheumatic mitral valve disease and permanent atrial fibrillation for several years. The thorax was opened by a median sternotomy, the mitral valve replaced, and the radiofrequency ablation performed with the use of the Cobra RF System (Boston Scientific, Boston, MA), starting with the isolation of the pulmonary veins and additional connecting lesions linking the mitral valve annulus and the back wall of the left atrium. Energy was applied for 20 seconds at 80°C. Furthermore, the left atrial appendage was isolated. The patient was in sinus rhythm for 10 days, and intermittent atrial fibrillation was treated with amiodarone and electrical cardioversion. The white blood cell count was continuously increasing up to 36,000 cells/mm³ on postoperative day 9 when dysphagia occurred. A chest CT (computed tomography) scan revealed mediastinal air and an esophageal leak at the level of the left atrium (water-soluble contrast medium and thin barium esophagograms). She was immediately reoperated and died the next day due to sepsis, severe pulmonary dysfunction, and uncorrectable coagulopathy. Histopathological examination confirmed the esophageal perforation and surrounding inflammation of the tissue. Gillinov advised to pay attention to the extent of ablation treatment, especially in very thin patients [19].

However, we changed our initial strategy using IRAAF after the first fatal events without success. Despite positioning some gauze between the posterior wall of the left atrium and the esophagus into the transverse sinus, we observed another case of esophageal perforation. Thus, direct contact may not be the only reason for such severe complications to occur. According to our experience, the first signs of an esophageal perforation are often those of an unspecific inflammation: an increase in white blood cell count and C-reactive protein level with fever, typically accompanied by neurological symptoms (similar to a transient ischemic attacks) that are caused by embolism of micro-air-bubbles. They demand a high degree of vigilance. Cranial CT does not necessarily give evidence of air embolism. The emboli are supposedly too small to be visualized.

From the initial 387 patients receiving ablation therapy in our hospital, 133 were operated using a lateral minithoracotomy and 3 of them had esophageal injuries like perforation or a fistula between the esophagus and the left atrium. These complications always occurred with some delay and never in the acute phase during the ablation procedure. It was impossible to identify any risk factors and there were no significant differences between patients with and without occurrence of these complications. Probably thermal damage leads to the inflammatory reaction with secondary perforation of the tissue. There was no relation to intraoperative transesophageal echocardiography as the echo probe was removed during the ablation procedure.

The lesions were performed with a handheld probe with 10-mm T-shaped electrode tip (Radios 504; Osypka GmbH, Grenzach-Wyhlen, Germany) in a unipolar mode with energy applied at 60°C for 20 seconds. The first lesion line was created from the mitral annulus to the left lower pulmonary vein (lower and upper ones were connected), followed by a lesion line between left and right upper pulmonary vein, and finally a line to the right lower vein orifice. Care was taken to not injure the inside of the pulmonary veins [20, 21]. This was a standard protocol and we did not find any relation of the lesion lines to the occurrence of severe complications.

Were there any patient-specific factors? For better understanding, the individual profiles are given below.

Patient I was a 42-year-old male suffering for 5 years from paroxysmal, drug-refractory atrial fibrillation. Because of his increasing symptoms, surgery was indicated after a singular percutaneous radiofrequency pulmonary vein isolation was unsuccessful. He had no other organic heart disease. On postoperative day 3, he developed fever and his white blood cell count increased. Echocardiography and chest CT scans showed a normal anatomy; after a course of antibiotics the unspecific inflammation parameters decreased. After 7 days, he suffered a 3-hour episode of transient ischemic attack postprandially. The next day these symptoms returned dramatically and he was referred to the operating room. The thorax was opened and a fistula between the esophagus and the left atrium was found. A partial resection of the esophagus was performed. Four days later the patient developed a pneumomediastinum. Another operation via a posterolateral thoracotomy showed a new fistula between the esophageal stump and the right main bronchus. A right pneumonectomy and further esophageal resection were necessary. Six weeks later the patient underwent gastroesophageal reconstruction. He was finally discharged with persisting neurological deficit.

Patient II was a 62-year-old female suffering from permanent atrial fibrillation and hemodynamically significant atrial septal defect. Six days after the IRAAF procedure she vomited blood and died

4 hours after a gastroscopy due to a severe cerebral air embolism as a result of the air insufflation.

The atrial fibrillation of patient III (59 yr, male) was for the last 3 years permanent and unresponsive to flecainide, propafenone, amiodarone, and sotalol, and relapsed after electrical cardioversions. Similar to other patients after radiofrequency procedure, he was in stable sinus rhythm and his early postoperative course was uneventful. On postoperative day 12, the patient developed nonspecific signs of an inflammation and neurological symptoms. A chest CT scan with water-soluble contrast medium revealed free air in the mediastinum between the esophagus and the left atrial wall due to an esophageal perforation. Six days later—like in case 1—signs of a new fistula appeared and he had to undergo an extensive resection once again. Recently, his upper intestinal tract has been reconstructed successfully.

Patient IV, a 36-year-old man, with paroxysmal atrial fibrillation was highly symptomatic and was referred for surgical treatment. A few years ago he had undergone a partial gastric resection owing to bleeding ulcers. On postoperative day 8, he had an episode of severe chest pain. A chest CT scan with water-soluble contrast medium showed esophageal perforation. He underwent successful resection and reconstruction [21].

Not being able to control these complications and with no clear factor being the just cause, we abandoned the use of radiofrequency energy for the treatment of atrial fibrillation.

Coronary artery stenosis due to different sources of ablation energy

Another severe complication proved to be related to different ablation techniques is new-onset coronary artery stenosis. This can be caused by direct or even indirect contact with the ablation probe.

In 1977, Mikat and coworkers published first experimental results of a study on mongrel dogs. They examined the effects of epicardial lesion lines after cryoapplication from -40 to $50°C$ over the bifurcation of the left anterior descending artery, followed by histopathological examination. The tissue responded with all signs of an acute inflammatory reaction, such as fibrosis and fat infiltration, necrotic medial and intimal cells, lympho-

cytes, macrophages, and red blood cells. Although the main arteries remained patent after 4 weeks, mural fibrosis with marked intimal thickening with atherome-like plaque formation with splitting and discontinuity within the internal elastic lamina was recognized. The pathological alterations have been reported until the last staining of the tissue was performed after 12 weeks [22].

Cryoablation is widely known to be a safe and efficient technique. Nevertheless, one clinical case report concerning coronary artery stenosis after cryotherapy is available in the literature [23]. In 1987, a 48-year-old patient underwent cryoablation ($-60°C$, 2 min) for Wolff–Parkinson–White syndrome. The postoperative period was uneventful. Six months later the patient was readmitted to the hospital owing to symptoms of angina. ECG demonstrated an ST-segment elevation in leads II, III, and aVF. Coronary angiography revealed occlusion of the circumflex coronary artery in segment 13, correlating directly to the site of cryoablation. The patient subsequently underwent successful percutaneous transluminal coronary angioplasty. No further evidence of coronary complications after cryotherapy has been reported till now.

Radiofrequency is supposed to provide much more aggressive ablation energy. The importance of clinical practice would lie in the analysis of the following four cases of coronary artery stenosis after cryoapplication, microwave ablation, and radiofrequency ablation for atrial fibrillation: one of them after a maze procedure, the second after a microwave ablation within the left atrium, and two children with Ebstein's anomaly. These four patients need to be analyzed [24, 25].

In 1996, Sueda and coworkers reported a case of maze procedure with the use of cryoapplication. A 68-year-old male patient had suffered from permanent atrial fibrillation for 6 years and had had a history of a cerebral infarct and peripheral arterial embolism. A cryoablation following the most classic pattern of maze lesions (including right atrioventricular (AV) groove and posterior mitral annulus site) was performed within 2 minutes of cryoapplication at $-60°C$. No complications occurred postoperatively. After 3 months the patient was readmitted to the hospital with signs of acute myocardial infarction. ECG showed an ST-segment depression in leads II, III, aVF, and V_4 to V_6. Coronary angiography confirmed the prior diagnosis and revealed an obstruction of the right coronary artery (segment 2) and the severe stenosis of the left circumflex coronary artery in segments 12 and 13, both corresponding to the site of cryoablation. One month later the patient underwent surgical coronary revascularization [24].

In 2001, Bertram and coworkers reported two cases of accidentally diagnosed asymptomatic coronary stenosis in children after Ebstein malformation correcting operation.

The first 6-year-old boy demonstrated symptomatic drug-refractory, paroxysmal supraventricular tachycardia. Two accessory pathways were ablated intraoperatively with radiofrequency energy. After 2 years, coronary artery stenosis was diagnosed.

In the second patient, the Ebstein's anomaly was accompanied by an atrial septal defect and the Wolff–Parkinson–White syndrome with recurrent paroxysmal supraventricular tachycardia episodes. At the age of 2.9, two accessory pathways were ablated successfully with the use of radiofrequency energy. Similar to the first case, coronary artery stenosis was revealed with a delay of 14 months. Routine coronary angiography detected a stenosis in the marginal branch of the right coronary artery [25].

Recently, reports on coronary artery stenosis after ablation surgery using microwave energy have been published [26]. A 62-year-old man with a severe rheumatic mitral valve stenosis suffered from permanent atrial fibrillation for 6 years. Multiple electrical cardioversions had been unsuccessful. Coronary arteries were normal. As a concomitant procedure to mitral valve replacement, the patient underwent single encircling ablation of the pulmonary veins with microwaves (Flex 4 probe, AFx Inc., for 90 sec with 65 W). The postoperative period was uneventful and the patient left the hospital in stable sinus rhythm. On postoperative day 90, he developed myocardial infarction treated successfully with double coronary artery bypass grafting [26].

Catheter and surgically induced pulmonary vein stenosis after unipolar radiofrequency ablation

Pulmonary vein stenosis is another severe complication related to ablation therapy. This complication most certainly is caused by lesion pattern lying directly within the thin-walled pulmonary veins. Manifested clinically with gradually developing dyspnea on exertion, nonproductive cough, hemoptysis, recurrent pulmonary infections, and all signs of pulmonary hypertension, severe stenosis of up to all four pulmonary veins is a life-threatening and potentially fatal complication. In 1998, Robbins and coworkers published two cases of this complication after percutaneous ablation therapy [27]. Two of 18 patients of a multicenter study suffered from permanent atrial fibrillation (for 3 yr) and paroxysmal atrial fibrillation (for 19 yr), respectively. Both were refractory to either antiarrhythmic drugs or multiple electrical cardioversions; thus, pulmonary vein ablation was indicated.

In those patients percutaneous radiofrequency ablation was performed with a target temperature of $55^{\circ}C$ after transseptal puncture and consisted of five lines within both atria. All four pulmonary veins (including not only the orifices but also the inside of the vessels), the roof of the left atrium, the interatrial septum, and the posterior wall linking the superior vena cava with the inferior one were involved. The patients' immediate postinterventional course remained uneventful until both started gradual development of worsening dyspnea on exertion and nonproductive cough after 3 months. They underwent a series of diagnostic procedures until the final diagnosis of pulmonary vein stenosis was made after several months. In the meantime, both patients presented with constantly increasing symptoms. Finally, they underwent successful curative balloon dilation with no signs of recurrence at 1-year follow-up [27].

Another patient with previous interventional ablation therapy was treated surgically at our institution. He was a 44-year-old male patient with previous history of permanent atrial fibrillation, hypertension, and hyperlipidemia, and had undergone successful intraoperative radiofrequency ablation of his atrial fibrillation.

Despite being in normal sinus rhythm, he presented with symptoms of shortness of breath and dyspnea on exertion. Angiography of his pulmonary veins revealed severe (90%) stenosis of both left pulmonary veins and an occluded right upper pulmonary vein.

He had operative repair of the pulmonary vein stenosis using bilateral pericardial patch plasty. The operation was performed through a median sternotomy. After arterial cannulation of the ascending aorta and venous cannulation of superior and inferior vena cava, the temperature was lowered to 24°C. The aorta was cross-clamped and 2 L of crystalloid cardioplegia solution was infused for cardiac arrest. The left atrium was approached through the right atrium with a transseptal incision. Inspection of the left atrium showed massive fibrosis and thickening of the left atrial wall. The orifices of the left upper pulmonary veins were concentrically stenosed for a length of 1 cm. The right lower pulmonary vein was not affected.

Due to postinflammatory reactions after treatment of atrial fibrillation with radiofrequency, there were dense adhesions in the area of the bilateral upper pulmonary veins intraoperatively. The pulmonary veins were dissected into the periphery, exceeding the bifurcation into smaller branches.

The stenosis was repaired using autologous pericardium as a patch plasty. The orifices of the upper pulmonary veins were then inspected endoscopically and a 14 mm Hegar dilator passed through easily. The left atrial roof was reconstructed and closed along with the atrial septum and the right atrium. Following deairing of both atria and rewarming, spontaneous sinus rhythm was achieved.

Postoperative course

Postoperative CT and MRT scans revealed normally sized upper pulmonary veins with no further stenosis. Twenty-four-hour Holter monitoring revealed episodes of atrial fibrillation for 9 and 15 hours of sinus rhythm. There was no evidence of ventricular arrhythmias. ECG at discharge showed sinus rhythm with a heart rate of 81 per minute. There was no occurrence of AV block or arrhythmias. The postoperative echocardiogram demonstrated normal dimensions of the left ventricle with an ejection fraction of 70%. The E/A ratio was 1.4. The valves showed normal function without any insufficiency or morphologic pathology.

The patient was discharged after 11 days postoperatively. The discharge medications included anticoagulation for 3 months.

Comment

The use of different ablation techniques and energy sources has simplified the surgical treatment of atrial fibrillation, leading to a widespread application of the method with good results [28]. However, these emerging techniques require thorough follow-up, especially in terms of possible complications. The aim of this chapter is to analyze the potentially life-threatening complications after the relatively new ablation treatments.

The incidents described often occur with delay in the initial procedure and are usually associated with specific symptoms. Knowing them can be very useful for further clinical practice.

Perforation of the esophagus or esophagoatrial fistula is associated with a specific clinical pattern. The neurological symptoms, especially similar to a transient ischemic attack in combination with nonspecific inflammatory signs like fever, leukocytosis, and C-reactive protein, demand awareness of the possibility of an esophageal injury and require an immediate and proper diagnostic process. A chest CT scan with water-soluble contrast medium or gastrograffin swallow is highly recommended. Gastroscopy should be strictly avoided because of the danger of air embolism. Pain and other symptoms are most often connected with food intake and swallowing and should remind us of possible perforation of the esophagus or an emergence of a new fistula between the esophagus and the left atrium.

The symptoms of the coronary artery stenosis are well known. Nevertheless, it would be highly advisable to be aware of such a possibility in patients after ablation, first of all for a surgeon performing the procedure, but also for those who admit a patient with angina to a hospital, especially when the age of a patient usually excludes the presence of coronary artery disease.

Pulmonary vein stenosis as an ablation complication touches a problem of the recognition and early diagnosis. The symptoms like dyspnea on exertion, nonproductive cough, hemoptysis, and recurrent pulmonary infections are highly unspecific and can occur with the very different grades of severity and dynamics. Most importantly, an early diagnosis plays a major role in these patients because of all the long-term, potentially nonreversible changes in the pulmonary circulation. Robbins raised a problem of lack of clinical manifestation of pulmonary vein stenosis that seems to occur when not all the vessels are involved [27].

In conclusion, the complications after ablation occur very differently as far as time after the procedure is concerned. Esophageal perforation occurs within days after surgery. Other complications, such as coronary artery stenosis and pulmonary vein stenosis, can occur with a delay of months or years.

Concerning the energy sources, radiofrequency currently seems to be the most aggressive stimulus for tissue damage. Most of the reported cases are in direct relation to the use of radiofrequency. However, other sources are associated with very similar tissue alterations and are also able to cause a severe complication.

Radiofrequency ablation seems to be dangerous because of the deep penetration to the surrounding tissue, which can lead to such dramatic events like esophagus perforation or esophagoatrial fistula with subsequent massive air embolism and stroke. Reports on pulmonary vein stenosis are also strictly related to that energy source. The conclusion of avoiding lesion lines directly within the pulmonary veins is widely accepted and applied.

The cases of reported coronary artery stenosis show that the use of cryotherapy must not lead to the deceptive and misleading imagination of total safety; an adequate measure of suspect for the occurrence of complications has to be maintained.

Manasse *et al.* reported coronary artery stenosis after microwave ablation as a result of probe misplacement [26]. However, considering recently reported coronary complications after ablations, a potential risk of microwave energy cannot be excluded. A retrograde perfusion of the coronary arteries via the coronary sinus, while ablating in the left atrium, could be an option to protect the vessels. Furthermore, a tailored anatomical approach on the basis of the left circumflex coronary anatomy has been proposed, with particular emphasis toward the lesions that cross the AV groove to reach the mitral valve annulus during the left atrial maze [29]. Particularly in the case of a strongly dominant right coronary artery when the circumflex ends with a ramus medianus or an early marginal branch, the mitral line is performed following the shortest route and reaches the posterior annulus between its mid portion and the anterolateral commissure. When the right coronary artery is mildly dominant, the circumflex artery usually gives rise to one or two marginal branches and dwells in the lateral portion of the posterior AV groove. In this case the ablation

connecting the mitral valve with the appendage is conducted to the medial portion of the posterior annulus with a curved shape in order to cross the AV groove perpendicularly. In a minority of patients with a dominant circumflex artery, the mitral ablation line is performed from the right pulmonary encircling and reaches the annulus close to the posteromedial commissure.

In conclusion, the population of patients with atrial fibrillation is growing. Surgery remains the most effective method to treat this kind of arrhythmia. Since the description of the maze procedure, a rising number of surgical approaches have been devised for the treatment of atrial fibrillation. During the past few years, a variety of energy sources such as radiofrequency, low temperature, microwaves, laser, and ultrasound systems have been described. The new methods are technically improved. However, they require thorough analysis, especially in terms of possible complications. Analyzing mentioned complication cases leads to better understanding of the problem and can be useful in the clinical practice.

References

1 Reardon M, Camm AJ. Atrial fibrillation in the elderly. *Clin Cardiol* 1996; **19**(10): 765–775.

2 Chatap G, Giraud K, Vincent JP. Atrial fibrillation in the elderly: facts and management. *Drugs Aging* 2002; **19**(11): 819–846.

3 Domanski MJ. The epidemiology of atrial fibrillation. *Coron Artery Dis* 1995; **6**: 95.

4 Grubb NR, Furnis S. Radiofrequency ablation for atrial fibrillation: science, medicine and the future. *BMJ* 2001; **322**: 777–780.

5 Lip GYH, Beevers DG. ABC of atrial fibrillation: history, epidemiology, and importance of atrial fibrillation. *BMJ—Educ Debate* 1995; **311**: 1361.

6 Kannel WB, Abbott RD, Savage DD, McNamara PM. Epidemiological features of chronic atrial fibrillation: the Framingham study. *N Engl J Med* 1982; **306**: 1018–1022.

7 Kannel WB, Wolf PA, Benjamin EJ *et al.* Prevalence, incidence, prognosis, and predisposing conditions for atrial fibrillation: population-based estimates. *Am J Cardiol* 1998; **82**: 2N–9N.

8 Brugada R, Tapscott T, Czernuszewicz GZ *et al.* Identification of a genetic locus for familial atrial fibrillation. *N Engl J Med* 1997; **336**: 905–911.

9 Walther T, Falk V, Walther C *et al.* Combined stentless mitral valve implantation and radiofrequency ablation. *Ann Thorac Surg* 2000; **70**: 1080–1082.

10 Sueda T, Nagata H, Orihashi K *et al.* Efficacy of a simple left atrial procedure for chronic atrial fibrillation in mitral valve operations. *Ann Thorac Surg* 1997; **63**: 1070–1075.

11 Allessie MA, Boyden PA, Camm AJ *et al.* Pathophysiology and prevention of atrial fibrillation. *Circulation* 2001; **103**: 769.

12 Gallagher MG, Camm AJ. Classification of atrial fibrillation. *Pacing Clin Electrophysiol* 1997; **20**: 1603–1605.

13 Haissaguerre M, Jais P, Shah DC *et al.* Spontaneous initiation of atrial fibrillation by ectopic beats originating in the pulmonary veins. *N Engl J Med* 1998; **339**: 659–666.

14 Shinagawa K, Shi YF, Tardif JC, Leung TK, Nattel S. Dynamic nature of atrial fibrillation substrate during development and reversal of heart failure in dogs. *Circulation* 2002; **105**: 2672.

15 Aronow WS. Management of the older person with atrial fibrillation. *J Gerontol A Biol Sci Med Sci* 2002; **57**(6): M352–M363.

16 Hindricks G, Mohr FW, Autschbach R, Kottkamp H. Antiarrhythmic surgery for treatment of atrial fibrillation—new concepts. *Thorac Cardiovasc Surg* 1999; **47**(suppl): 365–369.

17 Patwardhan AM, Dave HH, Tamhane AA *et al.* Intraoperative radiofrequency micropolar coagulation to replace incisions of maze III procedure for correcting atrial fibrillation inpatients with rheumatic valvular disease. *Eur J Cardiothorac Surg* 1997; **12**: 627–633.

18 Keane D. New catheter ablation techniques for the treatment of cardiac arrhythmias. *Card Electrophysiol Rev* 2002; **6**: 341–348.

19 Gillinov AM, Gosta P, Rice TW. Esophageal injury during radiofrequency ablation for atrial fibrillation. *J Thorac Cardiovasc Surg* 2001; **122**: 1239–1240.

20 Mohr FW, Fabricius AM, Falk V *et al.* Curative treatment of atrial fibrillation with intraoperative radiofrequency ablation: short term and midterm results. *J Thorac Cardiovasc Surg* 2002; **123**: 919–927.

21 Doll N, Borger MA, Fabricius A. Esophageal perforation during left atrial radiofrequency ablation: is the risk too high? *J Thorac Cardiovasc Surg* 2003; **125**: 836–842.

22 Mikat E, Hackel DB, Harrison L *et al.* Reaction of the myocardium and coronary arteries to cryosurgery. *Labor Invest* 1977; **37**(6): 632–641.

23 Watanabe H, Hayashi J, Aizawa Y. Myocardial infarction after cryoablation surgery for Wolff–Parkinson–White syndrome. *Jpn J Thorac Cardiovasc Surg* 2002; **50**: 210–212.

24 Sueda T, Shikata H, Norimasa M, Nagata H, Matsuura Y. Myocardial infarction after a maze procedure for idiopathic atrial fibrillation. *J Thorac Cardiovasc Surg* 1996; **112**(2): 549–550.

25 Bertram H, Bökenkamp R, Peuster M *et al.* Coronary artery stenosis after radiofrequency catheter ablation of accessory atrioventricular pathways in children with Ebstein's malformation. *Circulation* 2001; **103**: 538–543.

26 Manasse E, Medici D, Ghiselli S *et al.* Left main coronary arterial lesion after microwave epicardial ablation. *Ann Thorac Surg* 2003; **76**: 276–277.

27 Robbins IM, Colvin EV, Doyle TP *et al.* Pulmonary vein stenosis after catheter ablation of atrial fibrillation. *Circulation* 1998; **98**: 1769–1775.

28 Khargi K, Hutten BA, Lemke B, Deneke T. Surgical treatment of atrial fibrillation: a systematic review. *Eur J Cardiothorac Surg* 2005, **27**: 258-265.

29 Benussi S, Nascimbene S, Calvi S, Alfieri O. A tailored anatomical approach to prevent complications during left atrial ablation. *Ann Thorac Surg* 2003; **75**: 1979–1981.

Index